MODERN
PHARMACEUTICAL
INDUSTRY

A PRIMER

EDITED BY

THOMAS M. JACOBSEN, PharmD, MS, RPh
Associate Director, Medical Affairs
ViroPharma Incorporated

ALBERT I. WERTHEIMER, PhD, MBA
Director, Center for Pharmaceutical Health Services Research
School of Pharmacy at Temple University

JONES AND BARTLETT PUBLISHERS
Sudbury, Massachusetts
BOSTON   TORONTO   LONDON   SINGAPORE

World Headquarters

Jones and Bartlett Publishers	Jones and Bartlett Publishers	Jones and Bartlett Publishers
40 Tall Pine Drive	Canada	International
Sudbury, MA 01776	6339 Ormindale Way	Barb House, Barb Mews
978-443-5000	Mississauga, Ontario, L5V 1J2	London W6 7PA
info@jbpub.com	Canada	United Kingdom
www.jbpub.com		

Jones and Bartlett's books and products are available through most bookstores and online booksellers. To contact Jones and Bartlett Publishers directly, call 800-832-0034, fax 978-443-8000, or visit our website www.jbpub.com.

Substantial discounts on bulk quantities of Jones and Bartlett's publications are available to corporations, professional associations, and other qualified organizations. For details and specific discount information, contact the special sales department at Jones and Bartlett via the above contact information or send an email to specialsales@jbpub.com.

The authors, editor, and publisher have made every effort to provide accurate information. However, they are not responsible for errors, omissions, or for any outcomes related to the use of the contents of this book and take no responsibility for the use of the products and procedures described. Treatments and side effects described in this book may not be applicable to all people; likewise, some people may require a dose or experience a side effect that is not described herein. Drugs and medical devices are discussed that may have limited availability controlled by the Food and Drug Administration (FDA) for use only in a research study or clinical trial. Research, clinical practice, and government regulations often change the accepted standard in this field. When consideration is being given to use of any drug in the clinical setting, the health care provider or reader is responsible for determining FDA status of the drug, reading the package insert, and reviewing prescribing information for the most up-to-date recommendations on dose, precautions, and contraindications, and determining the appropriate usage for the product. This is especially important in the case of drugs that are new or seldom used.

Production Credits

Publisher: David Cella
Associate Editor: Maro Gartside
Production Manager: Julie Champagne Bolduc
Production Assistant: Jessica Steele Newfell
Senior Marketing Manager: Sophie Fleck
Manufacturing and Inventory Control Supervisor:
  Amy Bacus

Composition: Achorn International
Cover Design: Kristin E. Parker
Cover Image: ©†Kamil Fazrin Rauf/ShutterStock, Inc.
Printing and Binding: Malloy, Inc.
Cover Printing: Malloy, Inc.

Library of Congress Cataloging-in-Publication Data
Modern pharmaceutical industry : a primer / [edited by] Thomas M.
  Jacobsen, Albert I. Wertheimer.
    p. cm.
  Includes bibliographical references and index.
  ISBN-13: 978-0-7637-6636-8 (casebound)
  ISBN-10: 0-7637-6636-4 (casebound)
  1. Drug development. 2. Pharmaceutical industry. I. Jacobsen, Thomas M. II. Wertheimer, Albert I.
  [DNLM: 1. Drug Industry. 2. Drug Discovery. 3. Technology, Pharmaceutical. QV 736 M6896 2010]
  RM301.25.M635 2010
  615'.19—dc22

                                    2009012593

6048

Printed in the United States of America
13 12 11 10 09   10 9 8 7 6 5 4 3 2 1

This book is dedicated to my wife, Rebecca, and my children, Ryan, Matthew, and Lauren, for it is their love and support that brings a project like this to fruition. Also, for Mom and Dad—I wish you could have seen what I've accomplished.
—T. M. J.

To Joaquima and Lia, who permitted this endeavor at the expense of some family activities, and to Bill Helfand who introduced me to the pharmaceutical industry.
—A. I. W.

Brief Contents

Contents

CHAPTER 4 ■ Manufacturing and Production — 75

Foreword

Any book on today's pharmaceutical industry establishes an ambitious set of goals, and the chapters that editors Tom Jacobsen and Albert Wertheimer include in this volume do offer a wide range of topics, from discovery and formulation to postapproval and legal issues. It is a "primer" unlike anything I have seen since the early part of the past decade. Its subject matter goes beyond its title and rewards readers with valuable insights into three major industry segments—the innovative, generic, and self-medication industries—by current and recently retired practitioners and academics, an excellent mix of authors.

Among manufacturing industries, the pharmaceutical industry is the most significantly dependent upon the state of legal and regulatory measures and the practices of governments, from clinical development and patenting to regulatory approval, promotion, and postmarketing surveillance. These controlling political factors are uniquely additive to the general worker's health and safety as well as to the environmental laws and regulations that all manufacturers encounter. Many of these issues remain subject to review and frequent change. For example:

- The societal balance between the effectiveness of new drugs and the risks of adverse reactions reflected in the US Food and Drug Administration's and international agencies' decisions
- The scope of duration of patents, broadened internationally in recent years and lengthened in a number of developed countries
- The transparency and reporting of clinical trial results, generally toward greater transparency in reporting earlier trials more rapidly
- The ongoing debates about direct-to-consumer advertising of medicines in the United States and the growing urgency for better informed patients in Europe and Japan, especially in light of continuing restrictions of the access of patients in these regions to innovative medicines
- The regulatory boundaries set for prescription and over-the-counter medicines

- The trend toward the harmonization of technical documentation required for regulatory reviews not only among the original International Conference on Harmonisation (ICH) regions, but also beyond in Latin America and Southeast Asia

Globalization is a force that will continue to be a key element in the future of the pharmaceutical industry. Demands are placed on innovative companies to think globally in their marketing strategies, as most clearly evidenced by the AIDS "access-to-medicines" discussions at the World Health Organization and the World Trade Organization. Developing countries, such as China and India, are expanding their capacities in generic medicines to supply global markets while also aiming to become forces for the development of innovative medicines. The rate of patenting is accelerating rapidly in China, India, Korea, Singapore, and in others such that they, too, are beginning to see that they cannot rely solely on a "commodity" generic industry to survive as pharmaceutical product providers. To paraphrase R. A. Mashelkar—a leader in India's transition to a high-quality and innovative industry—in India, the issue is no longer "publish or perish" but "patent or perish."

The industry faces many challenges today, a number of them not new in nature but occurring today in wider geographic scale:

- Demands by regulatory authorities for more clinical trial data resulting in regulatory delays
- Challenges to intellectual property
- Parallel importation
- Circulation of substandard and counterfeit medicines
- Price controls
- Challenges of doing business in countries where corruption is prevalent

These issues never die, and, with the expansion of the industry into the global marketplace, they will become a constant pull on the attention of scientists and managers in the industry.

However, as the industry is highly regulated and constantly challenged to address political, regulatory, and legal challenges, it is—as the editors and authors of this book demonstrate—uniquely positioned to improve the global health standards of society by saving lives and improving the quality of lives around the world through developing and marketing innovative products of chemical and biological science as well as high-quality generic and over-the-counter medicines. The industry has and will continue to adapt to changes in science and politics. Indeed, as a mentor said to me in my early days, the pharmaceutical industry treats political and regulatory challenges to its operations in the same way that an oyster treats a grain of sand that it ingests: it creates a pearl.

—Dr. Harvey E. Bale, Jr.
Director General, International Federation of
Pharmaceutical Manufacturers and Associations
President, Pharmaceutical Security Institute

Preface

The idea for this book arose in 2004 during conversations with some new hires at a major pharmaceutical firm. The idea percolated during the following year until we, the editors, clearly decided that our assumption was a correct one. That assumption was that most people—even some who are employed in the pharmaceutical industry and in associated fields—often have a very limited and incomplete picture of the size, diversity, and activities of the necessary divisions or components in a contemporary pharmaceutical company.

We discovered that personnel in the manufacturing, quality assurance, or laboratory areas frequently knew almost nothing about their own company's activities regarding marketing, legal, and regulatory activities. And, similarly, persons in the sales and marketing divisions seemed to have incomplete information about what goes on in clinical development, manufacturing, and the R&D laboratories. So, in 2005, the final concept for the book was born. The most difficult part was not in the writing or organization of the book but in locating colleagues who were willing and able to contribute chapters in the areas of their expertise and experience. The "willing" part was not difficult, but the "able" component proved to be a real challenge. Time after time, our friends and colleagues told us that their employers would not approve of their involvement. We finally succeeded by using persons who, in many cases, had previously been in the industry, due to recent retirement or a job change to academia or elsewhere.

We need to insert a few words of caution. The functions of nearly all pharmaceutical companies are very similar. They need a human resources capacity, a legal department to write contracts and other documents, persons to interface with the regulatory authorities, scientists, and many others. But that is where the similarity ends. Each firm is organized somewhat differently, often because of their history. You should consider what you read in this book more as a prototype or typical organization instead of an accurate description of any one company in the industry.

And lastly, we want to express our great gratitude to the generous friends and colleagues who freely share their knowledge and experience with you. If there are any errors, we alone are responsible and apologize in advance. We hope that the book can be used by persons considering employment in the pharmaceutical industry and by those who want to learn more about "their industry" as well as students new to the industry.

After reading the book, you should understand how the industry does far more than merely synthesizing some white powder, compressing it into tablets, testing it on animals, and selling it. All comments from readers are welcome.

About the Editors

THOMAS M. JACOBSEN, PharmD, MS, RPh, has more than 15 years of industry experience in the areas of medical affairs, clinical research, regulatory affairs, microbiology, and analytical chemistry. In addition to his industry experience, Dr. Jacobsen has taught at the School of Pharmacy at Temple University and at the University of Pennsylvania. He completed his postdoctoral training at Temple University's Schools of Medicine and Pharmacy in infectious diseases and pulmonary/critical care medicine. Dr. Jacobsen lives in suburban Philadelphia with his wife and three children.

ALBERT I. WERTHEIMER, PhD, MBA, is a professor at the School of Pharmacy at Temple University and director of its Pharmaceutical Health Services Research Center. He is a former director of outcomes research and management at Merck and Company and a former vice president of First Health Services, a pharmacy benefit management firm. Previously, he held academic positions at the State University of New York at Buffalo and at the University of Minnesota. Dr. Wertheimer has served as a consultant or invited lecturer in more than 50 countries, and he is the author or editor of 25 books and nearly 400 scientific or professional journal articles.

Contributors

Anthony Ekpe, PhD
Senior Staff Scientist, Analytical Development, Consumer Care Division
Bayer Healthcare
Morristown, NJ

Adam George, PharmD
Clinical Scientist
Bristol-Myers Squibb
Lawrenceville, NJ

Steven Gelone, PharmD
Vice President, Clinical Development
ViroPharma Incorporated
Exton, PA

Kathleen Jaeger, BS, JD
Executive Director
Generic Pharmaceutical Association
Fairfax, VA

Sok Kang, PharmD
Senior Manager, Regulatory Affairs
Ono Pharmaceuticals
Princeton, NJ

Brian Kearns, BS, MBA
Chief Financial Officer
Lannett Company, Inc.
Philadelphia, PA

Tanya Knight-Klimas, PharmD
Senior Medical Communications Scientist
Wyeth Pharmaceuticals
Collegeville, PA

Harris Levinson, RPh
Development Engineer
GlaxoSmithKline
Parsippany, NJ

Steven M. Lonesky, RPh
Associate Director, Pharmaceutical Formulation
Teva Pharmaceuticals
Sellersville, PA

Patrick McDonnell, PharmD
Associate Professor of Clinical Pharmacy
School of Pharmacy at Temple University
Philadelphia, PA

Michael McGraw, PharmD, MS
Manager of Regulatory Affairs
Teva Pharmaceuticals
Horsham, PA

Richard F. Randall, BSc, PhD
President, Marketing and Sales Consulting
Tawelfan, Inc.
Bellevue, WA

James Russo, BS
Founding Executive Director
Partnership for Quality Medical Donations
Bernville, PA

MaryJean Sawyer, BS
Technical Documentation Manager, Consumer Care Division
Bayer Healthcare
Morristown, NJ

Michael F. Snyder, Esq
Volpe & Koenig, PC
Philadelphia, PA

David Spangler, JD
Senior Vice President, Policy and International Affairs
Consumer Healthcare Products Association
Washington, DC

Tully Speaker, PhD
Professor of Pharmacy and Toxicology Emeritus
School of Pharmacy at Temple University
Philadelphia, PA

Kristie Stephens, BS, RAC
Senior Regulatory Affairs Associate
Lannett Company, Inc.
Philadelphia, PA

Dennis Williams, RPh
Assistant Director, Oncology Regulatory Affairs
GlaxoSmithKline
King of Prussia, PA

Drug Discovery: New Compounds

Tully Speaker

■ Then and Now

Discussion of the generation of new drug compounds by the pharmaceutical industry must consider the topics of drug-receptor modeling, high-throughput screening, and candidate selection. These topics have driven most of the industry over the last two decades. Advances in these areas have developed remarkable, nay, amazing, new science and technology. But the dearth of new products now in most pipelines calls into question the corresponding allocation of effort and expenditures that have compounded by about 13% per year since 1970.[1,2] Yet it is entirely possible the near future will see the pipelines quickly fill. In light of that possibility, it is useful to consider how drugs have historically come about, how the new methods arrived, and what they do.

Long ago plant extracts were the sources of formulations effective in treating a limited number of serious conditions, for instance, opium tincture for pain, digitalis fluid extract for dropsy. The conditions were physiologically and/or pathologically defined, and formulations were developed from folklore with the likelihood of few hits and uncounted numbers of complex misses. In the 19th century, use of plant extracts as drugs began to give way to treatment with specific chemicals separated from the extracts. New chemicals patterned on isolated natural substances became drugs. Then, in the 1840s, volatile chemicals that came into use as general anesthetics made surgery less utterly barbaric. Gradually matching drug to the condition requiring treatment became more nearly possible. Clinical medicine gradually defined itself.

From the 1920s through the 1980s, rapid advances in chemistry, biology, and pharmacology were coupled with increasing reliance on careful clinical research. This coupling produced very effective, if not miraculous, drugs to treat infectious, inflammatory, cardiovascular, psychiatric, respiratory, and invasive diseases, even if the actual target for a drug or its mechanism of action were ill-defined. Retrospective consideration of the current best-selling 100 drugs shows the drug targets were selected on the basis of convincing published biological research extending to human studies. Analogies with bullets that magically found their targets or with keys to hidden locks romanticized the wide endeavor.[3]

■ Drug and Receptor

Drug-receptor modeling may be considered an outgrowth of the 19th- and 20th-century lock and key analogy as applied to drug and receptor, imaginative as that analogy may be. It is that outgrowth and much more. Existence of a number of what might be called keys was demonstrable. Administration of a specific drug in a defined dose could reasonably be relied upon to produce an effect more or less specific to that drug, for example, sleep, analgesia, wakefulness, emesis. Further, isolation and identification of specific physiologic neurotransmitters, acetylcholine by Loewi and Navratil[4] and norepinephrine by von Euler,[5] gave reason to believe a mechanistic description of drugs was feasible. Presumably locks that accepted these neurotransmitters existed.

Proof of the existence of drug receptors emerged only in the latter half of the 20th century. Demonstration of drug binding to specific cells and subcellular fractions was greatly facilitated by the availability of radiolabeled drug substances. Development of methods for the culture of mammalian cell lines and demonstration of specific drug–protein interactions served to show the locks of the lock and key theory really do exist. For example, the several types of steroid hormones independently bind with a specific cytoplasmic receptor protein. This binding causes the receptor to change shape and to dissociate from a preexisting intracellular complex with another protein. Dissociated, the receptor proteins diffuse from the cell cytoplasm into the nucleus where they associate with DNA to initiate protein formation.[6] Similarly, aspirin and other nonsteroidal anti-inflammatory drugs interact with cyclooxygenase enzymes, crippling them and preventing the enzymes from converting arachidonic acid to inflammatory and other mediators.[7]

■ Modeling Molecules

From the earliest days of chemistry, isolation of a substance in crystalline form was considered a requisite to recognizing and identifying a new solid chemical substance. Liquid substances were, if at all possible, converted to solid derivatives to demonstrate their unique identities. The wet, messy complexity of living things only very slowly gave way to recognition that order existed in the complexity, that chains of linked chemical reactions involving specific substances occurred in orderly processes.

In the 1920s, William Bragg began to study the paths of X-rays from essentially point sources as the rays passed through or were scattered by pure crystalline solids. He showed that such crystals allowed narrow beams of X-rays to travel uninterrupted along some paths relative to the crystal axes and were scattered by beams traveling along other paths in a manner analogous to lines of sight in an orchard planted in a regular grid pattern. From this he was able to infer and calculate the relative positions of atoms within the crystals studied. However, the manual measurements and calculations were very laborious.

Over the intervening decades, X-ray crystallography grew in sophistication and complexity so that by the 1960s Max Perutz had determined the crystal structure of myoglobin, a protein with, at that time, a staggering number of atoms in each molecule.[8] By the year 2000, both private and public funding supported X-ray crystallographic determination of structures of proteins from all the families for which amino acid sequences had been established. X-ray crystallography of proteins has benefitted immensely from development of highly sophisticated computing capability and automated equipment that: (1) serially adjusts the angle at which the X-ray beam impinges on the crystal being studied; (2) records the intensity and emergent angle of the beam; (3) calculates the position of the atoms in the crystal which scatter the beam; and (4) with these data map the three-dimensional structure of one or more of the molecules that comprise the crystal.

■ Picturing Molecules

Quite independently, beginning in the 1970s, computer programs able to represent the two- and later the three-dimensional structures of chemical substances were developed. These programs were based on the known composition and reactivity of individual substances, together with their NMR spectra and X-ray crystallographic structures. As the capability of these programs increased, representations of individual molecules could be moved about on the screen at will, rotation of functional groups about a bond could be displayed, and the interaction of pairs of compounds could be visualized.

Ideally, there is one more step before proceeding with drug-receptor modeling in silico. The drug is allowed to interact with and bind to the protein that acts as receptor for it, and then, it is hoped, the pair will crystallize in the bound state. If this in fact occurs, a new X-ray crystallographic study may show, atom for atom, both the drug and receptor in their bound relation to one another. It is more likely that the drug (key) being studied is not a perfect fit to the receptor (lock) and even more likely that the drug–protein complex will not crystallize.

It is possible to display the three-dimensional structure of the receptor protein and the putative drug on the same screen. A number of commercially available or proprietary programs allow the drug image to be nudged near the protein, to estimate the goodness of fit and to optimize it by repositioning the drug and/or by flexing the structures of drug and receptor. And, of course, if such an interaction can be studied with one putative drug, the same evaluation may be carried out with representations of other candidate drug molecules to identify a best fit.

It sounds simple, but programs to represent a structure in two or three dimensions quickly grow complex as more atoms are added and as the flexibility of a structure is displayed. Add a protein with 20,000 to 50,000 atoms and the demands on computer size and time become proportionally greater and therefore more expensive. It is possible to trade off either the sizes of the molecules to be visualized or the goodness of fit, but neither is a property willingly lost. Drug-receptor modeling is not limited to displaying the physical size and structure of molecules. Many programs allow use of colors and color intensities to represent the properties of parts of molecules, such as relative acidity or basicity, electron density, charge distribution, hydrophobicity or hydrophilicity, and solvent accessible surface. Massive computing power and machine time are simply expensive, as are molecular modeling programs capable of handling large molecules with high accuracy and speed.

This is not a text on computer graphics, but the elements of computer representation of molecules may be summarized briefly. The very smallest parts of an image, often referred to as *primitives*, are points, polygons, and vectors. Modeling programs combine these primitives into objects with a specific shape and coordinates in n-dimensional space. These coordinates thus are elements in n-dimensional mathematical matrices, constructs that computer modeling programs can very efficiently manipulate.

The objects are then transformed in object space into atoms and bonds, transformation being a mathematical operation that allows all the coordinates of all the vertices in an object to be changed simultaneously, as when a whole molecule appears to rotate or, more selectively, when atoms linked by a covalent bond rotate relative to one another. In the context of drug-receptor modeling, objects may be atoms, bonds between atoms, or whole molecular structures of candidate drugs. Similarly, but on a larger scale, macromolecular objects may represent proteins, nucleic acids, or membranes with which a candidate drug object may interact.

■ Picturing Interacting Molecules

Interaction between two objects represents a next level of graphic complexity. It requires that the object spaces of individual molecules be transformed into a world coordinate system. In the world coordinate system, matrices of individual "objects" are reassigned positions in a larger common matrix so that interacting molecules may be positioned relative to one another in the larger matrix. Few people can think in the n-dimensional space of the larger matrix, so in almost all modeling programs the n-dimensional matrix is mapped to represent a two-dimensional display space.

Further transformations are applied to allow the person using the program to select the apparent orientation of the images (turned left, right, or upside down) in "viewer" space and to add Western artistic perspective so that an apparently more distant "object" or parts of it may appear proportionately smaller than those that are closer. In commercially available programs, the transformations are carried out without intervention or (usually) awareness of them by the person using the program. Using the best of these programs is akin to watching a video cartoon or playing a computer game. Commercial products are expensive because they enlist high talent and funding.

■ Selection of Preferred Models

The purpose of drug-receptor modeling is to find optimized or best fits between one or more similar drugs and a receptor. (Better fit implies better drug.) This requires calculation of the energy of association between candidate drugs and the receptor. Each candidate drug can, within limits, rotate, flex, stretch and/or compress all the bonds between its atoms. So can the receptor. Thus, the energy with which each conforms to the association varies.

The energy to be considered is the Gibbs free energy DG. *Free* here means available, not necessarily without cost. DG is defined as the difference between the enthalpy or heat content DH and the absolute temperature T of the system multiplied by the entropy DS. In equation form this is written as follows:

$$DG = DH - TDS$$

The heat content is the sum of the energy required to assemble a real compound from essentially infinitely separated atoms (its heat of formation) and the average kinetic energy of its molecules. The entropy of a system is a measure of its tendency to occupy all possible states. For molecular bonds this corresponds to all the energy stored in bonds, analogous in simple terms to the energy stored in springs connecting two atom models as the springs (bonds) are rotated, flexed, compressed, or stretched.

Additional contributions to the free energy of an interacting system arise from electrostatic attractions between oppositely charged portions of molecules and from van der Waal's attractions between any two atoms when they are in very close proximity to one another. For practical considerations in drug-receptor interactions, temperature is assumed constant or nearly so; humans are nearly constant temperature systems.

The sum of these types of potential energy in any specific instance is sometimes referred to as an *empirical force field*. It is considered empirical because the energy terms come from experimental data and basic quantum mechanical calculations. Adapting empirical force field calculations to biological systems has led to gradual improvements and to an approximate consensus now applied in popular programs, notably CHARMM[9] and AMBER.[10]

The whole point of performing these calculations is to estimate those geometries of interacting molecules that reduce the energy of the pair. In the real world, molecules preferentially move to structural forms that reduce their energy. So, too, in silico. A computer program can align the image of a drug molecule in approximation to its presumed receptor and then repetitively adjust the alignment so that oppositely charged atoms more closely approach one another; pairs of electron-rich atoms stretch their bonds to share electron-poor hydrogen atoms with one another to form hydrogen bonds, hydrophobic sections of drugs twist enough to match up more fully with hydrophobic patches of the receptor surface; and, importantly, the drug molecule snuggles deeper into a groove or depression on the receptor surface. At each stage, the energy of the resulting alignment is estimated until, by sequential iterations, a minimum energy is found. The fit is optimized.

Evaluation of fit by energy calculation is central to current efforts to discover new medicinal agents. When, as is usually the case, more than one candidate drug structure is considered, the process is repeated for each to find the drug-receptor pair with the lowest interaction energy, the pair that is very likely to be the most active when tested in vivo. The process is not simple but once set in motion is more effective, simpler, quicker, and less costly than animal studies.

■ The Need for Crystals

The mathematical selection process leads to the one or the few candidate drug computer images of the set available for trial that optimally bind with the computer image of the receptor protein in silico. The process relies on the availability of a real crystal of the receptor protein with well-defined facets and sharp edges. The crystal need not weigh more than the ink needed to print this sentence, but the X-ray diffraction pattern generated from this target receptor protein is the basis for the seemingly three-dimensional computer image of the protein. It may seem a small matter, but the work of crystallizing a useful quantity of each new receptor protein in a reasonable amount of time has been and continues to be a major bottleneck in drug discovery.

At least partial resolution of this bottleneck emerged from a separate series of experiments directed to resolution of the structure of nucleic acids.

■ The Double Helix and All That

As many literate adults know, in 1953 Watson and Crick[11] won the race with Pauling to generate X-ray crystallographic data about deoxyribonucleic acid (DNA) and to interpret the findings to yield new knowledge. They found: (1) DNA exists primarily in the form of helical double strands; (2) the strands consist of chain-like structures in which the sugar deoxyribose and phosphate groups alternate; (3) one of four cyclic nitrogenous bases is attached to each sugar link; (4) the nitrogenous bases of the strands' hydrogen bond to one another in very specific pairings (adenine with thymine, guanine with cytosine); (5) the specific pairings of the nitrogenous bases render the two strands of the double helix anti-parallel and complementary to one another; and (6) the helices have right-handed twists.

These bits of knowledge soon led to further understandings. The complementarity of pairs of DNA strands provides a mechanism for highly accurate replication and transmission of genetic information from one cell to its progeny. In this process, the enzyme DNA polymerase untwists the paired strands and, using each as a template, assembles its complementary strand. Genetic information encoded in DNA as sets (codons) of three consecutive nitrogenous bases is transcribed to corresponding codons in ribonucleic acid (RNA). It is then translated into successive amino acids of protein. These proteins determine the properties and activities of each cell. Some of these proteins act as receptors with which drug molecules interact to exert their effects.

In the 1970s, new types of enzymes were recognized. One type, *restriction enzymes*, breaks apart the chain of alternating ribose and phosphate units of DNA of any organism.[12] Each restriction enzyme acts at one link in a highly specific sequence of four to eight nitrogenous bases attached to a sugar-phosphate chain thousands of links long. The chopped bits are sometimes referred to as *restriction fragments*. Another new type of enzyme found in the 1970s, *DNA ligases*, is able to assemble and integrate restriction fragments into DNA strands and so to generate recombinant DNA.[13]

■ Determining Nucleotide Sequences

It helps, in interpreting X-ray crystal data, if the sequence of nucleotides in a sample of DNA is known. By 1975, Sanger et al.[14] had developed the first successful DNA sequencing method. The technique involves cutting each of multiple replicates of the DNA to be sequenced into restriction fragments and using a reserved fraction of the original DNA molecules as templates on which ligases assemble exactly matching strands.

The method cleverly attaches a different fluorescent label to a small fraction of each of the four nucleotides to be linked together by ligases. Linking is in the order dictated by the template, successively attaching nonlabeled nucleotides until, by chance, a labeled nucleotide is added to the chain. The label gums up the works because the bulk of the label cannot be accommodated by the ligase as it attempts to add another nucleotide. Chain building stops at the fluorescent label. What results is a soup containing newly made bits of DNA all of which started at the same point but with ends bearing differently fluorescent nucleotides. Separating the strands electrophoretically by size allows the sequence to be determined in reverse.

In 1986, Hood et al. described a method to attach different fluorescent compounds, each specific to one of the four nucleotide types, to an entire strand of DNA, thus allowing more rapid sequencing.[15] This improvement allowed successive bases to be identified more easily and served as the basis for current high-speed sequencing machines, that is, the laser detection of fluorescently tagged nucleotides as DNA strands flow through capillary tubes, a development that now enables arrays of high-throughput machines to sequence tens of thousands of nucleotides per day.[16,17]

Restriction fragments containing a few thousand base pairs are relatively easily replicated by polymerase chain reaction (PCR) and sequenced by automated procedures. In the 21st century, PCR instruments that automatically replicate DNA are available for modest sums and tens of commercial laboratories compete in offering sequencing services. However, PCR machines have been known to make random mistakes in replication of DNA strands.

■ From DNA to Protein

Recall that a crystal of receptor protein is needed to produce the X-ray pattern on which the computer-generated image is patterned. Converting strands of DNA into a protein crystal involves several steps. First, the DNA sequence of interest, usually a restriction fragment, must be inserted into a suitable recombinant protein-expression system and the resulting system employed to make useful amounts of protein. The choice of expression system is not trivial. Obviously, expressing a human DNA segment in a human cell system is very likely to produce a protein that is correctly folded and posttranslationally modified, for example, by correct attachment of methyl groups and sugars. Mammalian expression systems generally produce low yields, are complex, and are comparatively costly. For many years addition of fetal bovine serum to the growth medium of mammalian systems has been widely used to aid cell growth. However, it is possible and generally preferable to avoid adding complex mixtures of small peptides, growth factors, trace lipids, bovine viruses, and prions to cultures intended to yield therapeutic proteins.

But most strains of human cells, or of nonhuman mammals for that matter, eventually die, just as whole humans and other animals do. Having a cell strain die out raises hob with an experiment. It is easier to plan with immortal cells.

Mammalian cells able to live indefinitely in culture are referred to as a *cell line* or as *immortalized cells*. They are derived from tumors or other cells that have been transformed. They resemble tumor cells but perform most posttranslational modifications in the same way normal cells do. There are many readily available immortalized mammalian cell lines that have remained stable for decades, but other cell types also have advantages.

Generating substantial quantities of recombinant DNA is best done in replicating cells by taking advantage of small double-stranded circles of DNA, called *plasmids*, found in bacteria, yeasts, and a few higher organisms. Plasmids are not chromosomal DNA, but are replicated when a cell containing them replicates. Plasmids can be isolated from other cellular components. To make recombinant DNA, isolated plasmids are cut with the restriction enzyme used to generate the restriction fragment of interest. Then, with the aid of a ligase, the fragment of interest and the cut circle are linked to make a larger circle. The ligase must be chosen to act at the same nucleotide sequence as had been cut, both to make the fragment and to open the original plasmid circle.

The new recombinant plasmids are transplanted or *transfected* into intact cells, for example, *Escherichia coli*, by mixing the cells and plasmids and exposing the mix to high concentrations of certain divalent cations, such as calcium. The efficiency of such transfection is very low and it is often advantageous to link into the plasmid another restriction fragment, one conferring resistance to a specific antibiotic to aid selection of the cells of interest. The mix of cells, most normal and a few doubly recombinant, is then grown in culture medium containing the antibiotic to which the transfected cells are resistant. The antibiotic kills off normal nonresistant cells. Each colony of cells that arises from a single doubly recombinant transformed cell, a colony from one, is called a *clone*. A clone carrying the restriction fragment of interest can thus replicate easily and produce the protein wanted for crystallization experiments or other scientific and economic ends.

Alternatively, cut plasmids and restriction fragments are mixed and the mix is transplanted into yeast cells. Inside yeast cells, the cut plasmid and fragment are linked by yeast DNA repair enzymes to make larger plasmids. Expression systems utilizing yeasts such as *Saccharomyces cerevisiae* or *Pichia pastoris*[18] are perhaps the most frequently used.

In addition, and more amenable to adaptation to high-throughput processes, continuous flow systems providing cell-free protein have been described. These offer the advantages of stable genetic sequences, most posttranslational modifications of mammalian systems, and minimal background protein secretion.[19,20]

Numerous other procedures for generating transfected cells may also be employed. Insect cell-baculovirus expression systems are not costly and can generate proteins in posttranslationally modified soluble form, but yields vary from one protein to the next. More important, although insect-derived proteins are close to, they are usually not identical in posttranslational modification to the corresponding human proteins.

■ Converting DNA Sequences to Genomes

The ability to generate substantial amounts of each of the many restriction fragments available from the DNA has allowed sequencing the entire genetic assembly (the genomes), of many types of organism (*E. coli*), microbes that live in the intestines (*Drosophila melanogaster*), fruit flies, and, in 2001, *Homo sapiens* (people).[21–23]

■ Structural Genomics

Structural genomics research applied to the human and other genome sequences allows identification of a huge number of proteins capable of serving as drug targets. In many instances, stretches of DNA sequence correspond to the known structure of specific proteins; in many others the genetic information represents proteins with unknown structure or function.

As data on the human genome have been acquired, it has become evident that the DNA sequences of people, although very much alike at the large scale, vary from what may be considered a consensus genome at numerous points (or else, for example, we would all have the same color of eyes or hair or all have the same allergies, and so forth). Most frequently, these variations take the form of single-nucleotide polymorphisms (SNPs), which generally do not result in readily distinguishable phenotypic differences, such as eye color or allergies. They are surprisingly frequent as well, occurring about once in every thousand consecutive nucleotides.[24]

SNPs almost always take the form of biallelic polymorphisms in which one purine is replaced by the other (adenosine/guanosine interchange) or one pyrimidine substitutes for the other (cytidine/thymidine interchange). Theoretically, any of the base pairings could substitute for another. These differences help allow differentiation/identification of individuals on the basis of their DNA, a method of some forensic interest. Of broader importance, the presence of a specific SNP or set of SNPs has been linked to human disorders. But sequencing accurate enough to provide better than 99.99% assurance of an individual human's genome is expensive. Stimulus to develop the needed speed and analytic accuracy is provided, at least in part, by a recent National Institutes of Health grant program to support workers attempting to sequence a complete mammalian genome at a cost below $100,000 and eventually $1000. One may expect some employers and insurance companies to encourage this work.

Regrettably, there are as yet very few associations of a specific gene with a specific disease. It is technically possible to examine each gene in a person to find whether or not it is relevant to a specific disease by comparison with the genes of large well-defined sets of people with that disease and a comparable well-characterized set of control individuals. Accurate determination of an individual's genome and accurate comparison of sequences with millions upon millions of nucleotides in nearly identical strings of genomic data from the sets of disease and control populations are required. That can be done.

Goldstein et al.[25] retrospectively examined some 42 sequence variants of genes for which response to a drug had been identified at least twice. They reported that half of these coded for the drug target protein or a metabolic pathway associated with the target. As a result it is fair to say there are data supporting the notion that genetically linked targets can serve as guides to a drug target. It is also fair to say genetic variants may provide targets for new drugs, but also to recognize genetic susceptibility does not necessarily identify individuals who will develop and need treatment for the disease flagged by the variant.

Other studies have associated diseases with variations in gene structure more specifically. By 2002, research in the fields of genetic epidemiology and statistical genetics led to high-throughput searches for genome–disease correlations and estimation of their statistical significance.[26–28]

It is not unreasonable to consider also that expression of the same SNP in a small fraction of the population may be the basis of an infrequent side effect in those taking a candidate drug in a phase 1 or later trial. When multiple variants of a gene appear to militate toward expression of the disease/condition, the group is commonly referred to as *susceptibility genes*. Practically speaking, the multiplicity inherent in a set of susceptibility genes does not render them efficient targets for single drugs nor for high throughput screening procedures to select candidate magic bullets, magic shotgun shot perhaps.

The enormous effort and expense of enlisting clinicians, defining uniform criteria for assessment and diagnosis, assembling libraries comprising clinical data on cohorts of sick people and healthy controls, collecting their DNA and individual genome data, codifying their responses to marketed drugs and drugs in phases 2 though 4, gathering informed consent agreements, and integrating these multidimensional data into a coherent assemblage are daunting. An example is a project begun in 1997 by GlaxoSmithKline in which, by 2005, some 80,000 patients and controls had been enrolled.[29]

■ Genomes to Proteomes

Conversion of the sequence information to an understanding of the posttranslational modification and folding processes represents another major step toward generating a receptor model. Messenger RNA mediates the translation of the complete DNA sequence to the corresponding sequence of amino acids linked as peptides and in so doing edits out *introns*, large noncoding parts of the DNA sequence. The resulting proteins may differ substantially from what was writ as the inheritance from the dividing parent cell: repetitive sequences are omitted as are introns, noncoding sequences scattered throughout the genome.

The edited sequence of all the DNA in a parent cell is generally referred to as the *expressed sequence* and the set of corresponding protein structures is identified as the *proteome*. In 2005, the National Institutes of Health announced awards of approximately $300,000,000 in a continuation of the Protein Structure Initiative, an effort to determine the proteomes of many organisms. The project, initiated in 2000, had by 2005 deciphered more than 1000 protein structures from genomic data and was expected to add another 5000 proteins to the database by 2010.

■ Purifying Proteins and Growing Crystals

Having generated the receptor(s) of interest, a next major step in growing protein crystals is developing a protein purification system. Highly purified protein is essential to produce a useful crystal because the presence of impurities impedes growth of a single large crystal and fosters growth of many small ones. Chromatographic separation techniques provide excellent separations and allow isolation of individual proteins.

However, relatively small differences between similar proteins significantly alter chromatographic behavior and could complicate or perhaps frustrate attempts to automate the separation process as a set of parallel systems. It is now commonplace to include in the expression system a handle or tag that allows facile identification and separation of the desired protein. Such tags include maltose-binding protein or other large proteins with strong affinities, but these necessitate cleavage of the tag and another separation step. A widely used small tag is a sequence of six histidines at the amino end of a protein. The tag latches onto nickel complexing polymer films or to beads that can be separated magnetically from a complex mix. Separation of the hexamer from the nickel with an imidazole reagent is straightforward.

There are several methods to induce a solution of a protein to form single large (a millimeter or more in length) crystals of protein. The protein is almost always in scarce supply, so small volumes of protein solution are the rule. One attempts to dissolve as much protein in as little solvent as possible, centrifuging to separate (and recover) undissolved material. The solvent is almost always water, but it may be a more complex system containing three or more other components in addition to the anticipated ligand: a co-solvent such as dimethylsulfoxide, low concentrations of highly soluble buffer and other salts, and a reducing agent to protect against air oxidation of the anticipated ligand.

All these methods involve gradually increasing the concentration of dissolved protein to a value above its solubility. Obviously, one might add more protein and stir the mix to dissolve the added bit. But stirring or other agitation favors formation of multiple small crystals, not the single crystal wanted. One may slowly cool a warm solution of protein and so at some temperature exceed the solubility of the protein. That must be done slowly to avoid setting up convection currents that disturb the mix. The most gentle and most likely to succeed method is vapor diffusion. Controlled evaporation of water in a closed chamber containing a nonvolatile desiccant gradually concentrates a protein solution. Alternatively, exposing the aqueous protein solution to a water-miscible volatile may allow the volatile to equilibrate with the water and so effectively reduce the amount of water available to dissolve the protein, in effect concentrating it. This latter method also requires careful thermal control.

Membrane proteins pose considerable challenges. Their cellular location in vivo puts them in extensive contact with both cytoplasmic and lipid layers; thus these proteins have both hydrophilic and lipophilic surfaces that do not readily stack one above another to form a crystal lattice. Use of a small co-solute that forms a lipidic cubic phase, for example, glyceryl monostearate, has allowed crystallization of a limited number of membrane proteins in the past decade.[30]

■ High-Throughput Systems for Growing Crystals

Optimizing conditions for growth of a single-protein crystal involves independently varying the types and concentrations of the several components of the mixture in which the protein is dissolved. Such optimization may best be pursued with the aid of any of several commercially available robotic systems. Typically, these robotic systems employ industry standardized plastic plates in which multiple flat bottom wells are molded in uniformly positioned sets of 96, 385, or 1536. These plates were initially developed for use in manual microtiter assays of microbial growth, enzymatic activity, immunoprecipitation, and so on.

By about 1990, clinical and industrial needs for performance of large numbers of repetitive tests led to development of automated instruments able to deliver small liquid volumes and to measure absorbance or emission of light by material in the wells.

The need for additional capabilities in conjunction with the human and other genome projects led to use of multiple quantitative additions of smaller volumes and to realization of throughput speeds of more than 50,000 samples per day. Increasing automation of delivery of crystallization solution components has been matched by successive reductions in the finished volumes of crystallization experiments. In 2006, the volume of mixed fluids needed in one well of a crystallization experiment was less than 100 microliters.

Detection of crystallization in exactly positioned liquids resting on the optically flat bottoms of experimental wells is monitored using microscopes fitted with digital image recorders. Such monitoring is as quick as taking a digital photograph. But crystal nucleation does not occur at some predictable time, and crystal growth to a discernible size is not an instantaneous process. Therefore, crystallization experiments must be monitored by capturing and analyzing a series of consecutive images. It is possible to screen many variables (co-solvent, salts, antioxidant, etc.) in parallel and so to identify the conditions likely to provide X-ray diffraction-quality crystals.

Once a set or a few sets of conditions that yield single crystals of receptor protein have been experimentally identified, it is reasonable to invest more protein in growing larger crystals for X-ray study. At least one milligram-sized crystal of the native protein is currently needed for crystallographic characterization. If several crystals of the protein are available, it is of interest to soak at least one briefly in a solution of the candidate ligand expected (hoped) to bind to it. If the crystal binds with the ligand, the resulting diffraction pattern will differ from its previous pattern, indicate binding, and may define the position at which the ligand binds to the protein.[31]

In some instances, brief soaking in ligand solution results in cracking of the crystal. This is usually taken as evidence that the binding interaction is very strong and that binding induces substantial conformational changes in the protein. These findings are useful guides in determining the extent to which other candidate congeners are likely to fit the binding site on the protein molecule.

In some rare cases, it is possible to cocrystallize the protein and a candidate ligand.[32] In such an instance, there is little doubt about the goodness of fit of the candidate ligand to the binding site on the protein.

■ New and Novel Proteins

The availability of nearly complete human genome sequence information (Build 35 is about 99% complete in 2006[33]) and methods for isolating corresponding individual proteins of unknown structure or function have resulted in recognition of some 2000 to 3000 genes and their corresponding proteins as possible drug targets. The consensus druggable protein appears to be one that presents folds in which drug-like chemicals can fit and that displays functional moieties with which those chemicals may interact. Proteins lacking such properties may have interesting features and/or generate important biological responses but probably are not pharmaceutically accessible in the near term.[34,35]

This abundance of druggable genes has been a mixed blessing for the pharmaceutical industry and has prompted solving of X-ray crystal structures in as rapid a manner as possible. The intent is to categorize the function of a new protein by comparison with protein structures of known function. High-throughput crystal growth and X-ray analysis are essential to rapid screening and development of new drug entities targeting new proteins. Newly recognized protein targets call for synthesis of many candidate drugs and efficient means to screen those many candidates for drug-like activity at receptors whose function is not yet known. All this costs a lot.

Moreover, identifying the function of a newly recognized protein may not produce a therapeutic effect or one that is clinically successful. It is tempting to reason one gene Æ one protein–Æ one target, but many receptors comprise heteromeric assemblies of subunits encoded by distinct genes. (For example, for the pharmacologist an ion channel in an intact animal may behave as a single target but a candidate drug binding to an isolated protein of the channel may not elicit a recognizable response.)

Certainly many successful drugs act at multiple targets, accounting for at least some side effects, but the clinical utility of these drugs results more from the net effect than from single receptor specificity.[36]

■ Fitting Drug to Receptor in Silico and Culling Misfits

When the structure of a drug binding site is known, usually from studies involving an active compound, it is frequently of interest to consider analogs of the active compounds that may have greater bioactivity, an exploitable secondary activity, or fewer unwanted side effects. Virtual screening using rapid automated fitting of drug to receptor becomes an attractive tool. It may be used to select probably active compounds from libraries of structures, such as those in a corporate compound collection, or to assemble candidate structures from a virtual catalog of structural parts.

And virtual screening may be used concurrently for negative selection, ruling out toxicophores or compounds with poor water solubility or poor oral bioavailability. Lipinsky's rule of five, which eliminated compounds that violated one or more of the rules, may be considered an early virtual screening method.[37] Those rules amount to categorical tests predicting good oral absorption and/or permeation if the compound being considered has fewer than 5 hydrogen bond donors; fewer than 10 hydrogen bond acceptors; a molecular weight of less than 500; and a logarithm of the octanol/water partition coefficient (logP) of less than 5.

More recently, Clark and Picket[38] observed that oral bioavailability of absorbed molecules is minimal if their polar surface areas exceed 100 to 140 square angstrom units, and Veber[39] suggests oral absorption of a compound is maximal if it has seven rotatable bonds. Pursuing this set of ideas, Congreve et al.[40] developed a rule of three (or six, depending on what one counts) for synthons, the carbon, oxygen, nitrogen, sulfur, and other skeletons of molecular fragments such as chains of atoms, ring structures, and the like. They based the rule on electron density maps generated from X-ray crystallographic studies of weakly interacting small structures. The rule of three suggests selecting synthons in which molecular weight contribution is less than or equal to 300; the number of hydrogen bond donors is less than or equal to 3 and of hydrogen bond acceptors less than or equal to 3; the calculated logarithm of the octanol/water partition coefficient is less than or equal to 3; the number of rotatable bonds is less than or equal to 3; and the polar surface area is less than or equal to 60 square angstrom units.

More than 20 computer programs collectively offer many thousands of synthon fragment images that may be clicked together in silico to form candidate structures similar to the known actives. The synthon skeletons can be fleshed out with hydrogens by using the Sybyl program and then "3D-ized" with Concord and/or Corina programs. Additional programs rank similarities between the guide structures and the candidate analogs.[41]

Linking synthons together to represent structures likely both to have bioactivity and to be synthetically feasible allows in silico estimation of the ability of the constructs to bind to a receptor site, to dock. Docking programs seek to find the best fits of ligands and receptor sites. Extensively used docking programs include FlexX,[42] DOCK,[43] and GOLD.[44] In most docking programs, the small molecule can be modified to allow conformational changes, but the protein receptor is held rigid.

Several strategies are applied to match ligand and receptor. In FlexX, the Ogston three-point attachment concept[45] is brought to bear; successive triplets (triangles) of points on each putative ligand in its several conformations are matched to triads of all possible interaction sites on the receptor. The fits are scored and recorded with the conformations in a table of triplets of interaction sites. The DOCK algorithm has evolved over more than 20 years. In DOCK, the receptor is envisioned as a pocket in which spherical loci of possible ligand interaction are located. The "goodness" of fit of at least four atoms of a putative ligand (or its disembodied parts) into these interaction spheres is scored and recorded in successive iterations accommodating possible orientations and conformations of the ligand. The GOLD program utilizes parallel algorithms that allow full ligand and partial receptor flexibilities and iteratively searches for hydrogen bonding and other energy-minimizing interactions.

Docking programs differ, sometimes importantly, in how the score, an estimate of the change in energy of association between ligand and receptor (the binding affinity), is computed. Two broad types of scoring calculations are used. They are what might be called empirical and knowledge-based. Empirical systems rely on measures of binding constants in known ligand-receptor systems chosen to include several sets of ionic, hydrogen, and hydrophobic bondings and corresponding entropy values. Knowledge-based scoring systems are derived from the Boltzman law and are used to calculate energies between attracting and repelling atom pairs.

The systems differ from one another in the number of ligand-receptor pairs, reference states, ranges of interacting distance, and other variables used in computing the scores. Scoring programs in current use include ChemScore, GoldScore, and DrugScore. Neither docking nor scoring programs are perfect; human perception still works. Fiorino[46] recently described finding three additional highly active compounds patterned on a known active by in silico docking and scoring augmented by in-person viewing of the results to eliminate false-negative scores.

It is not enough to identify molecules that might bind to receptors and estimate the goodness of fit. The actual chemical substances need to be in hand for testing. The in silico ability to assess the match of a molecular structure of a candidate drug with that of a binding site on a protein relatively accurately and quickly has been paralleled by the ability to prepare extensive sets or libraries of chemical substances that share a common scaffolding and likelihood of exerting biological activity. Two main approaches to the generation of chemical libraries have been pursued, combinatorial and parallel chemical synthesis.

■ High-Throughput Chemistry: Combinatorial Synthesis

If a chemical substance is found to have some desirable/useful biological activity, for example, it reduces elevated blood pressure or stops an infection, the finder of that activity is likely to hope to capitalize on it not only to benefit all humankind, but particularly the finder. And the finder will no doubt hope to find other chemicals that might share that activity in more potent or less toxic form. The finder will want to prepare those other related chemicals and test their activities.

Preparing those other related chemicals has for decades relied on the one-by-one synthesis of new related compounds, *analogs*. That changed in 1982 when Árpád Furka described combinatorial chemistry, a method to prepare a multiplicity of closely related substances, for example, peptides, essentially simultaneously.[47,48]

The essence of Furka's approach was to generate mixtures of chains of a given number of amino acids in every possible sequence and submit the mixtures for screening tests. (It may be noted that shortly before Furka's work was recorded, reports appeared describing tripeptide pituitary hormones and the pentapeptide endogenous opioid peptides Leu-enkephalin and Met-enkephalin.[49])

The choice of a peptide chain as the basis of the combinatorial structure allowed use of amino acids for each link and thus the advantage of having the same functional group, amino or carboxyl, to react at each increment in chain length. To facilitate handling, one end of each peptide chain was fixed at the carboxyl group to resin beads, and additions to the chain were made by so-called solid state synthesis. The carboxyl groups were attached with a bond type that could be easily cleaved under specific conditions but that was otherwise stable. Additionally, side products of a coupling reaction could be removed by pouring off the solvent and rinsing the beads bearing their attached peptide chains with fresh solvent.

At the start, the activated resin was divided into N1 equal portions (where N1 was the number of different amino acids available to react at one end, the acidic end, of the anticipated chain). The amino group of each of the amino acids was protected by attachment of a small blocking group that could be removed without disturbing other bonds. Each type of amino-protected amino acid was then allowed to react at its acidic end with one of the resin bead portions. After reaction the beads with pendant amino acids were unblocked to generate aminoacyl modified resins. An aliquot of each resin sample was reserved for subsequent use.

The remaining portions of the aminoacyl resins were carefully mixed, divided into N2 equal portions, allowed to react separately with one of the N2 types of protected amino acids to generate dipeptides, and then unblocked. As before, aliquots of each resin sample were reserved for subsequent use and the mixtures of dipeptides on each resin sample were cleaved for use in bioactivity tests.

Again, the remaining portions of the now dipeptide-bearing resin were carefully mixed, divided into N3 equal portions, allowed to react separately with one of the N3 types of protected amino acids to generate tripeptides, and then unblocked. As before, aliquots of each resin sample were reserved for subsequent use and the mixtures of tripeptides on each resin sample were cleaved as before.

This process was repeated until the desired n-length of peptide chain was realized. The sum of all the peptides formed S is as follows:

$$S = N1 \times N2 \times N3 \ldots \times Nn$$

a large number, but the number of coupling reactions C is comparatively small:

$$C = N1 + N2 + N3 \ldots + Nn$$

After all the planned amino acid chains had been attached to the sets of resin beads, equal samples of each set of beads were mixed and the peptides were cleaved from the resins to provide material for bioactivity testing.

A Combinatorial Example

If 10 amino acids were employed at each of 5 consecutive steps, the process would generate 100,000 differently sequenced chains of 5 amino acids, a cornucopia of possible new drugs but in a mixture of enormous complexity. Larger sets of starting compounds would of course produce yet more complex mixtures, but orderly ones. The utility of combinatorial largess did not become evident until the mixture was screened for biological activity.

If the peptide mixtures produced by the last synthetic step showed bioactivity, isolation and identification of the active peptide(s) were the next order of business. Each of the samples of resin to which the final peptide links had been attached, the samples one peptide shorter, were separately treated to release their respective peptides. Then, each of the freed peptide mixes was screened for biological activity in as quantitative a manner as feasible to determine the most active peptide mix and to assess how activity varied with the terminal amino acids. Finding active mixes narrowed the field of search.

Next, each of the samples of resin to which the penultimate peptide links had been attached was separately treated to release the respective two-unit-shorter peptide mixes. Each of these two-unit-shorter peptide mixes was likewise screened for biological activity in as quantitative a manner as feasible to determine the most active shorter peptide mix and to see how activity varied with the amino acid sequences.

This process was repeated with resin samples bearing successively shorter peptide chains until an amino acid sequence without activity was encountered. Reasoning backward from the longest active peptide chain allowed identification of the sequence associated with the measured activity. Clearly, expenditure of considerable resources for biological screening was key to unraveling the complexity of the synthetic mixtures.

To confirm the inferences arising from an experimental sequence such as described previously, it is always necessary to make the inferred compounds and to show that the resulting substances have the expected biological activity.

The logic of combinatorial synthesis is not limited in its application to peptide substances. It may equally be applied to oligosaccharides, oligonucleotides, and sequential polycondensates. Recent development of readily cleaved and broadly applicable linker groups to join resin beads (or films) to the molecular scaffold on which candidate drugs are constructed has increased the range and utility of combinatorial synthesis. Further, combinatorial synthesis typically employs reaction mechanisms that may be applied to a wide range of related compounds under essentially identical conditions (eg, Mitsonobu reaction, an intermolecular dehydration reaction between alcohols and acidic components to give stereospecific products,[50] and Suzuki coupling,[51] joining of two aromatic nuclei through reaction of an arylboronic acid and an aryl halide).

■ High-Throughput Chemistry: Parallel Synthesis

Most chemical syntheses have classically been carried out in solution phase with each reaction mixture in a separate vessel. That has not usually been a problem. The difficulties in synthesis have typically been separating excess reactant, side products, and solvents to purify the desired product. Typically, this separation, the *workup*, has involved adding a second solvent immiscible with the first, more or less selectively partitioning excess reactant, side products, and desired product between the solvents, separating and collecting the product-rich solvent phase, and evaporating the solvent from a residue, mostly of desired product. Often, the desired product required a further chromatographic purification. In short, running the reaction has not been the problem, isolating the product has. The process did not readily yield large numbers of closely related candidate drugs and neither was it amenable to automation.

That changed with the commercial availability of high-quality polymer polystyrene resin beads carrying, initially, ion-exchange sulfonic acid or quaternary ammonium groups and later other reactive functionalities such as isocyanate or aldehyde. These beads, especially ion-exchange beads, prepackaged sterile in 5-, 10-, 25-, and 100-mL hypodermic syringe tubes have greatly facilitated cleanup and solid phase extraction of urine samples in clinical laboratories. Such tubes are uniformly packed with resin or sorbent, typically occupying not more than half their volume, allowing all the sample to be added in one step. This application of tube processing was soon followed by its application to multiplexed parallel synthesis of small batches of compounds.[52–54]

The concepts involved are simple. In the simplest sort of application, a mixture from a completed small-scale reaction, for example, an amide synthesis mixture made using a slight excess of acidic reactant, is poured into a tube packed with a quaternary-ammonium fuctionalized resin bead. The excess acid is trapped by the resin and the product flows out dissolved in the initial reaction solvent. Any reaction solvent and contained product held up in the resin bed is eluted into clean receivers with an additional small volume of the initial reaction solvent. If 10 different acids are to be used in 10 similar reactions, 10 tubes and receivers are set up in parallel. If a hundred acids are to be used, a robotic system is desirable, but keeping track of the starting materials and labeling the receivers emerges as a task requiring attention.

Alternatively, a product may be held in a resin-packed tube while reaction solvent, excess reagent, and side products are rinsed away with more of the same solvent. Then, an appropriate solvent can elute the desired product. Obviously, separate tubes containing cation- and anion-exchange resins may be used in tandem, the first tube delivering into the second without intervention.

The variety of commercially available resin-supported functionalities useful as scavengers of unreacted components includes benzaldehyde for primary amines or hydrazines, benzylisocyanate for both primary and secondary amines and for alcohols, benzyltriethylammonium carbonate for carboxylic acids and phenols, triphenylphosphine for alkyl halides, and benzyltrisaminoethylamine for acid chlorides and isocyanates.

Variations in the packing of filtration tubes are useful and sometimes necessary. Polystyrene beads may disadvantageously swell in common halogenated solvents, so it may be useful to pack tubes with purified silica instead. Water and diluted acids or bases are easily retained by silica beds. Organic solvents added to such water-wetted columns readily equilibrate with the interstitial water, allowing selective partitioning of hydrophilic compounds into water retained in the silica bed and nearly complete elution of the organic phase.

Equipment for the separate steps in parallel synthesis protocols is available in almost all chemical synthesis laboratories but is not necessarily organized or integrated for parallel synthesis. Such equipment includes temperature-controlled heating blocks that accept multiple identical vessels, multiunit filtration racks, and nitrogen blow-down or heated centrifugal evaporators. Robotic systems offered by several manufacturers are adapted or adaptable to multisample processing.

Additionally, a number of liquid-handling systems may be adapted to parallel separation. Thus, it may be practical to generate many more candidate drugs a day using a parallel synthesis, or more accurately, a parallel separation approach. Refined automation of workup in place of the complex manipulations and high levels of eye–hand coordination that characterize classical product isolation are brought to bear in making parallel synthesis an economical way to prepare extensive libraries of candidate drugs. Robots are tireless.

Teflon 96-well plates in the format developed for microbiologic and enzymatic assays are of particular utility for high-throughput small-scale syntheses. Reaction mixtures in which precipitates form in one plate may be robotically pipetted to a second, filter-bottomed plate (eg, bottoms of glass fiber, microporous polypropylene, polyvinylidene fluoride, etc.) to capture the solid while the filtrates are collected in a third plate made in the same 96-well format.

■ Automated Cleanup

All the desired products from a group of parallel syntheses, even resin-based reactions, require workup to reduce impurities as much as practicable and, looking ahead, to lower the incidence of false positives when tested in biological systems. Selective resins might certainly be used to scavenge expected impurities and side products from reactions performed in 96-well plates. Resin beads, which quickly dry, develop high static charges, and scatter, are difficult to pack into even 10-mL tubes. Prepacked 96-well plates suited to parallel synthesis separations do not seem to be commercially available.

A high-throughput purification system adaptable to products of parallel syntheses is available, but there are none commercially available capable of purifying, quantitating, and tracking very large numbers of reaction mixtures, especially in the small volumes characteristic of the automatable 96-well format. Ideally, for a high-throughput system, each filtrate is separated/purified by high-performance chromatography before the individually collected fractions are characterized.

■ Product Characterization

Ultraviolet spectrophotometers able to utilize volumes of 1 μL became available in 2005 and with reference to a calibration file can estimate the amount of product(s) in a sample. These seem ideal for small-scale synthesis, but at this writing are not yet adapted to robotic sample handling or to automated data recording and tracking. Instead, it has become routine to characterize the structure and identity of major components in an aliquot of a chromatographic fraction with liquid chromatography/ mass spectrometry or electrospray/mass spectroscopy.

The technique of ambient mass spectroscopy or desorption electrospray ionization (DESI) is a very recent innovation in structure determination applicable to high-throughput analysis of very small sample sizes. Very briefly, electrically charged solvent droplets are sprayed in ambient air onto a succession of dried samples arranged in an array on a substrate such as a microscope slide. The charged droplets cause ions from the sample surface to be released and these ions are swept into the vacuum interface of a mass spectrometer where the ions (and daughter ions in a tandem instrument) are rapidly and sensitively analyzed.[55,56]

In short order, high-throughput synthesis generates an enormous amount of data that must be linked unambiguously to each reaction mixture and anticipated candidate drug. Commercial systems capable of tracking huge volumes of data arising from synthesis, separation, identification, and quantitation of products in one 96-well plate per day do not seem to be available. Large pharma has assembled these for in-house use; Everett et al. have described one such as at Pfizer UK.[57] It is evident that many new series of chemical substances may be generated much more rapidly than before the adoption of high-throughput systems.

◼ Structural Genomics Leads to Structural Proteomics

Structural genomics research applied to the human and other genome sequences allows identification of a huge number of proteins capable of serving as drug targets. In many instances, stretches of DNA sequence correspond to the known structure of specific proteins; in many others, the genetic information represents proteins with unknown structure or function.

The transition from structural genomics to structural proteomics calls on the traditional larger scale separation of proteins by chromatography or two-dimensional gel electrophoresis followed by mass spectroscopic identification of the proteins. An application of this information can provide a differential basis for comparison of expression during the maturation of an organism/culture or in the development of a disease. This traditional procedure provides a chance to monitor the associated proteins as the process unfolds. The information in an inventory of an organism's proteins and their functions is also useful in its own right.

◼ Target Selection Through Structural Proteomics

Elucidation of the proteomes of many microorganisms has allowed assembly of this information in a series of flow diagrams separately displaying the individual metabolic pathways of each of numerous species of microbes. This information may be displayed as a diagram for each organism in which the sequences of enzymatic substrates and products are shown as a series of loci, each substance appearing only once. The enzymes catalyzing conversion of substrate to a first and then successive products are represented by arrows. Thus, the web-like diagrams show not only the metabolic routes but also metabolic junctions. It is immediately evident on examination of such diagrams that some few enzymes act as choke points because they are the only means by which a given organism can generate an essential product if it is not available in the environment.

These diagrams may be used in conjunction with information on the rates at which substrates are converted by enzymes to their respective products under various conditions. So informed, one can use these flow diagrams in various modeling approaches, notably incorporating constraint-based flux-balances, and successfully use these to calculate deletion phenotypes and either optimal or fatal growth conditions.

The constraint-based flux-balance approach has been applied to a number of microbes. Notable among these are *E. coli, Helicobacter pylori*, and *Saccharomyces cerevisiae*. The result is identification of a metabolic core of essential reactions for each organism, reactions that never stop, in any of thousands of simulated environments.

Core reactions appear to be evolutionarily conserved and always active. An analogous study of more than 700 *Salmonella enterica* enzymes in a smaller number of environments identified 15 absolutely essential enzyme reactions.

Noncore reactions are species specific and may be considered conditionally active, that is, functioning as may be advantageous depending on nutrient supply or balance.

Core reactions, the unconditionally essential reactions, serve as targets of antibiotics that interfere with bacterial metabolism, for example, trimethoprim, fosfomycin, cycloserine.[58–60] If the core reactions are considered choke points, they identify the microbial metabolic fluxes that are particularly vulnerable to antibiotics.

It follows that coupling knowledge of the proteome and corresponding metabolic fluxes of other microbes, such as the *Mycobacterium avium* complex, would allow an informed search for agents capable of blocking unconditionally essential pathways in such organisms, and thereby offer a means of blocking further emergence of drug-resistant strains.

However, as Rene Dubos[61] pointed out in 1942 and again in 1952, microbes inevitably develop drug resistance and the more quickly if overused, a caution almost universally unheeded by a pressured medical community with few alternatives.

■ High-Throughput Binding Studies

It must be self-evident that most biological functions of cells do not involve DNA itself but protein molecules ultimately derived from DNA. It follows that preparation of protein microarrays analogous to DNA microarrays would be useful in screening for biological activity. Microarrays of individual protein receptors printed on glass slides provide a convenient and automatable format with which to assess protein interaction with candidate ligands or other small proteins.[62] Printed fresh, they are excellent tools.

As an alternative to printing, protein microarrays have been prepared by transferring multiply protonated proteins selected from mixtures on the basis of mass and charge and gently depositing them on solid or liquid-coated surfaces. Mass spectra of proteins from the resulting arrays have been shown to match those of the authentic compounds, and the arrayed proteins retain their bioactivity.[63]

Unfortunately, protein array components have short working lifetimes. Even frozen in place, proteins have widely different stabilities, a weakness that limits the utility of such arrays. Neither is it feasible to dry the arrays; proteins dried in contact with vitreous surfaces are quickly denatured. Nonetheless, the idea of protein microarrays is highly attractive for high-throughput screening.

Just as a large number of essentially identical cells may be transfected with many replicates of the same plasmid to generate substantial quantities of one protein, it is possible to transfect a large number of essentially identical cells with a large number of different plasmids. Such a procedure can result in a large number of differently transfected cells, each expressing a different protein.

The process depends on the availability of copy DNA (cDNA) probes. These probes are specific nucleotide sequences that bind only to their complementary DNA to form duplex strands. cDNAs may be prepared using restriction enzymes as described earlier. Alternatively, cDNA may be prepared using *reverse transcriptases*, viral enzymes able to reverse transcribe single-stranded messenger RNA to the corresponding single-stranded DNA. This alternative process is sometimes called *retro-synthesis*.

cDNA is often radioactively or fluorescently labeled as an aid in detecting the probe when it is incorporated into a plasmid in an array. cDNA, however made, can be incorporated into plasmids, essentially as previously described. Microscope slides may be robotically printed with cDNA-containing plasmids suspended in gelatin solution to generate microarrays in a manner analogous to preparation of DNA microarrays. Gelling of the gelatin solution fixes the plasmids in place on the slide. The resulting plasmid microarrays can have densities of 5000 to 10,000 spots per slide. Thus, whole genomes may be represented on a small number of slides.

Adding a lipoidal transfection agent such as polyethylenimine converts the plasmid microarray to one of lipoidal DNA complexes. Adding a suspension of adherent mammalian cells on top of the spots quickly results in a new microarray in which each spot contains about 25 to 100 transfected cells. Each so transfected slide represents a living microarray. Because the cells are placed on the plasmids rather than the plasmids on the cells, this process is sometimes referred to as *reverse transfection* and the array is called a *transfected cell array* (TCA).

Because each of the few transfected cells in each spot expresses only one protein and the spots have been printed at discrete locations, the transfected cell array may be considered a kind of microarray displaying many different proteins. If the cells in the array are those of eukaryotic (nucleated cell) origin, posttranslational modification (eg, glycosylation) of the expressed proteins may be expected. Using several cell lines allows one to distinguish posttranslational modifications characteristic of the lines and possibly to recognize protein–protein interaction.[64,65]

■ Assemble a Mouse

Transgenic and/or knockout mice have traditionally been used in genetically based gain- or loss-of-function studies. Their use entails very high costs for commercial strains and/or lengthy periods of in-house animal care for home-grown strains. Additionally, using such designer mice is complicated by their similarity to normal mice; they generally do not display a readily evident alteration in phenotype that might be associated with certainty to the mutated gene.

Transfected cell arrays may also be utilized to reduce the costs and lengthy care needed to use such mice. Transfected cell arrays may be constructed to exhibit specific genetic RNA interference (RNAi), and thus to generate dozens of phenotypes in a single array. No one spot in the array is equivalent to a whole genetically modified mouse. The array may be thought analogous to those holiday toys for children that bear the label "Some assembly required."

RNA interference, first described in nematodes,[66] is initiated by the action of the enzyme Dicer on long double-stranded RNA (dsRNA) cutting it into bits called *short interfering duplex RNA* (siRNA). A resulting snippet of siRNA associates with certain cytoplasmic proteins to form an RNA-induced silencing complex (RISC) the anti-sense strand of which guides the RISC to corresponding messenger RNA. RISC acts on the mRNA, slicing it into smaller segments that are then readily lysed by nucleases in the cytoplasm. A knockout organism results.

Mammalian cells are more finicky; they do not respond as well to siRNA prepared from long dsRNA as do nonmammalian cells. dsRNA longer than 30 nucleotide triads (nt) stimulates a lethal interferon response. But, mammalian siRNA strands between 21 and 15 nt work well to silence gene expression and can either be transfected or introduced into cells as synthetic agents. In contrast to nonmammalian cells, neither replication of siRNA nor its interference with gene expression is heritable in mammalian cells; the siRNA effect is itself silenced as cells repeatedly divide and the siRNA becomes diluted in the growing culture.

This problem has been overcome by developing plasmid constructs that contain a so-called short hairpin RNA (shRNA) along with drug resistance coding sequences that allow stable transfection and the ease of antibiotic-based cell selection.[67–69] Furthermore the duration of siRNA effectiveness has been increased through use of retrovirus and lentivirus as expression vectors.[70]

Movement of siRNA techniques from multiwell screens to transfected cell arrays has been relatively slow and applied only to small sets of genes coding for specific proteins to date. However, it is reasonable to expect the technical advantages developed and refined for high-throughput DNA microarray systems will accrue to transfected cell arrays, for example, use of smaller volumes of reagents, robotic spot printers, automated array scanning systems, and commercial availability of siRNA libraries to make TCAs cost effective. In parallel, computational tools to identify the genomic targets of siRNAs have become available.[71–72]

An immediate advantage of cDNA spotted microarrays is that they may be stored for extended periods before use in a screen or to replicate/confirm a prior screen. Additionally, only a relatively few cells are used to prepare a microarray, in general providing economy of scale and an advantage if the biological system is in short supply. More generally, cell microarrays are well suited to high-throughput screening for specific activities, such as interference with kinase signaling pathways. The cDNAs are printed at specific locations on each slide so that the cDNA at a spot and its corresponding expressed protein are known; the target protein of an active drug can be traced and identified rapidly. Their corresponding amino acid sequences can thus be learned.

■ High-Throughput Screening: G-Protein-Coupled Receptors

Of the currently 100 best-selling drugs, about a quarter act through G-protein-coupled receptors (GPCR). These include opioid agonists to block pain, b2 adrenoceptor agonists to control asthma, histamine receptor antagonists to suppress peptic ulcers, and angiotensin receptor antagonists to reduce hypertension. Together they represent a large share of the world pharmaceutical market.

Yet these drugs target only about 30 of the approximately 750 receptors in the GPCR superfamily of the human genome. About 400 others are considered likely to be of interest as drug targets. Natural ligands are known for roughly half of these putative drug targets. These GPCRs (and other receptors) for which no ligand has been identified are often referred to as *orphan receptors* and appear to offer opportunities for development of new drugs.

On the basis of sequence homology, GPCRs are usually grouped in three sets. The largest set, Group A, contains receptors for catecholamines, chemokines, glycoproteins, lipids, neuropeptides, and nucleotides. Group B includes receptors for other peptide ligands, and Group C encompasses metabotropic receptors for ligands such as gamma-aminobutyric acid and calcium ion.

Structure of G-Protein-Coupled Receptors

All GPCRs are large membrane-bound filamentous proteins in which eight hydrophilic lengths alternate with seven hydrophobic segments. By convention, the hydrophobic segments are serially numbered starting with the segment nearest the very hydrophilic carboxylic acid end. The acid end and the first hydrophobic segment normally position themselves at the interface between the cytoplasm and the cell membrane. The acid end is in the cytoplasm, the hydrophobic segment in the oily membrane; the free energy change drives the system. The amino end extends into the extracellular medium.

In successive adjustments of free energy, the hydrophobic segments become aligned side by side spanning the oily membrane between the interfaces. The hydrophilic lengths form loops alternately projecting past the external interface into the surrounding medium or through the internal interface and into the cytoplasm. Tracing these in order, the hydrophilic length connecting segments 1 and 2 is in the surrounding medium, the one connecting segments 2 and 3 in the cytoplasm, the length between 3 and 4 in the surrounds, that between 4 and 5 again in the cytoplasm, and so on. The filamentous GPCR is said to assume a sinusoidal disposition, snaking back and forth through the cell membrane.

The arrangement of hydrophobic segments in the membrane is yet more complicated. They approximate a cylindrical shape in which the hydrophobic segments are wrapped around to form a barrel-like assembly. The segments are positioned like barrel staves, parallel to the cylindrical axis with segments 1 and 7 aligned side by side.

The whole assembly resembles a transmembranal pore in which the exposed terminal amino group and hydrophilic extracellular loops form a binding site for large ligands; smaller ligands bind deeper into the barrel structure. In the barrel-like structure, the terminal carboxyl group of every G-protein-coupled receptor protein is positioned near the intracellular loop between the sixth and seventh transmembranal strands.

The loop between segments 6 and 7 usually serves as the binding site for G proteins. There are three G-protein subunits, usually identified as a, b, and g, assembled as a heterotrimer. More than a dozen closely related types of G proteins have been recognized, each with quite specific activities.

A number of individual ligands bind at more than one type of G-protein-coupled receptor. Ligand binding causes subunits of the G-protein heterotrimer to dissociate and to activate nearby membrane-bound enzymes that generate so-called second messengers. One major type of thus activated enzymes catalyzes conversion of purine triphosphates into the corresponding cyclic purine monophosphate (cyclic adenylmonophosphate or cyclic guanylmonophosphate). Another is a family of phospholipases that release phospholipid-derived esters (diacylglycerol or inositol triphosphate). The second messengers in turn activate protein kinases that trigger a cellular response. For example, inositol triphosphate triggers release of calcium ion from bound intracellular stores. The calcium then binds to calmodulin and kinases activating yet another set of intracellular enzymes by phosphorylation.

It may be seen that taking into account the sheer number and variety of G-protein-coupled receptor proteins, the nearly promiscuous ligand binding at these receptors, the variety of G-protein types, and the range of second messengers, disentangling their mechanisms and functions allows wide scope for development of new drug entities.

But G-protein-coupled receptor processes are not haphazard. The structures of the receptor proteins are known or knowable and in the intricate ballet of second messengers the same steps are traced in each repeated performance.

An example of one strategy to identify ligands for orphan receptors is the linking of a restriction fragment bearing the genetic sequence for the orphan receptor into a plasmid and its transfection into cells. The resulting expression systems are then exposed to a set of compounds that in nature might serve as ligands for the orphan receptor. Binding of a candidate ligand to the GPCR is monitored by measuring second messenger–induced effects.

The expression system needs to be chosen with care. It should supply G proteins, membrane-bound enzymes activated by G proteins, and the wherewithal to generate second messengers. These needs may be met with any of several well-characterized cell lines, notably Chinese Hamster Ovary (CHO), Human Embryonic Kidney (HEK), *Xenopus laevis* oocytes, or *Saccharomyces cerevisiae*.

Monitoring Transfection

Further, in a well-controlled experiment seeking ligands for the orphan, it is necessary to be sure the plasmid has been expressed in all the cells to be used. It may happen that not all cells in a culture will be transfected. Failure to generate second messenger effects might not mean the absence of an effective ligand, but rather that the plasmid DNA was not transfected and expressed as a surface protein.

It is relatively simple to enlarge the plasmid slightly to carry a tag of convenience. The DNA sequence coding for a protein such as hemagglutinin can serve as such a tag. Linking it to the N-terminal sequence of the orphan receptor restriction fragment builds it into the plasmid. As cells carrying the plasmid grow and divide, the tag is displayed at the surface of the cell together with the amino group of the receptor when both proteins are expressed.

The presence of the tag, and thus of the GPCR too, may be established and assured by adding a fluorescently labeled hemagglutinin antibody to the cell culture. So labeled, transfected cells may be separated from nonfluorescent cells and collected with a fluorescence-activated cell sorter. The population of transfected cells may be grown to numbers needed for high-throughput screening in multiwell plates.

To screen for the ligand(s) binding to G-protein receptors one needs not only to generate the second messengers but also to have a way to recognize them should they appear. In a mammalian cell-based screen, there is almost always release of second messengers.

Some dyes, such as fura-2, fluoresce when they bind calcium. If such a dye in the form of its neutral lipophilic ester is added to a resting cell culture, the ester diffuses across plasma membranes and, once in the cytoplasm, is hydrolyzed to the corresponding acid. The resulting negatively charged acid now cannot diffuse back out of the cell. Though it does not fluoresce itself, it can form a stable fluorescent complex with calcium but not other ions. The change in cytoplasmic concentration of free calcium ion in response to ligand binding may thus be monitored by measuring fluorescence at a wavelength characteristic of the fura-2-calcium complex.[73,74]

Additional assays based on more specific imaging of the cell, of the GPCR, or of another interacting protein have been developed. These assays are based on movement of the protein within the cell or on a change in spectral properties resulting from the binding of ligand to receptor[75,76] and, because they provide more information, are often called *high-content assays*.

A green autofluorescent protein (GFP, derived from the jellyfish *Aequoria victoria*) when attached to the cytoplasmic acid end of a b2 adrenoceptor has been shown to move with the receptor from the cell surface. After binding the ligand, the receptor is internalized in an acidic endosome and subsequently recycled to the surface. Movement of the GFP-GPCR conjugate is evidence of ligand binding[77] and can be followed by pseudoconfocal imaging systems adapted to monitor multiwell plates.

If a laboratory can enlist the skills needed to culture and transfect melanophores, these cells can serve in a screen selecting ligands for orphan GPCRs. *Melanophores*, cells from the nearly pigment-free frog *Xenopus laevis*, contain melanosomes, intracellular organelles carrying the dark brown/black pigment melanin.

Binding of a candidate ligand to an orphan receptor expressed in a melanophore may traduce a signal that dissociates the a subunit of the guanine nucleotide binding protein from the heterotrimer. If the trimer is thus broken up, the enzymes adenylate cyclase and phospholipase C become activated and the second messengers cyclic adenosine monophosphate (cAMP) and diacylglycerol are formed. A melanocyte responds to cAMP by dispersing its melanosomes quite uniformly throughout the cell, quickly causing it to appear darker. Melanosomes in a cell aggregate if adenylate cyclase is inhibited and the cell thus appears to become lighter. The response is sensitive, occurs within minutes, and is readily monitored colorimetrically. Constituative activity serves as an indicator of successful transfection. *Xenopus* melanocytes are readily adaptable to growth in multiwell plates and high-throughput screening of orphan GPCRs for candidate ligands.

Complex as G-protein-coupled receptor screening assays may seem, they are readily adaptable to 96-well or denser plates and well within the capabilities of commercially available automated systems that can perform 100,000 screens per day. The strength of this approach derives from direct targeting of the disease phenotype as a mechanistic study using relevant cell models.

■ Validating Target Receptors

Identification of a class of ligands or a new ligand in a class that binds to an orphan GPCR is exciting. But it is important to connect (or to use the *mot de jour*, validate) the newly found receptor with a disease for which a marketable drug is needed. Receptor validation is a series of steps in which the cumulative weight of evidence is the relevant measure.

A first step is attempting to match the genomic sequence of the presumed orphan receptor with sequences of known receptor function, but matching, although a clue, does not guarantee the expected function. Similarly, finding a ligand that activates a receptor provides another item of evidence. Steps matching the orphan receptor to an endogenous ligand and in vitro to a receptor that varies expression in health and disease offer stronger validation. So too does matching the orphan to the expression of the receptor in healthy and diseased animal models and humans. Perhaps the last steps in validating a candidate receptor are refining the initial set of candidate ligands to an optimized candidate and to advance the ligand as a drug that is effective in clinical treatment of the disease. Validation that begins as high-throughput screening gradually changes to low-throughput clinical experiments extending over days to months and longer.

Validation is tricky business. For example, high-throughput screening coupled with an understanding of the global metabolic fluxes in an infectious organism may allow efficient design, synthesis, and validation of a new antimicrobial. It is not certain that these combined capabilities would today anticipate drug action on unintended targets, for example, aminoglycosides on the eighth cranial nerve and ability to hear.

It is immensely helpful, but not necessary, to understand the origins of a disease condition to find and validate drugs that benefit the patient. For example, though essential hypertension has been recognized for decades, its genetic or other origins remain uncertain. Useful drugs for its treatment appear to act by indirect targeting. Quick-paced technologies validated at each step have allowed development of effective therapies using angiotensin-converting enzyme inhibitors, calcium channel blockers, and a 1-adrenergic antagonists.

There is, however, another set of drug targets to which high-throughput methods do not now seem amenable. Many complex disease conditions, such as depression and schizophrenia, do not readily admit study of the phenotypic cell isolated from the intact organism. It is possible these and others may arise from single nucleotide polymorphisms.

Huge libraries have been developed by the pharmaceutical industry. These catalog synthons, chemical entities, X-ray diffraction and mass spectrometric data, ligand activities, known and orphan receptors, drug effects and side effects in many diseases, diagnostic criteria, clinical histories, treatment outcomes, patient-specific genomes, and patient-specific SNP cohorts. Holdings in these libraries have been correlated, mostly in the physical sciences. The computational power needed to integrate these entire libraries is enormous and the costs staggering. At successive stages validation will be both essential and challenging.

■ References

1. Booth JB, Zemmel R. Prospects for productivity. *Nat Rev Drug Discov*. 2004;3:451–456.

2. Chapman JT. Drug discovery—the leading edge. *Nature*. 2004;430:109.

3. Zambrowicz BP, Sands A. Knockouts model the 100 best drugs: will they model the next 100? *Nat Rev Drug Disc*. 2003;2:38–51.

4. Loewi O. Pflugers Arch. *Gesamte Physiol*. 1921;189: 239–242.

5. von Euler US. *Handbuch der Experimentellen Pharmakolgie*. Heidelberg, Germany: Springer-Verlag; 1946:186–230.

6. Chan L, O'Malley BW. Mechanism of action of sex hormones. *N Engl J Med*. 1976;294:1322–1328, 1372–1381, 1430–1437.

7. Vane JR. Inhibition of prostaglandin synthesis as a mechanism of action for aspirin-like drugs. *Nat New Biol*. 1971;231:232–235.

8. Perutz M. Early days of crystallography. *Meth Enzymol*. 1985;114:3–18.

9. Brooks BR, Bruccoleri RE, Olafson BD, States DJ, Swaminathan S, Karplus M. CHARMM: a program for macromolecular energy, minimization, and dynamics calculations. *J Comp Chem*. 1983;4:187–217.

10. Weiner SJ, Kollman, PA, Nguyen DT, Sase DA. An all atom force field for simulations of proteins and nucleic acids. *J Comp Chem*. 1986;7:230–252.

11. Watson JD, Crick FH. A structure for deoxyribonucleic acid. *Nature*. 1953;421:397–398.

12. Pingoud A, Jeltsch A. Structure and function of type II restriction endonucleases. *Nucleic Acid Res*. 2001;29:3705–3727.

13. Barany F. The ligase chain reaction in a PCR world. *PCR Methods Appl*. 1991;1:5–16.

14. Sanger F, et al. Nucleotide sequence of bacteriophage phiX 174. *J Mol Biol*. 1977;125:225–246.

15. Strauss EC, Kabori JA, Siu G, Hood LE. Specific primer directed sequencing. *Anal Biochem*. 1986;154:353–360.

16. Dovichi N. Development of a DNA sequencer (letter). *Science*. 1999;285:1016.

17. Zhou G, Kamahori MH, Okano K, Harada K, Kambara H. Miniaturized pyrosequencer for DNA analysis with capillaries to deliver deoxynucleotides. *Electrophoresis*. 2001;22:3497–3504.

18. Cregg JM, Cereghino JL, Shi J, Higgins DR. Recombinant protein expression in *Picia pastoris*. *Mol Biotechnol*. 2000;16:23–52.

19. Kigawa T, et al. Cell-free production and stable isotope labeling of milligram quantities of proteins. *FEBS Lett*. 1999;442:15–19.

20. Stewart L, Clark R, Behnke C. High throughput crystallization and structure determination. *Drug Disc Today*. 2002;7:187–196.

21. Venter JC, et al. The sequence of the human genome. *Science*. 2001;291:1304–1351.

22. International Human Genome Sequencing Consortium. Initial sequencing and analysis of the human genome. *Nature*. 2001;409:860–921.

23. Ewing B, Green P. Analysis of expressed sequence tags indicates 35,000 human genes. *Nat Gen*. 2000;25:232–234.

24. Brookes AJ. The essence of SNPs. *Gene*. 1999;234:177–186.

25. Goldstein DB, Tate SK, Sisodiya SM. Pharmacogenetics goes genomic. *Nat Rev Genet*. 2003;4:937–947.

26. Van Eerdewegh P, et al. Association of the ADAM32 gene with asthma and bronchial hyper responsiveness. *Nature*. 2002;418:426–430.

27. Giallourakis C, et al. IBD5 is a general risk factor for inflammatory bowel disease: replication of association with Crohn disease, and identification of a novel association with ulcerative colitis. *Am J Hum Genet*. 2003;73:205–211.

28. Martin E, et al. Association of single-nucleotide polymorphisms of the tau gene with late onset Parkinson disease. *JAMA*. 2004;286:2245–2250.

29. Roses AD, Burns DK, Chissoe S, Middleton L, St. Jean P. Disease specific target selection: a critical step down the right road. *Drug Disc Today*. 2005;10:177–189.

30. Landau EM, Rosenbusch JP. Lipidic cubic phases: a novel concept for crystallization of membrane proteins. *Proc Natl Acad Sci USA*. 1996;93:1452–1455.

31. Gill AG, et al. Identification of novel p38 alpha MAP kinase inhibitors using fragment-based lead generation. *J Med Chem*. 2005;48:414–426.

32. Card GL, et al. A family of phosphodiesterase inhibitors discovered by cocrystallography and scaffold based drug design. *Nat Biotechnol*. 2005;23:201–207.

33. International Human Genome Sequencing Consortium. Finishing the euchromatic sequence of the human genome. *Nature*. 2004;431:931–945.

34. Hopkins AL, Groom CL. The druggable genome. *Nat Rev Drug Disc*. 2000;1:727–730.

35. Orth AP, Batalov S, Perrone M, Chanda SK. The promise of genomics to identify novel therapeutic targets. *Expert Opin Ther Targets*. 2004;8:587–596.

36. Roth BL, Sheffler DJ, Kroeze WK. Magic shotguns versus magic bullets: selectively non-selective drugs for mood disorders and schizophrenia. *Nat Rev Drug Disc*. 2004;3:353–359.

37. Lipinsky CA, Lombardo F, Dominy BW, Feeney PJ. Experimental and computational approaches to estimate solubility and permeability in drug discovery and development settings. *Adv Drug Deliv Rev*. 1997;23:3–25.

38. Clark DE, Picket SD. Computational methods for prediction of drug-likeness. *Drug Disc Today*. 2000;5:49–58.

39. Veber DF, Johnson SR, Cheng HY, Smith BR, Ward KW, Kopple KD. Molecular properties that influence oral bioavailability of drug candidates. *J Med Chem*. 2002;45:2615–2623.

40. Congreve M, Carr R, Murray C, Jhoti H. A "rule of three" for fragment-based lead discovery. *Drug Disc Today*. 2003;8:876–877.

41. Schneider J, Bohm H-J. Virtual screening and fast automated docking methods. *Drug Disc Today*. 2002;7:64–70.

42. http://www.ercim.org/publication/Ercim_News/enw29/kramer.html.

43. http://dock.compbio.ucsf.edu/44. http:// www.ccdc.cam.ac.uk/products/life_sciences/gold/45. Ogston AG. Specificity of the enzyme aconitase. *Nature*. 1951;167:693.

46. Forino JM, Jumg D, Easton JB, Houghton PJ, Pellechia M. Virtual docking approaches to protein kinase B inhibition. *J Med Chem*. 2005;48:2278–2281.

47. http://www.archiv bmn.com/sup/ddt/.CCHUN.pdf for the Hungarian original text.

48. Furka A, Sebestyen F, Asgedom M, Dibo G. General method for rapid synthesis of multi-component peptide mixtures. *Int J Peptide Protein Res*. 1991;37:487–493.

49. Hughes J, Smith TW, Kosterlitz HW, Fothergill LA, Morgan BA, Morris HR. Identification of two related pentapeptides from the brain with potent opiate agonist activity. *Nature*. 1975;258:577–580.

50. Mitsunobu O, Masaaki Y. Preparation of esters of carboxylic and phosphoric acid via quaternary phosphonium salts. *Bull Chem Soc Japan*. 1967;40:2380–2382.

51. Miyaura N, Yanagi T, Suzuki A. The palladium-catalyzed cross-coupling reaction of phenylboronic acid with haloarenes in the presence of bases. *Synth Commun*. 1981;11:513–519.

52. Shuker AJ, Siegel MG, Mathews DP, Weigel LO. The application of high throughput synthesis and purification to the preparation of ethanolamines. *Tetrahedron Letts*. 1997;38:6149–6152.

53. Gayo LM, Suto MJ. Ion-exchange resins for solution phase parallel synthesis of chemical libraries. *Tetrahedron Letts*. 1997;38:513–516.

54. Lawrence RM, Biller SA, Fryszman OM, Poss MA. Automated synthesis and purification of amides: exploitation of automated solid phase extraction in organic synthesis. *Synthesis*. 1997;5:553–558.

55. Takats Z, Wiseman JM, Gologan B, Cooks RG. Mass spectrometry sampling under ambient conditions with desorption electrospray ionization. *Science*. 2004;306:471–473.

56. Cooks RG, Ouyang Z, Takats Z, Wiseman JM. Ambient mass spectrometry. *Science*. 2006;311:1566–1570.

57. Everett J, Gardner M, Pullon F, Smith GF, Snarey M, Terrett N. The application of non-combinatorial chemistry to lead discovery. *Drug Disc Today*. 2001;6:779–785.

58. Almaas E, Oltvai ZN, Barabasi A. The activity reaction core and plasticity of metabolic networks. *PLoS Comput Biol*. 2005;1(7):e68.

59. Almaas E, Kovacs B, Vicsec T, Oltvai ZN, Barabasi A. Global organization of metabolic fluxes in the bacterium *Escherichia coli*. *Nature*. 2004;427:839–843.

60. Becker D, Selbach M, Rollenhagen M, Ballmaier M, Meyer TF, Mann M, Bumann D. Robust Salmonella metabolism limits possibilities for new antimicrobials. *Nature*. 2006;440:303–307.

61. Dubos R, Dubos J. *The White Plague, Tuberculosis, Man and Society*. Boston: Little, Brown; 1952.

62. MacBeath G, Schreiber S. Printing proteins as microarrays for high throughput function determination. *Science*. 2000;289:1760–1763.

63. Outang Z, Takats Z, Blake TA, Gologan B, Guymon AJ, Wiseman JM, Oliver JC, Davisson VJ, Cooks RG. Preparing protein microarrays by soft landing of mass selected ions. *Science*. 2003;301:13251–13254.

64. Ziauddin J, Sabatini DM. Microarrays of cells expressing defined cDNAs. *Nature*. 2001;411:107–110.

65. Chang FH, Lee CH, Chen MT, Kuo CC, Chiang YL, Hang CY, Roffler S. Surfection, a new platform for transfected cell arrays. *Nucleic Acids Res*. 2004;32:e32.

66. Fire A, Xu S, Montgomery MK, Kostas SA, Driver SE, Melo CC. Potent and specific genetic interference by double stranded RNA in *Caenorhabditis elegans*. *Nature*. 1998;391:806–811.

67. Brummelkamp TR, et al. A system for stable expression of short interfering RNAs in mammalian cells. *Science*. 2002;296:550–553.

68. Paul CP, Good PD, Winer I, Engelka DR. Effective expression of small interfering RNA in human cells. *Nat Biotechnol*. 2002;20:4497–4500.

69. Paddison PJ, Caudy AA, Bernstein E, Hannon GJ, Conklin DS. Short hairpin RNAs (shRNAs) induce sequence specific silencing in mammalian cells. *Genes Dev*. 2002;16:948–958.

70. Scherr M. Modulation of gene expression by lentiviral-mediated delivery RNA interference. *Cell Cycle*. 2003;2:251–257.

71. Lewis BP, Shih IH, Jones-Rhoades MW, Bartel DP, Burge CB. Prediction of mammalian microRNA targets. *Cell*. 2003;115:787–798.

72. Rajewsky N, Socci ND. Computational identification of microRNA targets. *Dev Biol*. 2004; 267:529–535.

73. Poenie M, Alderton J. Changes of free calcium levels with stages of the cell division cycle. *Nature*. 1985;315:147–149.

74. Szekeres PG. Functional assays for identifying ligands at orphan G-protein-coupled receptors. *Recept Channels*. 2002;8:297–308.

75. Conway BR, Demarest KT. The use of biosensors to study GPCR function: applications for high content screening. *Recept Channels*. 2002;8:321–341.

76. Milligan G. High-content assays for ligand regulation of G-protein-coupled receptors. *Drug Des Today*. 2003;8:579–584.

77. Barak LS, et al. Internal trafficking and surface mobility of a functionally intact b2-adrenergic receptor-green fluorescent conjugate. *Mol Pharmacol*. 1997;51:177–184.

Pharmaceutical Formulation

Steve Lonesky and Harris Levinson

■ Preclinical/Preformulation Testing

Once you have discovered a new drug, it's the formulator's goal to learn as much as possible about the active portion of the drug during this early phase of development. Absorption, distribution, metabolism, and elimination (ADME) studies need to be performed on animals. You need to learn the following information about the drug before you can dose it in humans.

- *Absorption.* The following factors can influence drug absorption:

  - *Solubility.* Knowing the drug's solubility over a wide pH range is paramount. FIGURE 2-1 shows a simplified diagram of the digestive tract.
  - *Partition coefficient.* This is a measure of the active's lipophilicity, which indicates its ability to cross cell membranes. Because human cells are constructed of phospholipid bilayers, lipophilicity contributes to the drug's rate and extent of absorption.
  - *Permeability.* This is the measure of a drug's passive diffusion through the intestinal wall. The higher the permeability, the greater the drug's absorption will be.

- *Distribution.* Solubility and lipophilicity also play a major role in drug distribution as described previously.
- *Protein binding.* Drugs can bind to proteins, mainly albumin, based on acidity or basic properties. If a drug is highly bound, its half-life can be greatly increased because the bound drug cannot permeate into body issues and be metabolized and eliminated.
- *Metabolism.* The liver is the main organ involved in drug metabolism. Metabolism is the conversion of a drug from a lipid-soluble form to a more water-soluble form so that it can be eliminated. A long list of enzymes can metabolize a drug by chemical reduction, oxidation, or hydrolysis. Cytochrome P450 plays a major role in this process.
- *Excretion.* Excretion can occur through the following pathways:

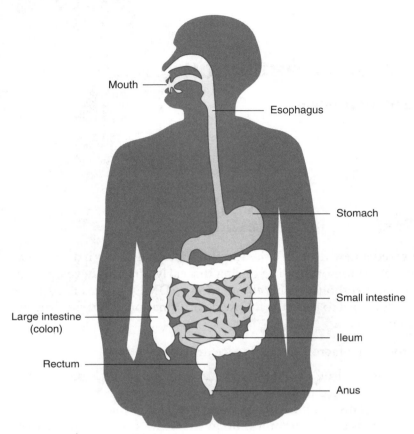

FIGURE 2-1 Anatomy of the digestive tract.

- ○ *Kidneys.* Once a drug is metabolized to a more water-soluble form, it can be excreted by the kidneys. The pH of the urine can affect the rate of excretion through the kidneys. Intentional acidification of the urine can promote the excretion of toxins and unwanted drugs.
- ○ *Bile.* Some drugs pass through the liver unchanged and can be excreted in bile.

Toxicity studies can be performed on mice, rats, dogs, or even monkeys to ensure safety before introduction in to humans.

Once the drug passes the 6 to 7 pH of the mouth, pH of the digestive system decreases as it enters the stomach. The stomach's pH is typically 1 to 5 (1–2 in the fasting state and 2–5 in the fed state). The pH then increases through the small intestine, which usually ranges in pH between 5 and 7. The digestive tract terminates at a pH of about 5.5 to 8 in the colon. The drug's solubility range allows you to know where it will dissolve in the intestinal tract and thus when it will be absorbed.

The dissociation constant (pKa) is the measure of the amount of drug that is non-ionized at a given pH. A drug needs to be neutral/nonionized to be absorbed in the digestive tract. You can predict absorption and the area of absorption based on the pKa value.

Drug stability is tested through forced degradation studies. Subjecting the drug to various conditions can predict future interactions. Typical stressing agents include, but are not limited to, heat, acid, base, peroxide, and light.

■ Dosage Form Design: Choosing a Dosage Form

The first step in dosage form design is to determine the drug's site of absorption. For drugs that are intended to be absorbed systemically, the dosage form needs to dissolve in the mouth, stomach, or intestines. Some absorption occurs in the buccal (oral) cavity (mouth) of very soluble actives. This site is usually reserved for conditions that require rapid onset of relief such as migraine headaches. Very little absorption, if any, occurs in the stomach. That leaves the intestines as the main site for drug absorption.

Some drugs can irritate the stomach or degrade at a pH between 2 and 3. It is advantageous to protect such drugs during passage into the small intestine. If the drug is meant to exert its action in the colon, the dosage form has to remain intact until it enters the colon. This can be achieved by coating the dosage form with an enteric coating that dissolves at a pH between 5.5 and 7, which is typical of the colon.

The second step is to determine the drug's dosing interval based on the half-life of the drug. The half-life is the amount of time needed for half of the dose to be metabolized and eliminated. A relatively short half-life may require dosing 3 or 4 times a day whereas a longer half-life may require only 1 or 2 doses per day.

Several options are available when introducing a drug product into the body via the oral route of administration:

- *Tablets:*
  - *Orally disintegrating (ODTs) and sublingual.* These tablets dissolve in the mouth, making the drug available for absorption in the buccal cavity or farther down the digestive tract.
  - *Immediate release (IR).* These tablets dissolve in the stomach for immediate absorption.
  - *Modified release (MR).* These tablets dissolve slowly to delay or prolong drug absorption.
  - *Effervescent.* These tablets liberate CO_2 and yield oral solutions for quick absorption.

- *Capsules:*

  - *Hard shelled.* Typically made of gelatin, these capsules can also be made of hypromellose (formally known as hydroxypropyl methylcellulose). Hard capsules can be filled with liquids, powders, granules, mini-tablets, or any combination of the last three.
  - *Soft gelatin.* Active is introduced as a solution or suspension between two ribbons of soft gelatin and sealed to form a soft gel.

- *Powders or granules:*

  - *Powders for oral suspension (POS).* Powders are stored in dry form for reconstitution prior to dispensing.
  - *Powder packets.* Powder is stored in small pouches or sachets for administration in dry form or for suspension or solution prior to administration.

- *Liquids:*

  - *Oral solutions.* Active is in solution for quick absorption.
  - *Suspensions.* Active is in solid form suspended in a liquid vehicle.

Formulation Basics

For the sake of this text, we concentrate on solid dosage forms. More specifically, we focus on the most prevalent dosage forms: tablets and capsules. There are three basic ways to make tablets and capsules:

- Direct blend
- Wet granulation
- Dry granulation/roller compaction

Deciding on one of these techniques depends on some basic information regarding the active you want to deliver:

1. *Is the active compressible by itself?* Simply try to compress the material using a hand press and a set of tablet tooling. If a compact is formed, the active is at least somewhat compressible. In this situation, you can try a direct compression process. Mix this active with other compressible excipients (inactive ingredients) and compress into tablets. Microcrystalline cellulose, lactose, and dibasic calcium phosphate come in compressible grades that form tablets nicely. If the active is not compressible and is not sensitive to moisture, then a wet granulation technique can be employed. In wet granulation, the active, alone or with other excipients, is mixed with water and energy is exerted on the materials to

create granules through agglomeration. If the active is not self-binding, a binder such as povidone or hypromellose can be added to the formulation to aid in granule formation. Once the granules are formed, the moisture is removed to yield a more compressible powder.

2. *Does the active flow by itself?* A vast majority of actives do not flow by themselves. For compressible actives that do not flow well, you need to choose an excipient to increase flow. A glidant, such as colloidal silicon dioxide, can help ensure that the final blend adequately flows into the tabletting or encapsulation machine. If the active does not flow or compress well, a wet granulation route should be used.

3. *Is the active moisture sensitive?* If the drug degrades in the presence of water or other solvents, a direct blend technique is desired. If the active is both moisture sensitive and is poorly compressible, a roller compaction method can be used. During roller compaction, also known as dry granulation, the active is mixed with excipients and is passed between two compression rolls to form a "compact" or "ribbon." The resulting compact is passed through a mill to reduce its particle size to optimize flow and uniformity. This process makes the material denser and changes its surface structure to promote compression into a tablet or filling into a capsule.

4. *What percentage is the active of the final dosage form weight?* Direct blending is best suited for actives that are present in quantities of approximately 25% or more. For actives present at less than 25%, wet granulation is desired to ensure homogeneity. Even though it is not preferred for low-dose actives, direct compression can be used if the drug is moisture sensitive. In this case, special care needs to be taken to choose ingredients of the correct particle size, shape, and density. This will ensure that the drug is equally distributed, or homogeneous, throughout the blend, which will result in the correct dose being delivered to the patient.

5. *Is the drug sensitive to compression forces?* If the act of compression causes degradation or changes its physical or chemical form, direct blending is the desired process followed by encapsulation instead of tablet compression.

6. *Does the resulting tablet or capsule disintegrate in water?* If the disintegration time of the immediate release (IR) product is excessive, addition of a disintegrant, such as croscarmellose sodium or sodium starch glycolate, can speed the breakup of your dosage form. Disintegrants swell when contacted with water, thus helping to rupture the tablet or capsule.

Before employing one of the techniques described, it is advantageous to check compatibility of your active with various materials that you may want to use to obtain your final dosage form. Compatibility studies (sometimes called binary studies) can be performed at room temperature or at accelerated temperature and/or humidity. Because some interactions do not present themselves at room temperature, high temperature and humidity are recommended. Simply mix your active with potential inactive ingredients to identify possible interactions that may lead to degradation of the active. Pick a ratio that will best represent your final dosage form. For example, magnesium stearate, a lubricant, and colloidal silicon dioxide, a glidant, both contain basic functional groups and can cause degradation of some actives. Compression of the binary mixtures on a hand press can get the ingredients in intimate contact and further simulate the final dosage form.

Problem Formulations

Because drug absorption depends greatly on water solubility, poorly soluble actives pose a huge challenge for formulators. The following subsection describe some basic solutions to overcome solubility issues.

Particle Size Reduction

Reducing the active's particle size increases the surface area of the active to promote dissolution. This can be achieved by milling or grinding. The extent of particle size reduction depends on the degree of solubility of the active. For minor solubility issues, simple milling will suffice. Reducing the active particle size from 1000 μm (microns) down to 200–500 μm can have a profound impact on dissolution of your active.

For extreme cases, micronization may be necessary. Micronization is typically considered to be reduction of particle size down to below 10 μm. This increases the surface area exponentially. In extreme cases, particle size reduction can even be taken a step farther down to the submicron or nanometer range.

Addition of a Surfactant

Addition of a surfactant, such as sodium lauryl sulfate (SLS), can promote dissolution of a poorly soluble active. A surfactant works by reducing the surface tension between the active and the surrounding fluid. This allows for increased wetting of the solid, which increases dissolution of the drug.

Creation of a Solid or Molecular Dispersion

Dispersions can significantly increase the solubility of your drug. A solid dispersion is formed when a poorly soluble crystalline active is dissolved along with a stabilizing polymer such as hypromellose or povidone. The mixture is then dried, and the resulting material is more soluble than the starting active. This is possible because the active is converted from a highly ordered crystalline form to a random amorphous form. This amorphous form has a higher energy state, resulting in rapid drug dissolution.

Degradation Issues

The most common type of degradation is hydrolysis. Some drugs may break down when contacted with water. Silica-based or clay-based desiccant systems can adsorb excess moisture and protect the dosage form against hydrolysis. Molecular sieves are stronger adsorbers that can be used in the case of extremely moisture sensitive drugs.

Some drugs, such as mesalamine, are sensitive to oxygen. Steps to protect this molecule from oxygen must be employed. Simple antioxidants, such as ascorbic acid and tocopherol (vitamin E), can be used to slow or reduce/eliminate the oxidation process. Special packaging can be employed to minimize the effects of oxygen as well. Oxygen scavenger packets can be placed in the bottle to sequester residual oxygen once the bottle is sealed. In the most extreme cases, the head space (empty space) in a bottle can be purged with nitrogen to displace the oxygen before the container is sealed.

■ Stability Testing

Once you have a formulation that shows some promise, you must check whether it will remain consistent over time. Chemical, as well as physical, changes can occur when an active is put in intimate contact with fillers, binders, lubricants, capsule shells, and so forth. Capsule contents can form a hard plug over time if any of the components are hygroscopic. Binders, such as hypromellose and povidone, can absorb moisture when exposed to excessive humidity. Starch, which can be used as a binder and a disintegrant, is hygroscopic and will absorb water. Empty capsule shells themselves can contain up to 16% water that can contribute to this phenomenon.

Some excipients, such as polyethylene glycol (PEG), have been proven to cause cross-linking with gelatin to delay release of drugs in capsule form. Because gelatin can be used as a binder, cross-linking, even though less common, can occur in tablets as well. Tablet formulations that contain sugar can harden over time, delaying drug release.

When testing stability of your product, the International Conference on Harmonisation (ICH) recommends testing pharmaceutical dosage forms at the following room temperature and accelerated conditions:

- 40/75—40°C and 75% relative humidity (RH)
- 30/60—30°C and 60% RH
- 25/60—25°C and 60% RH (controlled room temperature)

The final product needs to be tested after 4, 8, and 12 weeks at 40/75. Product is also placed at 30/60 as a backup in case the 40/75 data are unacceptable. If the product is acceptable after 12 weeks at 40°C and 75% RH, it is assumed that the product should be stable for 2 years at controlled room temperature. You must back this up with actual testing for 2 years at controlled room temperature.

Some simple tests can be employed to monitor physical changes that may indicate a stability problem:

- *Tablet or capsule weight.* An increase in the weight of a dosage form can indicate moisture absorption. Excessive water uptake can lead to stability issues for your active if degradation is hydrolysis driven. A loss in weight can reveal that maybe too much desiccant is being used in the packaging.

- *Change in appearance and feel.* Discoloration (ie, speckles) can indicate degradation of your active and possible interaction between ingredients. If the color of an active "bleeds through" the coating, more coating may be required or a physical change in the active has occurred. Tackiness can indicate a problem with active melting or coating issues.

Some of these changes can alter drug release:

- *Tablet hardness.* A decrease in tablet hardness can indicate a physical change and interaction between the ingredients that can lead to a change in drug dissolution. Softening of a tablet or capsule can show excessive water uptake, active sublimation, or formation of a eutectic mixture. An increase in tablet hardness can lead to an increase in disintegration time.
- *Disintegration.* The time it takes for a tablet to disintegrate can let you know if the tablet is changing over time. An increase in disintegration time can slow down the drug's dissolution, which in turn can delay absorption.

Pilot Batches

After a formulator/formulation scientist has developed a laboratory scale product and/or process, the next step toward commercialization is to scale it up in a pilot plant setting. The purpose of pilot batches is to confirm that the data, information, and observations obtained for smaller laboratory bench-top scale batches are reproducible in larger pilot scale manufacturing. Because not all formulations/processes behave the same at all manufacturing scales, one of the other main objectives of pilot plant manufacturing is to define any changes to the formulation or process that must be made when the product is produced on a larger scale. Laboratory scale batches are typically on the order of 1 to 5 kg in batch size, whereas pilot scale batches typically range from about 10 to 100 kg in batch size, depending on the working capacity of the pilot plant equipment.

Solid dosage forms (tablets), which are the most predominant form of pharmaceutical products, are discussed in this section along with the issues attached to scale-up processing. Typically, other dosage forms such as liquids (solutions or suspensions) have inherently fewer scale-up problems. Pharmaceutical processes involved in solid dosage form manufacturing of tablets generally fall into two distinct categories:

1. Granulated products
2. Directly compressible products

Granulated products are traditionally manufactured using a series of equipment pieces also known as the equipment train. For granulated products, the following is a typical equipment train used for tablet processing:

- Granulator (high shear, low shear, top spray)
- Dryer (fluid bed or tray drying)
- Milling (oscillating, impact, or conical)
- Blending (twin shell blending or tote/bin blending)
- Compression (rotary tablet press)
- Tablet coating (film or sugar)

The main advantage of granulating products is that a more consistent product is produced and it is easy to incorporate materials whether they are active ingredients or functional excipients. The main disadvantage of granulated products is the increased cost in capital equipment because they generally are more complex to produce as a result of a long equipment train. This complex train of equipment also leads to an increase in the time it takes to manufacture because these types of products require an increased process complexity. One must consider material movement between pieces of equipment in the train and how this will be handled (manually or by some form of mechanical transfer). Bearing in mind how the product will be handled on a larger manufacturing scale, it may be prudent to evaluate the effect of mechanical material transfer, if it is feasible in each specific pilot plant setting.

For direct compression products, the following is a typical equipment train used for processing:

- Blending (twin shell blending, tote/bin blending, or sigma/ribbon blade mixing)
- Compression (rotary tablet press)
- Tablet coating (film or sugar)

The main advantage of direct compression products is that they are relatively easy to produce because of a straightforward manufacturing process/equipment train, which generally provides a reduction in the overall processing time. The disadvantage of this type of process is that the product quality and reproducibility are much more dependent on the raw material. Therefore, it is essential that the raw material vendors provide consistent raw materials that meet your specifications. If the raw material specifications are not set appropriately, this can lead to processing problems or finished product testing issues such as segregation. As the raw materials push the high and low ends of the specification, this may yield product failures as the ability to process the raw materials is diminished.

There are other types of niche pharmaceutical dosage forms that utilize unique types of processing equipment required for their specific dosage form requirements, such as these:

- Liquids (solutions and suspensions)
- Hard-boiled "candy" lozenges
- Transdermal patches
- Deramatologic (creams, gels, ointments, solutions, or shampoos)

- Suppositories
- Injectible sterile products
- Quick/fast-melting wafers
- Continuous processes (reserved for very large scale products)
- Film casting

Because these dosage forms are not the most prevalent in the United States, this discussion focuses on tablets, the most commonly utilized dosage form. For most large pharmaceutical companies, tablet production is the most prevalent dosage form produced.

For existing types of manufacturing equipment, there is no issue with finding equipment that is utilized for traditional pharmaceutical solid dose processing. It should be noted that when going from the equipment you have in the laboratory to that available in your specific pilot plant, there may be differences with respect to equipment design and specifications for each individual type of process. For example:

- *High-shear granulation.* Change in configuration (top driven or bottom driven), size, number and placement of chopper blades, configuration of mixing or impeller blade, or the tip speed of blade
- *Tray drying.* Volume of air, size, number and area of trays, drying temperatures
- *Fluid bed drying.* Bed height, volume of air, drying temperatures
- *Milling.* Types of mill, oscillating, conical, air, jet
- *Blending.* Blender size, shape, configuration, use of extended blender leg
- *Tablet compression.* Turret speed, dwell time, feed frame speed, gravity or force fed feeders, pre- and main compression capabilities, insertion depth, use of tapered dies, use of coated tooling
- *Tablet coating.* Air volume, pattern and atomization spray settings, spray rate, type of spray nozzle
- *Facility.* Ability to condition incoming air, mechanical material transfer

To scale up processing in a pilot plant, strive to use equipment of similar design at both laboratory and pilot scale so as to minimize variables that could lead to non-reproducible results.

However, for new or novel dosage forms, or other processes done at laboratory scale, similar or identical pieces of pilot scale available may not be available. In some cases, the process may be so unique or innovative that pilot plant (and larger scale) equipment does not yet exist or is not readily available for purchase without significant customization. In these types of cases, it is necessary to work with a process equipment manufacturer to design and develop or configure a suitable piece of manufacturing equipment that meets the requirements set forth by the development formulation scientists and process engineers. Although working with existing pharmaceutical equipment manufacturers is helpful because they are familiar with CGMPs, be sure not to overlook the opportunities available in other manufacturing disciplines for equipment that may have similar manufacturing attributes. Food manufacturing has a great deal of similarity to pharmaceutical processing because both utilize powders as a predominant base material.

As a generalization, pilot batches should intentionally be approximately one-tenth the scale used for commercial manufacturing scale. When scaling up to pilot scale there may be subtle or significant differences with respect to the type and design and manufacturer of the process equipment. There may even be differences within a specific manufacturer's line for equipment as the scale of the equipment increases in size.

One consideration that should be made at the start of pilot scale work is the processing time. This should be taken into consideration because the eventual intention is to manufacture at a commercial plant and the processing time has a significant impact on the operational efficiency of manufacturing plants. Although the goal should be to make a very robust formulation/process, if it comes at the expense of an extended processing time, the manufacturing plant or contractor may reject the process. Or it may get translated into higher labor costs for the production. Processes that are overly complex or lengthy will decrease the plants' operating efficiency and ability to manufacture other products because most processing equipment throughout the plant is shared with other products/processes. Reasonable attempts should be made to keep processing times and equipment utilization to a minimum when developing a process.

It is very likely that a process developed at smaller laboratory scale by the formulation scientist may undergo significant changes to the formulation or process at pilot scale. If the project does not already have a process engineer assigned to it (either from R&D or from the manufacturing plant), this is an ideal time to bring one into the project team. The process engineer can bring some helpful insights that the formulation scientist may not be aware of, such as follows:

- Availability of pilot plant and manufacturing plant equipment
- Design and process capabilities of pilot plant or manufacturing plant equipment
- Familiarity with various or similar types of processes

The availability of materials, especially new chemical entities (NCEs), are generally very limited because they are made in small chemical synthesis batches and are expensive to produce. Depending on the NCE, there may only be hundreds of grams or a few kilograms of material available for use. In this case, experimentation may be limited and a well-planned experimental design must be designed to conserve material. Contrary to this, the development of many over-the-counter (OTC) medicines are relatively inexpensive when compared to NCEs and the cost will not generally figure in largely to the experimental plan, so a more thorough evaluation is more easily obtained.

■ Granulation

The formulator and/or process engineer should be prepared to make alterations to the process based on findings that occur during this experimental pilot plant phase. There are some well-documented areas where adjustments are typically required to reproduce results found at smaller scale. In the area of high shear granulation, changes typically made at pilot scale include the amount of granulating fluid required to achieve the desired granulation endpoint. This can be a somewhat dramatic change. An increase in batch size by 10 times (5-kg lab scale to 50-kg pilot scale) will generally require a significant reduction in the amount of granulation fluid used. This reduction may be on the order of 10–20% or more. This is due to increased efficiency of the manufacturing equipment at the larger scale and the overall bed height.

This generalization may not hold true for all materials or formulations and some formulations may actually require more granulating fluid to achieve a suitable granulation. The same reductions will generally apply when increasing from pilot scale to full-scale manufacturing. The granulation endpoint will eventually be based on some type of measurement (such as power draw, kW). However, some smaller pieces of equipment may not have suitable meters, so this scale may be the first opportunity a scientist has to measure the impact of changes made on the formulation/process. Consequently, a large part of the determination of the granulation endpoint may be based on visual and tactile cues. It is prudent at this stage to also stress the process to see where the limits lie and how robust the process is. It is a lot easier, faster, and less costly to do this experimentation at pilot scale rather than at larger manufacturing scale.

Drying

Drying of a granulation may or may not see significant changes. The most notable area will be the drying time, which is predominantly a function of the amount of air flow the dryer is capable of handling. The drying time is directly related to the volume of air flow, so this will be the parameter with the most impact on the process. Also, seasonal changes in processing air humidity for unconditioned air should be taken into account. Depending on the robustness of the formulation, one may see an increase in the fine material produced during processing. This increase may be caused by increased attrition within the fluid bed dryer resulting from greater product movement.

If the granules produced during granulation are not robust enough, particles may wear off or break to generate material of a smaller particle size. This is not an issue if tray drying is used. Tray dryers may be used at this scale; however, when the product is moved to larger scale manufacturing, it is not typical to use tray dryers because of the lengthy time of drying cycles. It is recommended to try and mimic the equipment used at larger scale to evaluate any changes. It is also important to check on the air handling of the equipment to note if the specific unit has capabilities for the treatment of incoming air. Air that has been pretreated (dehumidified) will have more drying capability than untreated (unconditioned/ambient) air and will affect the processing time.

Milling

Milling operations may significantly affect the scale-up process. Different types of mills have significantly different attrition and may result in significantly different particle size distributions. Other factors include the screen sizes available. Sometimes those available at pilot scale may differ slightly from those used at smaller lab scale. Factors such as mill speed need to be taken into account and may impart more attrition at higher mill speeds. It is important to try and match the mill type, mill screen size, and mill speed that you intend to use at production scale.

Blending

Blending operations are a bit more predictive. There have been significant studies done to determine the appropriate changes required to scale up a blending process for units configured as a V-blender. Because the material moves a somewhat consistent distance during the rotation of the blender, the distance particles travel is easily calculated and based on the size of the blender, so one can calculate an approximate blending time. This should be confirmed by utilizing blend optimization where batches are blended at lower and higher than anticipated blending times.

Confirmation of the data is best done by taking blend samples (typically, 1–3 times the finished dosage unit). Replicates are also easily taken at the same time should a retest of the blend sample be required. The predominant type of blend sampling is done via thief sampling, which intrinsically creates problems by trying to achieve a "static" sample from within a powder bed. Blend sampling results are also affected by static charge of materials and the ability of material to flow into the sampling cavity. Whenever possible, blend sampling should be limited to only one operator to minimize any variations caused by sampling error. Blend sampling should be designed to try and simulate the most difficult blending situations, such as sampling areas near dead spots or near the axis of rotation.

Scale-Up

After a scientist (formulation scientist, process engineer, or both) has developed a pilot plant scale product/process, the next step toward commercialization of the product/process is to scale it up in a full-scale manufacturing plant. The purpose of scale-up batches is to confirm that the data, information, and observances obtained at smaller pilot plant scale is reproducible at full-scale manufacturing and to define any changes that need to be made at this larger scale.

Typically, scale-up batches are initially done as "feasibility" or experimental batches. Feasibility trials can be performed as a single batch to confirm that the process scale-up goes as expected and there are no unexpected surprises at this phase. However, it is usually prudent to plan to have enough raw materials and plant time allocation to make additional batches should processing parameters need to be altered or should the scientist wish to make additional batches to see if the process is reproducible. Feasibility batches may or may not be done at full manufacturing scale.

The cost of the active ingredient and the raw materials affect the size and number of batches to be made at this scale. One factor that also plays a role is the manufacturing schedule of the plant or contractor where manufacturing will take place. If equipment needed for the feasibility trial is in the part of a plant that is heavily in demand for other products/processes, it may be difficult to gain access to that area because the plant will need to displace its current marketed products to accommodate the plant trial. These types of feasibility trials are often used for experimental purposes only because there are usually changes required within the process that need to be further explored.

Raw materials or active ingredients utilized at this stage often do not require full characterization or testing to be used for these types of large-scale experiments. These factors will usually limit feasibility batches being used for purely "experimental" work rather than for human consumption, registration, or clinical trials.

If the active ingredient being used in your product is new to a manufacturing facility, you may be required to perform a cleaning validation of the active ingredient. The purpose of this is to prove that after manufacturing products using this active ingredient is completed, the carryover of material is lower than the permissible levels.

Some limits that have been mentioned by industry representatives in the literature or in presentations include analytical detection levels such as 10 ppm, biological activity levels such as 1/1000 of the normal therapeutic dose, and organoleptic levels such as no visible residue or odor reside (when using flavors in the process).

There are many factors that affect the success of a feasibility trial:

- Similarity in design of the equipment that was used during the laboratory and pilot plant phases of development
- Changes required in the process
- Fluid volume required for granulation
- Granulation drying time
- Size of milling screens
- Mixing/blending times
- Changes in tablet press tooling

After a feasibility trial is successfully completed (and any corresponding changes made to the formulation and/or process), a qualification trial is often required. A qualification trial serves to reproduce the findings, data, and observances seen during feasibility batches. Material produced at this stage generally has more refined specifications for materials and testing requirements are significantly more than those for feasibility batches. As a result, material produced during these types of trials may be used for human use or clinical trials if the batches are produced under Good Manufacturing Practice (GMP) conditions.

Several technical transfer issues may arise during these trials that may require some changes to be made. One area to pay special attention to is material transfer. Typically, at laboratory and pilot scales, material transfers are done by hand. However, at large scale the volume of material is usually too large to move manually and technology is utilized to facilitate the manufacturing process. You may see the use of drum lifters, drum inverters, screw feeders, vibratory hoppers, or vacuum transfer units. The use of vacuum transfer units can be especially problematic if you have a material that has a tendency to segregate. This is possible with materials that have wide particle size distributions or with materials that have a two or more peaks in their particle size distribution. The use of any vibratory system during the process may induce a percolation effect where smaller particles are driven down in between larger particles, causing the powder bed to segregate. Visually this will be seen by looking at the top of the powder bed, and you will see what visually appear to be the larger particles rising to the top of the powder bed.

Overages of materials may also be needed at this stage because the type of material transfer is quite different from that used at smaller scales. As a result, some of the processes used for material transfer may cause selective material loss. To compensate for this an overage may be added with sufficient justification to determine the appropriate overage needed for your specific process. Overages should not be added without specific justification. CGMPs require that formulations are formulated to 100% of label claim.

Process Validation

Process validation principles that are described here are applicable to any drug product that is administered to either humans or animals. A process validation guideline can be found in Section 10.90 (21 CFR 10.90). Process validation is a required part of current good manufacturing practices (CGMPs) for pharmaceuticals. These requirements can be located in 21 CFR, specifically in Parts 210 and 211. We discuss process validation aspects and the concepts that are a significant part of a validation program. Specific requirements of process validation vary depending on such factors as the nature of the specific product (such as dosage form) and the nature of the specific process (granulation, direct compression, liquid manufacturing, etc.).

It is important to understand some of the basic terminology used within the process validation field. Following are some of the most commonly used terms relating to process validation:

- *Installation qualification.* An equipment trial that establishes confidence that the processing equipment is capable of consistently operating within the established limits and tolerances. This step is typically performed when new equipment is installed to adequately prove that it is suitable for its intended use or purpose. This is normally performed by the site where the equipment is being installed.

- *Process performance qualification.* A processing trial that establishes confidence that the process is effective and is reproducible.
- *Performance qualification.* A process trial that establishes confidence that the finished product produced by a specific process meets the testing requirements for its intended use.
- *Prospective validation.* A process validation trial conducted before a new product is released for its intended use to establish that the predetermined results can be achieved on a consistent basis. Typically, this is performed on three consecutive batches.
- *Validation.* Establishing documented evidence that a specific process will consistently produce a product meeting its predetermined specifications and quality.
- *Validation protocol.* A definitive written plan that describes how the validation will be performed, including the test criteria, sampling intervals and requirements, product characteristics, production equipment, and acceptable limits for test results.
- *Stressed or worst-case conditions.* A set of conditions encompassing the high and low extremes of the processing limits that pose the greatest chance of process or product failure. Such conditions may or may not induce product or process failure.

General Concepts

Assurance of product quality is derived from careful attention to a number of factors including selection of quality parts, equipment, and materials; adequate product and process design; control of the process; and in-process and end-product testing. Because of the complexity of the products, routine finished product testing alone often is not sufficient to ensure product quality. Some finished product tests have limited sensitivity. In some cases, destructive testing would be required to show that the manufacturing process was adequate, and in other situations finished product testing does not reveal all variations that may occur in the product.

The basic principles of quality assurance have as their goal the production of articles that are fit for their intended use. These principles are defined in the following statements:

- Quality, safety, and effectiveness must be designed and built into the product.
- Quality cannot be inspected or tested into the finished product.
- Each step of the manufacturing process must be controlled in a way to maximize the probability that the finished product meets all quality and design specifications.

Process validation is a key element in ensuring that these quality assurance goals are met. It is through careful design and validation of both the process and process controls that the manufactured products that are produced in consecutive lots meet the predetermined acceptable criteria.

The FDA defines process validation as follows:

Process validation is establishing documented evidence which provides a high degree of assurance that a specific process will consistently produce a product meeting its pre-determined specifications and quality characteristics.

It is required that a written validation protocol is approved prior to commencing any validation batch manufacturing. This protocol specifies the manufacturing procedures, the required testing/sampling intervals, and specifically identifies the locations to be tested and what testing data will be collected. A protocol should specify the required number of repeated process runs (typically three consecutively) to prove that the process is reproducible. The test conditions for these runs should encompass stressed conditions at the upper and lower process limits, which possess the potential to create a process or product failure. The process validation documentation should include information on the suitability of materials and the performance and reliability of equipment and systems.

Key process variables should be monitored and documented. Analysis of the data collected from monitoring will establish the variability of process parameters for individual runs and will establish whether or not the equipment and process controls are adequate to ensure that product specifications are consistently met.

Finished product and in-process test data can be of value in process validation, particularly in those situations where quality attributes and process variability can be readily measured. Where finished (or in-process) testing cannot adequately measure certain attributes, process validation should be derived primarily from qualification of each system used in production and from consideration of the interaction of the various systems.

CGMP Regulations for Finished Pharmaceuticals (The Current Codified CGMP Regulations, CFR Parts 210 and 211)

Section 211.100—*Written procedures; deviations*—which states, in part: A requirement for process validation is set forth in general terms:

There shall be written procedures for production and process control designed to assure that the drug products have the identity, strength, quality, and purity they purport or are represented to possess.

Several sections of the CGMP regulations state validation requirements in more specific terms. An excerpt from a section is as follows:

Section 211.110, *Sampling and testing of in-process materials and drug products.*

(a) Control procedures shall be established to monitor the output and validate the performance of those manufacturing processes that may be responsible for causing variability in the characteristics of in-process material and the drug product.

Preliminary Considerations

A manufacturer should evaluate the factors that affect product quality when designing and undertaking a process validation study. These factors may vary considerably among different products and manufacturing technologies and could include, for example, component specifications, air and water handling systems, environmental controls, equipment functions, and process control operations. No single approach to process validation will be appropriate and complete in all cases; however, the following quality activities should be undertaken in most situations.

During the research and development (R&D) phase, the desired product should be carefully defined in terms of its characteristics, such as physical, chemical, and performance characteristics. It is important to translate these product characteristics into meaningful specifications that will serve as a basis for description and control of the product.

Documentation of changes made during development will provide traceability that can later be used to pinpoint solutions to future problems.

The product's end use should be a determining factor in the development of product (and component) characteristics and specifications. All pertinent aspects of the product that have an impact on safety and effectiveness should be considered. These aspects include performance, reliability, and stability. Acceptable ranges or limits should be established for each characteristic to set up allowable variations. These ranges should be expressed in measurable terms.

The validity of acceptance specifications should be verified through testing and challenge of the product on a sound scientific basis during the lab scale, pilot plant scale development, and production phase.

Elements of Process Validation

Prospective Process Validation

Prospective process validation includes those considerations that are made before a new product is introduced or launched or when there is a significant change in the manufacturing process that may affect the product's characteristics, such as uniformity or identity. The following are considered as key areas of prospective process validation.

- *Equipment and process.* The equipment and process should be designed and/or selected so that product specifications are consistently achieved.
- *Equipment installation qualification.* Installation qualification identifies that the various pieces of processing equipment are capable of consistently operating within established limits and tolerances.

After process equipment is designed (using design qualification), it should be verified that it is capable of operating satisfactorily within the operating limits required by the process. This portion of validation includes examination of the equipment design, determination of equipment calibration, equipment maintenance, adjustment requirements, and identification of critical equipment features that could potentially affect the process or the product. Any information gathered from these qualification studies should be used to establish written procedures covering equipment calibration, maintenance, monitoring, and controls.

When assessing the suitability of a specific piece of processing equipment, it is insufficient to rely entirely on the manufacturer's representations or specifications. Practical engineering principles should be the first step in the equipment suitability assessment. It is important that equipment qualification simulate actual production conditions, including those that are worst-case situations.

Equipment tests and challenges should be repeated several times to ensure reliable, accurate, and reproducible results. All acceptance criteria must be met during the test or challenge. If any of the tests performed show that the equipment does not perform within its specifications, an investigation should be performed to identify the root cause of the test failure. Corrections should be made where appropriate and additional testing runs performed to adequately verify that the equipment performance is within the stated specifications. Variability of the equipment that is seen between and within runs can be used as a selection criteria basis for determining the number of testing trials required for the subsequent performance qualification studies.

Once the equipment configuration and performance characteristics are established and qualified, they should be documented. The installation qualification should include a review of pertinent maintenance procedures, repair parts lists, and calibration methods for each piece of equipment. The objective is to ensure that all repairs can be performed in such a way that will not affect the characteristics of material processed after the repair. In addition, special postrepair cleaning and calibration requirements should be developed to prevent inadvertent manufacture of a nonconforming product. Planning during the qualification phase can prevent confusion during emergency repairs that could lead to use of the wrong replacement part.

Process: Performance Qualification

The purpose of equipment performance qualification is to provide rigorous testing to demonstrate the effectiveness and reproducibility of the process. In entering the performance qualification portion of validation, the process specifications should be established and have been proven acceptable through laboratory trials and that the equipment has been deemed acceptable on the basis of proper installation qualification studies.

Each process should be defined and described with sufficient specificity so that employees understand what is required. Parts of the process that may vary so as to affect important product quality should be challenged. In challenging a process to assess its adequacy, it is important that challenge conditions simulate those that will be encountered during actual production, including worst-case conditions. The challenges should be repeated enough times to ensure that the results are meaningful and consistent.

Each specific manufacturing process should be appropriately qualified and validated. There is an inherent danger in relying on what are perceived to be similarities between products, processes, and equipment without appropriate challenge.

Formal Review

After actual production material has passed product performance qualification, a formal review should be performed to evaluate the following:

- Comparison of the product specifications and the actual qualified product
- Determination of the validity of test methods used to determine compliance with the product specifications
- Determination of the adequacy of the specification change control program

There should be a quality assurance system in place that requires revalidation whenever there are changes in formulation, equipment, or processes that could affect the product or its characteristics. Also for changes in raw material supplier, the manufacturer should consider differences in the raw material properties.

One way of detecting the kind of changes that should initiate revalidation is the use of tests and analysis methods that are capable of measuring these variable characteristics. Such tests and methods usually yield specific results that go beyond the mere pass/fail basis, thereby detecting variations within product and process specifications and allowing determination of whether a process is slipping out of control.

The quality assurance procedures should establish the circumstances under which revalidation is required. These may be based upon equipment, process, and product performance observed during the initial process validation. It is desirable to designate individuals who have the responsibility to review product, process, equipment, and personnel changes to determine if and when revalidation is needed.

The extent of revalidation depends upon the nature of the changes and how they affect the different aspects of production that were previously validated. It may not be necessary to revalidate an entire process. It may only be necessary to revalidate specific subprocesses that have been altered. Take the time to assess the nature and extent of the change and to determine the potential effects as part of the revalidation effort.

Documentation

It is essential that the validation program is documented and that the documentation is properly maintained. Approval and release of the process for use in routine manufacturing should be based upon a review of all the validation documentation, including data from the equipment qualification, process performance qualification, and product/package testing, to ensure compatibility with the process.

■ Suggested Reading

Ansel's Pharmaceutical Dosage Forms and Drug Delivery Systems, 8th ed., by Loyd V. Allen, Howard C. Ansel, and Nicholas G. Popovich.

Encyclopedia of Pharmaceutical Technology, Vol. 18, by James Swarbrick (Ed.).

Fundamentals of Early Clinical Drug Development: From Synthesis Design to Formulation, by Ahmed F. Abdel-Magid and Stephane Caron.

Handbook of Pharmaceutical Excipients, by Raymond C. Rowe, Paul J. Weller, and Paul J. Sheskey.

Handbook of Pharmaceutical Manufacturing Formulations, by Sarfaraz K. Niazi.

Handbook of Pharmaceutical Manufacturing Formulations: Compressed Solid Products (Vols. 1–6) by Sarfaraz K. Niazi (Ed.).

Handbook of Preformulation: Chemical, Biological, and Botanical Drugs, by Sarfaraz K. Niazi.

Pharmaceutical Dosage Forms: Tablets, 2nd ed., Vol. 2, by Herbert A. Lieberman and Schwartz L. Lachman.

Pharmaceutical Salts: Properties, Selection, and Use, by P. Heinrich Stahl (Ed.), Heinrich Stahl, and Camille G. Wermuth (Ed.).

Pharmaceutical Unit Operations: Coating, by Kenneth E. Avis (Ed.), Steven Strauss, Rong-Kun Chang, and Atul J. Shukla (Ed.).

Remington: The Science and Practice of Pharmacy, by David B. Troy (Ed.) and University of the Sciences in Philadelphia (USP) Staff.

Analytical Testing and Development

Anthony Ekpe and Mary Jean Sawyer

CHAPTER 3

■ Method Development

The need to develop and validate the analytical method is encountered by analytical chemists in the regulated industries on a daily basis. The scope of each development depends on the intended purpose, but the approach remains the same whether the method is for quantitation of major component or for trace impurity.

Although there exist different types of chromatographic separations, our focus is on reversed phase high-performance liquid chromatography (HPLC) method development for organic compounds with ultraviolet/visible (UV/Vis) wavelength absorbable chromophores. Most types of pharmaceutical compounds fall within this category.

Prior to starting method development, it is necessary to establish goals of the method. The question to answer might be, Is the method going to be for measurement of the major component (active ingredient) or for minor component(s) (impurity or impurities) or for both? In essence, is it going to be a stability-indicating method that will be validated according to the Food and Drug Administration/International Conference on Harmonisation (FDA/ICH) guidelines? Of equal importance that should not be ignored is the sample information. The information gathering should include the sample matrix, solubility of components in water/organic solvent mixture, chemical structure, polarity of the compound, molecular weight, and dissociation constant (pKa) as well as UV spectra in acidic, basic, and neutral environments.

The number of experiments to be performed could be highly reduced just by gaining full knowledge of the sample composition up-front. The resulting effect is the choice of separation and type of column selection is made easier. In the like manner, by defining the purpose of the method before the first experiment is performed, and coupled with the sample information, these could lead to scientifically sound selection of wavelength of detection and the initial composition of the mobile phase.

■ Column Selection

The choice of column for the initial set of experiments is typically based on the number of compounds that require quantitative separation. Generally, separation of component/retention varies inversely with chain length of the bonded phase (Retention: CN < C_4 < Phenyl < C_8 < C_{18}); and C_8 is the column of choice for the initial set of experiments. The advantage of C_8 as column of first choice is manyfold. It offers the advantage of shorter run time than C_{18} column, is widely available, has stable stationary phase, and is stable over a wide pH range. When the intended use of the method is for separation and quantization of multicomponents such as major components and their respective impurities, C_8 may not provide enough plate number (N) for adequate separation of all the components; then, C_{18} column should be the column of first choice.

Whether the goal of separation is for qualitative identification of compounds or for quantitative determination of the major components with or without trace impurities, the beginning of method development proceeds in the same way for all the cases. Example is use of standard diameter column (150 mm in length, 4.6 mm internal diameter, and 5 mm particle sizes).

■ Mode of Detection

Before the first sample is injected during HPLC method development, the detector of choice must be capable of detecting all sample of interest with UV scanning capability. Availability of a photo diode-array detector in modern HPLC instruments makes this the detector of choice.

The preferred wavelength for quantitative detection of compound can be obtained directly from the UV scan of the separation. An individual UV spectrum of well-characterized reference material with known purity and injected separately should be obtained if the composition of the sample is known and also available. This approach will help in confirming the elution profile of the sample.

■ Mobile Phase Selection

The separation and run time of reversed phase HPLC depends on the organic composition of the mobile phase or its solvent strength. Generally, a strong solvent strength that equates to a high proportion of organic solvent in the mobile phase always results in a decrease retention and shorter run time than with the low-solvent-strength mobile phase. For a stepwise process of method development, 50% water/methanol should be the combination of first choice in an isocratic mode of separation. This organic ratio allows for increase or decrease of the solvent strength depending upon the retention and run time. The separation achieved in the first set of experiments will lead to further optimization of the method.

The following are some practical considerations based on the outcome of the first set of experiments[1]:

1. If there is inadequate separation between components, one should consider one or a combination of the following: (a) changing the length of the column, (b) changing particle size of the stationary phase, and (c) switching the column to a C_{18} column or different bonded phase.

2. If a different elution order is desired to separate unrelated components, a change to a different bonded phase such as a phenyl or cyano column may be considered.

3. For separation of both acidic and basic compounds in the same sample mixture, use of buffer in the mobile phase to control pH and retention time should be considered.

4. Use of column temperature and change from an isocratic method of elution to gradient should be considered if there is adequate separation of components with long run time. A change in temperature of the column is similar to an increase of organic composition of the mobile phase. As the temperature increases, the relative retention time of the components decreases, without compromising the resolution and with improved peak shape.

■ Method Optimization

The separation achieved in the first set of experiments is usually less than adequate. Optimization of the method must be carried out to improve peak resolution, peak shape, and other parameters to meet the set goals. The process amounts to performing another set of experiments in which one parameter is varied at a time while holding others constant.

The variable parameters include some mentioned previously, such as use of ion pairing reagent, buffer, and column temperature, wavelength of detection, mobile phase composition, and change from isocratic mode of separation to gradient. Although the process is slow and time consuming, it helps in understanding how each of the variables affect the method. This approach was used in the separation of sample mixture containing both acidic and basic compounds (acetaminophen, 4-aminophenol, benzoic acid, and phenylephrine). See FIGURE 3-1.

■ Effect of Buffer

Selecting an appropriate buffer salt for the mobile phase is very critical when developing the method for the separation of the sample mixture containing both acidic and basic compounds. The purpose of the buffer is to control the pH of the mobile phase. The selection of buffer salt is based on the pKa of the separating compound. Maximum pH control of the mobile phase occurs at a pH that is equal to the pKa of the buffer salt. Some of the most commonly used buffers are listed in TABLE 3-1.

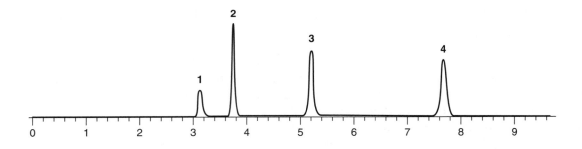

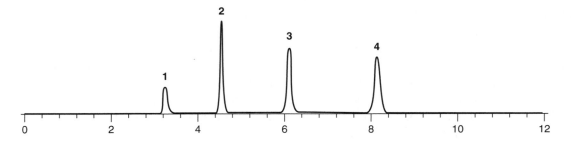

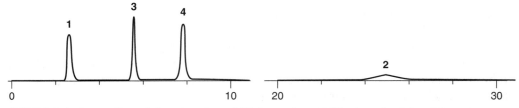

FIGURE 3-1 Separation of 4-aminophenol (1), benzoic acid (2), phenylephrine (3), and acetaminophen (4). *Conditions*: column, C18, 3 μm, 150 * 4.6 mm, mobile phase: 50 mM potassium phosphate buffer + 0.15% sodium butanesulfonic acid/methanol (90/10, pH); 40°C, flow rate 1.0mL/minute (a) pH 6.5, (b) pH 6.0, (c) pH 3.0. Brand A.

TABLE 3-1	List of Some Commonly Used Buffers With Their pKa Values	
Buffer	pKa	Buffer Range
Acetate	4.8	2.5–5.5
Citrate	3.1	2.0–4.0
	4.7	3.5–4.5
	5.4	4.5–6.5
Phosphate	2.1	1.0–3.0
	7.2	6.0–8.0
	12.3	11.2–13.2
Triethylamine	11.0	10–12.0

The concentration of buffer in the range of 25 to 50 mM is usually enough to provide buffering capacity. Higher concentration may result in the precipitation of the salt in the presence of organic solvent in the mobile phase.

As shown in Figure 3-1, in the separation of 4-aminophenol, acetaminophen, benzoic acid, and phenylephrine, the retention time of benzoic acid is highly affected by the pH of the mobile phase. As the benzoic acid loses a proton and becomes ionized with increasing pH of the mobile phase, its retention time decreases. The retention time of the other components remains relatively the same.

■ Column-to-Column Equivalency

Method optimization would not be completed without establishing column-to-column equivalency. This is essential for developing a robust, rugged, and reproducible method. Similar columns from the same or different suppliers can cause significant changes in retention time because of variation in plate number, band symmetry, and selectivity, especially when separating polar basic compounds. Unwanted interaction between basic compounds and acidic silanol group on the surface of silica-based stationary phases is the major cause of poor column efficiency and selectivity. Clearly, for the separation of 4-aminophenol, acetaminophen, benzoic acid, and phenylephrine in FIGURE 3-2, the third column in the experiment showed different selectivity, and thus is not equivalent to the other two columns. A fully reacted and end-capped column from different vendors tends to minimize the effect.

■ Effect of Temperature

Changing column temperatures also effects retention time. In FIGURE 3-3 note the differences in retention time of the compounds at 40°C compared to 25°C.

■ Effect of Ion Pair Reagent

Addition of an ion pair reagent to the mobile phase for reverse phase HPLC separation requires more experimental work to be done for optimization of retention. The advantage gained is for better control of retention and selectivity of polar compounds.

The most commonly used ion pair reagents fall into two main classes:

- Tetraalkylammonium salts, such as tetrabutylammonium and cetyltrimethylammonium salts, are for acidic compounds. Interaction with acidic compounds results in an increase of ionized acids and other anions.
- Alkyl sulfonic acid salts (C_4–C_8 sulfonic acid salts) and sodium dodecyl sulfate are for increased retention of protonated bases and other cations.

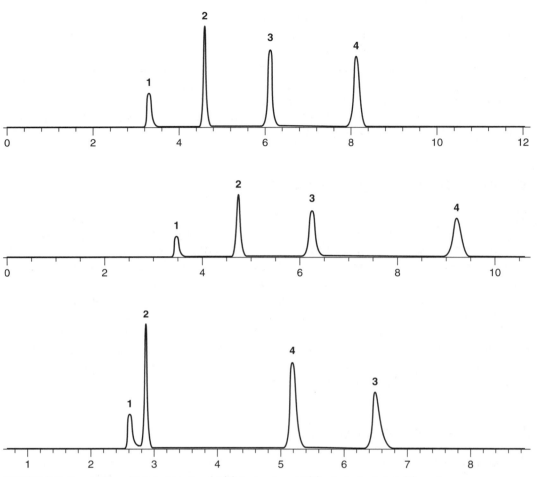

FIGURE 3-2 Separation of 4-aminophenol (1), benzoic acid (2), phenylephrine (3), and acetaminophen (4). *Conditions*: column, C18, 3 μm ,150 * 4.6 mm, mobile phase: 50 mM potassium phosphate buffer + 0.15% sodium butanesulfonic acid/methanol (90/10, pH 6.0); 40°C, flow rate 1.0mL/minute.

The alkyl sulfonate and tetrabutylammonium salts are the most frequently used reagents because of their low UV absorption at 210 nm. These reagents work by electrostatic and hydrophobic interactions between the ionic samples and the ion pair reagent. An interchange of any of the ion pair reagents with a different chain length within the same class (eg, hexanesulfonic acid for butane sulfonic acid salt, as shown in FIGURE 3-4) does not produce the same retention time effect. To reduce complexity of a method, ion pair reagents should be used in a method only to achieve specific objectives such as to have better control over retention range of polar compounds.

Once the analytical method for analysis has been developed, a regimented series of testing is performed to ensure the method is valid. A method that is valid can be used

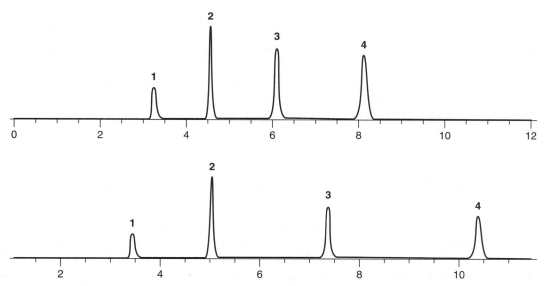

FIGURE 3-3 Separation of 4-aminophenol (1), benzoic acid (2), phenylephrine (3), and acetaminophen (4). *Conditions*: column, C18, 3 μm, 150 * 4.6 mm, mobile phase: 50 mM potassium phosphate buffer + 0.15% sodium butanesulfonic acid/methanol (90/10, pH 6.0); 40°C and 25°C, flow rate 1.0mL/minute.

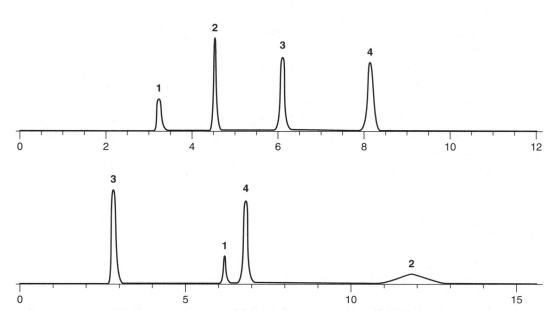

FIGURE 3-4 Separation of 4-aminophenol (1), benzoic acid (2), phenylephrine (3), and acetaminophen (4). *Conditions*: column, C18, 3 μm, 150 * 4.6 mm, mobile phase: 50 mM potassium phosphate buffer + 0.15% sodium butanesulfonic acid/methanol (90/10, pH 6.0); or 50 mM potassium phosphate buffer + 0.15% sodium heptanesulfonic acid/methanol (90/10, pH 6.0); 40°C, flow rate 1.0mL/minute.

routinely to test for the stability of excipients, active pharmaceutical ingredients APIs, and finished dosage forms. The FDA requires that all methods of analysis be validated and that the information be presented when applying for a new drug substance and drug products.

The primary guidances to follow when validating the method are located in the United States Pharmacopeia General Chapter [905], the FDA Guidance to Analytical Procedures and Methods Validation, the FDA "Reviewer Guidance, Validation of Chromatographic Methods," and the ICH guidance Q2B.[2–4] All these references are similar in criteria. TABLE 3-2 highlights the different validation characteristics of various types of tests.

The FDA and other health authorities require the following general information to be summarized in the final validation report:

a. Data demonstrating suitable accuracy, precision, and linearity over the range of interest (ca. 80% to 120% of the label claim). Data demonstrating specificity of the methods and determination limits for degradation products or impurities should be included. These degradation products or impurities should be adequately identified and characterized.

b. Data demonstrating recovery from the sample matrix where the nature of the product so indicates.

c. Data demonstrating that neither the fresh nor degraded placebo interferes with the proposed method.

d. Legible reproductions of representative chromatographs and instrumental recordings.

e. Data characterizing day-to-day, laboratory-to-laboratory, analyst-to-analyst, and column-to-column variability. These data may be included to provide a further indication of reproducibility and, in a limited sense, ruggedness.

f. A degradation schematic for the active ingredient in the dosage form, where possible (eg, products of acid/base hydrolysis, temperature degradation, photolysis, and oxidation).

g. System suitability tests (as defined in the current USP–NF [621])[2]:

    1. Number of theoretical plates
    2. Tailing factor
    3. Relative retention
    4. Capacity factor
    5. Resolution
    6. Relative standard deviation

In practice, each method submitted for validation must include an appropriate number of system suitability tests defining the necessary characteristics of that system. Other parameters may be included at the discretion of the applicant or the agency.

TABLE 3-2	Recommended Validation Characteristics of Various Types of Tests				
Type of Tests/ Characteristics/ Performance Factors	Identification	Testing for Impurities		Assay Dissolution (Measurement Only) Content/Potency	Specific Tests
		Quantitative	Limit		
Specificity	+[2]	+	+	+[5]	+[4]
Linearity	-	+	-	+	-
Range	-	+	-	+	-
Accuracy	-	+	-	+	+[4]
Precision					
Repeatability	-	+	-	+	+[4]
Precisions					
Intermediate					
Precision	-	+[1]	-	+[1]	+[4]
Limit of					
Detections	-	-[3]	+	-	-
Limit of					
Quantitations	-	+	-	-	-
Robustness	-	+	-[3]	+	+[4]

Notes:

⁻ Signifies that this characteristic is not normally evaluated.

⁺ Signifies that this characteristic is normally evaluated.

[1] In cases where reproducibility has been performed, intermediate precision is not needed.

[2] Lack of specificity for an analytical procedure may be compensated for by the addition of a second analytical procedure.

[3] May be needed in some cases.

[4] May not be needed in some cases.

[5] Lack of specificity for an assay for release may be compensated for by impurities testing.

The effect of adjustments in mobile phase composition on retention times should be included in the method. Any precolumns or guard columns must be described. The rationale for their use should be logically explained and justified.

Examples of common problems that can delay the acceptance of a successful validation include the following:

a. Failure to include a sample of a critical impurity, degradation product, or internal standard necessary to assess the adequacy of the method.

b. Failure to list complete specifications, or the selection of unsuitable specifications, such as the following:

   1. Unsubstantiated or overly broad ranges (broader than investigational data can support)
   2. Specifications that do not account for assay limitations

c. Failure to provide sufficient detail, or unacceptable choice of procedures, reagents, or equipment, such as the following:

   1. Use of placebo blanks
   2. Use of arbitrary arithmetic corrections
   3. Use of instrumentation not commercially available without a full description of components and their assembly
   4. Use of single-source chromatographic columns, equipment, or reagents without full specifications to permit duplication
   5. Use of specialized tools or equipment that is not commercially available for sample preparation
   6. Use of an internal standard or other reagent that is not commercially available
   7. Failure to provide system suitability tests for chromatographic systems
   8. Differing content uniformity and assay procedures without showing equivalency factors for defining corrections as required by the USP XXI [905]

d. Failure to submit complete or legible data:

   1. Failure to label chromatograms and spectra as to sample identity
   2. Failure to label x-axis and y-axis as appropriate

When writing the analytical procedure the following information should be considered. The guideline as issued under 21 CFR 10.90. An applicant (or sponsor) may rely upon the guideline in the presentation of data, assembly of information, and submission of materials to the FDA, concerning specifications and methodologies as required by 21 CFR 314.50, or may follow a different approach. When a different approach is chosen, a person is encouraged to discuss the matter in advance with the FDA to prevent the expenditure of money and effort on preparing a submission that may later be determined to be unacceptable.

Some individual drug products may not require submission of all the information described in the guideline. In other cases, additional detail may be needed to provide a rational, scientific foundation for proposed specifications and methodologies. Generally, however, the provisions of 21 CFR 211.194(a)(1) and (2) are descriptive of the kinds of information to be submitted.

This section covers definitions of some of the most common terms used in analytical development from a regulatory perspective.

■ Definitions

- *Regulatory specifications:* Regulatory specifications are the defined limits within which physical, chemical, biological, and microbiological test results for a drug substance or drug product should fall when determined by the regulatory methodology. For compendial articles, the specifications in the current edition of the United States Pharmacopeia–National Formulary (USP–NF) are those legally recognized under Section 501(b) of the Federal Food, Drug, and Cosmetic Act and are used by the agency when determining compliance with the act.
- *Regulatory methodology:* Regulatory methodology is the procedure or set of procedures used by the FDA to ascertain whether or not the drug substance or drug product is in conformance with the approved regulatory specifications in the new drug application NDA. Generally, a regulatory assay will be stability indicating. For USP–NF articles, the analytical test methods in the compendial monograph are those legally recognized under Section 501(b) of the act and are used by the agency when determining compliance with the act. However, compendial methods may require validation to establish their suitability for specific drug products.
- *Regulatory methods validation:* Regulatory methods validation is the process whereby submitted analytical procedures are first reviewed for adequacy and completeness and then are tested as deemed necessary in FDA laboratories. Depending in part on the quality of submitted data, validation may range from step-by-step repetition of an assay procedure to more elaborate studies that include assessment of accuracy, precision, sensitivity, and ruggedness of the method.

■ Stability Testing

The purpose of stability testing is to provide evidence on how the quality of a drug substance or drug product varies with time under the influence of a variety of environmental factors, such as temperature, humidity, and light, and to establish a retest period for the drug substance or a shelf life for the drug product and recommended storage conditions.[5–8]

Drug Substance

Information on the stability of the drug substance is an integral part of the systematic approach to stability evaluation.

Stress testing of the drug substance can help identify the likely degradation products, which can in turn help establish the degradation pathways and the intrinsic stability of the molecule and validate the stability indicating power of the analytical procedures used. The nature of the stress testing will depend on the individual drug substance and the type of drug product involved.

The testing should include the effect of temperatures (in 10°C increments, for example, 50°C or 60°C above that for accelerated testing); humidity (eg, 75% relative humidity or greater), where appropriate; oxidation; and photolysis on the drug substance. The testing should also evaluate the susceptibility of the drug substance to hydrolysis across a wide range of pH values when in solution or suspension. Photostability testing should be an integral part of stress testing.

Examining degradation products under stress conditions is useful in establishing degradation pathways and developing and validating suitable analytical procedures. However, such examination may not be necessary for certain degradation products if it has been demonstrated that they are not formed under accelerated or long-term storage conditions. Results from these studies will form an integral part of the information provided to regulatory authorities.

The stability studies should be conducted on the drug substance packaged in a container closure system that is the same as or simulates the packaging proposed for storage and distribution. Stability studies should include testing of those attributes of the drug substance that are susceptible to change during storage and are likely to influence quality, safety, and/or efficacy. The testing should cover, as appropriate, the physical, chemical, biological, and microbiological attributes. Validated stability-indicating analytical procedures should be applied.

At the accelerated storage condition, a minimum of three time points, including the initial and final time points (eg, 0, 3, and 6 months), from a 6-month study is recommended.

Drug Product

The design of the formal stability studies for the drug product should be based on knowledge of the behavior and properties of the drug substance, results from stability studies on the drug substance, and experience gained from preformulation studies. The likely changes on storage and the rationale for the selection of attributes to be tested in the formal stability studies should be stated.

Although normal manufacturing and analytical variations are to be expected, it is important that the drug product be formulated with the intent to provide 100% of the labeled amount of the drug substance at the time of batch release. Variance to this may complicate data handling of the stability study.

Stability testing should be conducted on the dosage form packaged in the container closure system proposed for marketing (including, as appropriate, any secondary packaging and container label).

Stability studies should include testing of those attributes of the drug product that are susceptible to change during storage and are likely to influence quality, safety, and/or efficacy. The testing should cover, as appropriate, the physical, chemical, biological, and microbiological attributes, preservative content (eg, antioxidant, antimicrobial preservative), and functionality tests (eg, for a dose delivery system).

Analytical procedures should be fully validated and stability indicating. Whether and to what extent replication should be performed will depend on the results of validation studies.

Shelf life acceptance criteria should be derived from consideration of all available stability information. It may be appropriate to have justifiable differences between the shelf life and release acceptance criteria based on the stability evaluation and the changes observed on storage. Any differences between the release and shelf life acceptance criteria for antimicrobial preservative content should be supported by a validated correlation of chemical content and preservative effectiveness demonstrated during drug development on the product in its final formulation (except for preservative concentration) intended for marketing. A single primary stability batch of the drug product should be tested for antimicrobial preservative effectiveness (in addition to preservative content) at the proposed shelf life for verification purposes, regardless of whether there is a difference between the release and shelf life acceptance criteria for preservative content.[9–12]

For testing frequency at the accelerated storage condition, a minimum of three time points, including the initial and final time points (eg, 0, 3, and 6 months), from a 6-month study is recommended. Where an expectation (based on development experience) exists that results from accelerated testing are likely to approach significant change criteria, increased testing should be conducted either by adding samples at the final time point or by including a fourth time point in the study design. Photostability testing should be conducted on at least one primary batch of the drug product. The standard conditions for photostability testing are described in ICH Q1B.

When testing at the intermediate storage condition is called for as a result of significant change at the accelerated storage condition, a minimum of four time points, including the initial and final time points (eg, 0, 6, 9, 12 months), from a 12-month study is recommended.

Reduced designs (ie, matrixing or bracketing), where the testing frequency is reduced or certain factor combinations are not tested at all, can be applied if justified.

Glossary of Terms for Analytical and Method Development

Listed below are definitions commonly used in analytical and method development in the pharmaceutical industry.

- *Accelerated testing:* Studies designed to increase the rate of chemical degradation or physical change of a drug substance or drug product by using exaggerated storage conditions as part of the formal stability studies. Data from these studies, in addition to long-term stability studies, can be used to assess longer-term chemical effects at nonaccelerated conditions and to evaluate the effect of short-term excursions outside the label storage conditions such as might occur during shipping. Results from accelerated testing studies are not always predictive of physical changes.

- *Bracketing:* The design of a stability schedule such that only samples on the extremes of certain design factors (eg, strength, package size) are tested at all time points as in a full design. The design assumes that the stability of any intermediate levels is represented by the stability of the extremes tested. Where a range of strengths is to be tested, bracketing is applicable if the strengths are identical or very closely related in composition (eg, for a tablet range made with different compression weights of a similar basic granulation, or a capsule range made by filling different plug fill weights of the same basic composition into different-sized capsule shells). Bracketing can be applied to different container sizes or different fills in the same container closure system.
- *Climatic zones:* The four zones in the world that are distinguished by their characteristic, prevalent annual climatic conditions. This is based on the concept described by W. Grimm.[13]
- *Container closure system:* The sum of packaging components that together contain and protect the dosage form. This includes primary and secondary packaging components if the latter are intended to provide additional protection to the drug product. A packaging system is equivalent to a container closure system.[14]
- *Dosage form:* A pharmaceutical product type (eg, tablet, capsule, solution, cream) that contains a drug substance generally, but not necessarily, in association with excipients.
- *Drug product:* The dosage form in the final immediate packaging intended for marketing.
- *Drug substance:* The unformulated drug substance that may subsequently be formulated with excipients to produce the dosage form.
- *Excipient:* Anything other than the drug substance in the dosage form.
- *Expiration date:* The date placed on the container label of a drug product designating the time prior to which a batch of the product is expected to remain within the approved shelf life specification, if stored under defined conditions, and after which it must not be used.
- *Formal stability studies:* Long-term and accelerated (and intermediate) studies undertaken on primary and/or commitment batches according to a prescribed stability protocol to establish or confirm the retest period of a drug substance or the shelf life of a drug product.
- *Intermediate testing:* Studies conducted at 30°C/65% RH and designed to moderately increase the rate of chemical degradation or physical changes for a drug substance or drug product intended to be stored long-term at 25°C.
- *Long-term testing:* Stability studies under the recommended storage condition for the retest period or shelf life proposed (or approved) for labeling.
- *Mass balance:* The process of adding together the assay value and levels of degradation products to see how closely these add up to 100% of the initial value, with due consideration of the margin of analytical error.

- *Matrixing:* The design of a stability schedule such that a selected subset of the total number of possible samples for all factor combinations is tested at a specified time point. At a subsequent time point, another subset of samples for all factor combinations is tested. The design assumes that the stability of each subset of samples tested represents the stability of all samples at a given time point. The differences in the samples for the same drug product should be identified as, for example, covering different batches, different strengths, different sizes of the same container closure system, and, in some cases, different container closure systems.
- *New molecular entity:* An active pharmaceutical substance not previously contained in any drug product registered with the national or regional authority concerned. A new salt, ester, or noncovalent bond derivative of an approved drug substance is considered a new molecular entity for the purpose of stability testing under this guidance.
- *Retest date:* The date after which samples of the drug substance should be examined to ensure that the material is still in compliance with the specification and thus suitable for use in the manufacture of a given drug product.
- *Retest period:* The period of time during which the drug substance is expected to remain within its specification and, therefore, can be used in the manufacture of a given drug product, provided that the drug substance has been stored under the defined conditions. After this period, a batch of drug substance destined for use in the manufacture of a drug product should be retested for compliance with the specification and then used immediately. A batch of drug substance can be retested multiple times and a different portion of the batch used after each retest, as long as it continues to comply with the specification. For most biotechnological/biological substances known to be labile, it is more appropriate to establish a shelf life than a retest period. The same may be true for certain antibiotics.
- *Shelf life* (also referred to as *expiration dating period*)*:* The time period during which a drug product is expected to remain within the approved shelf life specification, provided that it is stored under the conditions defined on the container label.
- *Specification, release:* The combination of physical, chemical, biological, and microbiological tests and acceptance criteria that determine the suitability of a drug product at the time of its release.
- *Specification, shelf life:* The combination of physical, chemical, biological, and microbiological tests and acceptance criteria that determine the suitability of a drug substance throughout its retest period, or that a drug product should meet throughout its shelf life.
- *Stress testing (drug substance):* Studies undertaken to elucidate the intrinsic stability of the drug substance. Such testing is part of the development strategy and is normally carried out under more severe conditions than those used for accelerated testing.
- *Stress testing (drug product):* Studies undertaken to assess the effect of severe conditions on the drug product. Such studies include photostability testing (see ICH Q1B) and specific testing of certain products (eg, metered dose inhalers, creams, emulsions, refrigerated aqueous liquid products).

■ Dissolution Test for Solid Dosage Forms

The dissolution test is used to determine the dissolution rate of active pharmaceutical ingredients in solid dosage forms (eg, tablets, capsules, and suppositories). For any active ingredient in solid pharmaceutical dosage form to be available for absorption, it must first be released into the biological medium. The processes which the solid form of dosage undergoes before dissolution or release includes wettability of the dosage form, penetrating ability of the dissolution medium, the swelling process, the disintegration of the active into granules, deaggregation of the granules into fine particles, and finally the dissolution and release of the drug into the microenvironment for absorption. To a small extent, dissolution of drug may occur from the intact dosage form after the penetration of the dissolution medium. The rate at which this occurs depends on the composition and method of preparation of the dosage form and may be the rate-limiting step in the bioavailability of the drug for systemic absorption. This can be altered by the formulator.

Dissolution testing of solid dosage forms provides critical means of evaluating formulations from development to end of shelf life. Dissolution testing is routinely used in the following area and should be performed on individual tablets/capsules to observe intralot variability:

- During the early product development phase, it serves as a means of screening formulations leading to the development of the optimal dosage form.
- The test is commonly used as a quality assurance/quality control (QA/QC) tool to measure batch-to-batch equivalence and surrogate for human clinical testing.
- A well-designed dissolution method can be used to predict physiochemical properties of the drug, thus correlating the in vitro process to in vivo absorption.

Of the types of apparatus commercially available, either the basket apparatus (apparatus 1) or the paddle apparatus (apparatus 2) or, in special cases, the flow-through cell apparatus are the most commonly used systems.

Apparatus 1

The apparatus 1 assembly consists of the following: a covered cylindrical vessel made of glass, a metallic drive shaft fabricated with stainless steel, a cylindrical basket made of stainless steel, and a water bath or heating jacket that maintains the dissolution medium at $37°C \pm 0.5°C$.

Apparatus 2

The apparatus 2 assembly consists of a vessel identical to that described for the basket apparatus (apparatus 1), a vertical metallic shaft with attached blade that serves as stirrer, and a water bath or heating jacket that maintains the dissolution medium at $37°C \pm 0.5°C$.

Flow-Through Apparatus

The flow-through apparatus consists of a reservoir for the dissolution medium, a pump that forces the dissolution medium upward through the flow cell, a flow cell, and a water bath or heating jacket that maintains the dissolution medium at $37°C \pm 0.5°C$.

Factors That Influence Dissolution Testing

The dissolution rate of drug dosage forms can be classified in four main classes:

1. *Physiochemical properties of the drug.* The physiochemical properties of the drug substance play a critical role in controlling its dissolution rate. Dissolution test medium is in most cases aqueous base such as buffer and purified water, so dissolution of drug substance in this medium is one of the major factors that govern its dissolution rate. Other factors such as particle size, crystalline nature, amorphic state, state of hydration, free acid, free base or salt form, eutectic, and polymorphic form of the drug substance contribute to variability of dissolution rate if not well controlled.

2. *Product formulation.* The dissolution rate of active ingredient in sold dosage form can directly be influenced when mixed with various excipients and by the manufacturing processes. These excipients include diluents, binders, lubricants, granulating agents, surfactants, disintegrants, and coloring agents. Manufacturing processing parameters, such as blending time, sequence of addition of ingredients, method of granulation, water content and density of granules, size of tablets and their hardness, all contribute to the dissolution rate of solid dosage product.

3. *Dissolution testing devices.* For reliable and accurate dissolution measurement of drug substance, the dissolution testing devices must be set up precisely. Extreme care should be taken to minimize vibration of the unit, wobbling of the shaft. These affect the flow pattern and the hydrodynamic properties of the dissolution medium. For dissolution rate data to be reproducible and reliable, the flow patterns of the medium must be consistent from test to test.

   With most automated sampling systems and newer fiber optic in-situ analysis techniques currently in operation, a filter-tipped or filter optic probe is immersed in the dissolution medium throughout the duration of the dissolution testing. The size of the probe can also affect the hydrodynamics of the system, resulting in erroneous dissolution rate.

4. *Dissolution test parameters.* Several factors associated with dissolution test parameters affect test-to-test reproducibility of dissolution rate. Factors such as temperature, pH, nature and composition, volume, and viscosity of the dissolution medium affect reliability of dissolution measurement. Dissolved air present in the dissolution medium is one of the major sources of error in dissolution measurement processes. With the change in temperature, the dissolved air may be released in the form of bubbles, causing unreliable dissolution measurement.

■ References

1. Snyder LR. In: Snyder LR, Kirkland JJ, Glajch JL, eds. *Practical HPLC Method Development*. 2nd ed. New York, NY: Wiley-Interscience; 1997.

2. US Pharmacopeia Convention. *United States Pharmacopeia–National Formulary (USP–NF)*. Rockville, Md: US Pharmacopeia; 2008.

3. International Conference on Harmonisation (ICH). *Guidance to Industry*. Rockville, Md: Center for Drug Evaluation and Research; 1996.

4. ICH. *ICH Q2B Guideline: Validation of Analytical Procedures Methodology*. Available at: www.fda.gov/Cder/Guidance/1320fnl.pdf. Accessed December 1, 2008.

5. ICH. *ICH Q1A (R2) Stability Testing of New Drug Substances and Products*. Available at: http://www.fda.gov/cber/gdlns/ichstab.pdf. Accessed December 1, 2008.

6. ICH. *ICH Q1B Guideline: Photostability Testing of New Drug Substances and Products*. Available at: http://www.ikev.org/haber/stabilite/kitap/30%201.2%20%20Stability%20Workshop%20ICH%20Q1B%20C.pdf. Accessed December 1, 2008.

7. ICH. *ICH Q1D Bracketing and Matrixing Design for Stability Testing of New Drug Substances and Products*. Available at: http://www.emea.europa.eu/pdfs/human/ich/410400en.pdf. Accessed December 1, 2008.

8. ICH. *ICH Q5C Quality of Biotechnological Products: Stability Testing of Biotechnological/Biological Products*. Available at: http://www.ich.org/LOB/media/MEDIA427.pdf. Accessed December 1, 2008.

9. ICH. *ICH Q6A Specifications: Test Procedures and Acceptance Criteria for New Drug Substances and New Drug Products: Chemical Substances*. Available at: http://www.emea.europa.eu/pdfs/human/ich/036796en.pdf. Accessed December 1, 2008.

10. ICH. *ICH Q6B Specifications: Test Procedures and Acceptance Criteria for Biotechnological/Biological Products*. Available at: http://www.emea.europa.eu/pdfs/human/ich/036596en.pdf. Accessed December 1, 2008.

11. ICH. *ICH Q3A Impurities in New Drug Substances*. Available at: http://www.fda.gov/cber/gdlns/ichq3a.pdf. Accessed December 1, 2008.

12. ICH. *ICH Q3B (R2) Impurities in New Drug Products*. Available at: http://www.fda.gov/CbER/gdlns/ichq3br.pdf. Accessed December 1, 2008.

13. Grimm W. Storage conditions for stability testing—long-term testing and stress tests. Part I. *Drugs Made in Germany*. 1985;28:196–202.

14. Grimm W. Storage conditions for stability testing—long-term testing and stress tests. Part II. *Drugs Made in Germany*. 1986;29:39–47.

Manufacturing and Production

Dennis Williams and Sok Kang

In this chapter, we provide a basic overview of the manufacturing process of pharmaceutical products. The manufacture of pharmaceuticals is a very complex process that is subject to extensive regulatory oversight. Consequently, each of the topics discussed in this chapter could easily be a chapter or even a book by itself; however, the topics here are provided in sufficient detail to provide a general understanding of the process. To aid in this process, we periodically use an example of the manufacture of a fictitious drug called Good Drug tablets.

■ Active Pharmaceutical Ingredient (Drug Substance)

The active pharmaceutical ingredient (API) is manufactured by chemical synthesis, extraction, cell culture/fermentation, recovery from natural sources, or any combination of these processes. Essentially, the API or drug substance is the main ingredient responsible for the drug product's effect. For the purposes of this section, the focus is the chemical synthesis of a small molecule drug substance or API used to manufacture Good Drug product.

The manufacture of the API used in the production of drug (medicinal) products begins with *starting materials*. Starting materials consist of a raw material, an intermediate, or an API that is incorporated as a structural fragment in the overall structure of the API. An API starting material can be purchased from one or more suppliers under contract or commercial agreement or produced in-house. API starting materials normally have defined chemical properties and structure.

The company should designate and document the rationale for the point at which production of the API begins. For the synthesis process of Good Drug, this is known as the point at which API starting materials are entered into the process.

From this point on, appropriate Good Manufacturing Practice (GMP) should be applied to these intermediate and API manufacturing steps. This includes the validation of critical process steps determined to affect the quality of the API. Please note that the process step, which the company chooses to validate, does not necessarily define the particular step as critical.

The stringency of GMP in API manufacturing usually increases as the process proceeds from early steps to final steps, purification, and packaging. Physical processing of APIs, for example, micronizing, a process to manipulate the particle size, should be conducted in accord with GMP.

■ Manufacturing Equipment

Equipment used in the manufacture of intermediates and APIs should be of appropriate design and adequate size, and suitably located for its intended use, cleaning, sanitation (where appropriate), and maintenance. Equipment should be constructed so that surfaces that contact raw materials, intermediates, or APIs do not alter the quality of the intermediates and APIs beyond the official or other established specifications.

Production equipment should only be used within its qualified operating range. Major equipment (eg, reactors, storage containers) and permanently installed processing lines used during the production of an intermediate or API should be appropriately identified.

Any substances associated with the operation of equipment, such as lubricants, heating fluids, or coolants, should not contact intermediates or APIs so as to alter the quality of intermediates or APIs beyond the official or other established specifications. Any deviations from this practice should be evaluated to ensure that there are no detrimental effects on the material's fitness of use. Wherever possible, food-grade lubricants and oils should be used.

A set of current drawings should be maintained for equipment and critical installations (eg, instrumentation and utility systems).

■ Storage and Distribution

All materials used for the manufacture of the API should be stored under appropriate conditions (eg, controlled temperature and humidity when necessary). Proper records should be maintained of these conditions if they are critical for the maintenance of material characteristics. In addition, systems should be in place to prevent the unintentional use of quarantined, rejected, returned, or recalled materials, or separate storage areas should be assigned for their temporary storage until the decision as to their future use has been made.

■ General Controls

All specifications, sampling plans, and test procedures should be scientifically sound and appropriate to ensure that raw materials, intermediates, APIs, and labels and packing materials conform to established standards of quality and purity. Specifications and test procedures should be consistent with those included in the registration/filing. There can be specifications in addition to those in the registration/filing. Specifications, sampling plans, and test procedures, including changes to them, should be drafted by the appropriate organizational unit and reviewed and approved by the quality unit.

Appropriate specifications should be established for APIs in accord with accepted standards and consistent with the manufacturing process. The specifications should include control of impurities (eg, organic impurities, inorganic impurities, and residual solvents). If the API has a specification for microbiological purity, appropriate action limits for total microbial counts and objectionable organisms should be established and met. If the API has specification for endotoxins, appropriate action limits should be established and also met.

In the event when out-of-specifications (OOS) are obtained, these results should be investigated and documented according to a defined procedure. These procedures should include analysis of the data, assessment of whether a significant problem exists, allocation of the tasks for corrective action, and conclusions. Any resampling and/or retesting after OOS results should be performed according to a documented procedure.

Primary reference standards should be obtained, as appropriate, for the manufacture of APIs. The source of each primary reference standard should be documented. Records should be maintained of each primary reference standard's storage and use in accordance with the supplier's recommendation. Primary reference standards obtained from an officially recognized source are normally used without testing if stored under conditions consistent with the supplier's recommendations.

When a primary reference standard is not available from an officially recognized source, an in-house primary standard should be established. Appropriate testing should be performed to establish fully the identity and purity of the primary reference standard. Appropriate documentation of this testing should be maintained.

Secondary reference standards should be appropriately prepared, identified, tested, approved, and stored. The suitability of each batch of secondary reference standard should be determined prior to first use by comparing against a primary reference standard. Each batch of secondary reference standard should be periodically requalified in accord with a written protocol.

An impurity profile describing the identified and unidentified impurities present in a typical batch produced by a specific controlled production process should normally be established for each API. The impurity profile should include the identity or some qualitative analytical designation (eg, retention time), the range of each impurity observed, and classification of each identified impurity (eg, inorganic, organic, solvent).

The impurity profile is normally dependent upon the production process and origin of the API. Impurity profiles are normally not necessary for APIs from herbal or animal tissue origin.

The impurity profile should be compared at appropriate intervals against the impurity profile in the regulatory submission or compared against historical data to detect changes to the API resulting from modifications in raw materials, equipment operating parameters, or the production process. Appropriate microbiological tests should be conducted on each batch of intermediate and API where microbial quality is specified.

Authentic certificates of analysis should be issued for each batch of intermediate or API on request. Certificates should list each test performed in accordance with compendial or customer requirements, including the acceptance limits and the numerical results obtained (if test results are numerical). In addition, certificates should be dated and signed by authorized personnel of the quality unit and should show the name, address, and telephone number of the original manufacturer.

A stability program should be established to test and monitor on an ongoing basis the stability characteristics of APIs, and the results should be used to confirm appropriate storage conditions and retest or expiry dates. The test procedures used in stability testing should be validated and be stability indicating.

Stability samples should be stored in containers that simulate the market container. For example, if the API is marketed in bags within fiber drums, stability samples can be packaged in bags of the same material and in small-scale drums of similar or identical material composition to the market drums.

Typically, the first three commercial production batches should be placed on the stability monitoring program to confirm the retest or expiry date. However, where data from previous studies show that the API is expected to remain stable for at least 2 years, fewer than three batches can be used. Thereafter, at least one batch per year of API manufactured (unless none is produced that year) should be added to the stability monitoring program and tested at least annually to confirm the stability. However for APIs with short shelf-lives, testing should be done more frequently.

■ Validation

The company's overall policy, intentions, and approach to validation, including the validation of production processes, cleaning procedures, analytical methods, in-process control test procedures, computerized systems, and persons responsible for design, review, approval, and documentation of each validation phase, should be documented.

The critical parameters/attributes should normally be identified during the development stage or from historical data, and the necessary ranges for the reproducible operation should be defined. This should include the following information:

- Defining the API in terms of its critical product attributes

- Identifying process parameters that could affect the critical quality attribute of the API
- Determining the range for each critical process parameter expected to be used during routine manufacturing and process control

Basically, validation should extend to those operations determined to be critical to the quality and purity of the API.

The number of process runs for validation should depend on the complexity of the process or the magnitude of the process change being considered. For perspective and concurrent validation, three consecutive successful production batches should be used as a guide, but there may be situations where additional process runs are warranted to prove consistency of the process (eg, complex API processes or API processes with prolonged completion times). For retrospective validation, generally data from 10 to 30 consecutive batches should be examined to assess process consistency, but fewer batches can be examined if justified.

Not only does the synthesis for the API have to be validated, the cleaning procedure during and after the manufacture should be validated. In general, cleaning validation should be directed to situations or process steps where contamination or carryover of materials poses the greatest risk to API quality. For example, in early production it may be unnecessary to validate equipment cleaning procedures where residues are removed by subsequent purification steps.

The cleaning validation protocol should describe the equipment to be cleaned, procedures, materials, acceptable cleaning levels, parameters, parameters to be monitored and controlled, and analytical methods. The protocol should also indicate the type of samples to be obtained and how they are collected and labeled.

Sampling should include swabbing, rinsing, or alternative methods (eg, direct extraction), as appropriate, to detect both insoluble and soluble residues. The sampling methods used should be capable of quantitatively measuring levels of residues remaining on the equipment surfaces after cleaning. Swab sampling may be impractical when product contact surfaces are not easily accessible because of equipment design and/or process limitations (eg, inner surface of hoses, transfer pipes, reactor tanks with small ports or handling toxic materials, and small intricate equipment such as micronizers and microfluidizers).

Validated analytical methods having sensitivity to detect residues or contaminants should be used. The detection limit for each analytical method should be sufficiently sensitive to detect the established acceptable level of the residue or contaminant. The method's attainable recovery level should be established. Residue limits should be practical, achievable, verifiable, and based on the most deleterious residue. Limits can be established based on the minimum known pharmacologic, toxicologic, or physiologic activity of the API or its most deleterious component.

Analytical methods should be validated unless the method employed is included in the relevant pharmacopoeia or other recognized standard reference. The suitability of all testing methods used should nonetheless be verified under actual conditions of use and documented.

■ Master Production Instructions

To ensure uniformity from batch to batch, master production instructions for each intermediate and API should be prepared, dated, and signed by one person and independently checked, dated, and signed by a person in the quality unit.

Master product instructions should include the following information:

- The name of the intermediate or API being manufactured and an identifying document reference code, if applicable.
- A complete list of raw materials and intermediates designed by names or codes sufficiently specific to identify any special quality characteristics.
- An accurate statement of the quantity or ratio of each raw material or intermediate to be used, including the unit of measure. Where the quantity is not fixed, the calculation for each batch size or rate of production should be included. Variations to quantities should be included where they are justified.
- The production location and major production equipment to be used.
- Detailed production instructions, including the following:
  - Sequences to be followed
  - Ranges of process parameters to be used
  - Sampling instructions and in-process controls with their acceptance criteria, where appropriate
  - Time limits for completion of individual processing steps and/or the total process, where appropriate
  - Expected yield ranges at appropriate phases of processing or time
- Where appropriate, special notations and precautions to be followed, or cross-references to those.
- The instructions for storage of the intermediate or API to ensure its suitability for use, including the labeling and packaging materials and special storage conditions with time limits, where appropriate.

■ Batch Production Records

Batch production records should be prepared for each intermediate and API and should include complete information relating to the production and control of each batch. The batch production record should be checked before issuance to ensure that it is the correct version and a legible, accurate reproduction of the appropriate master production instruction. If the batch production record is produced from a separate part of the master document, that document should include a reference to the current master production instruction being used.

These records should be numbered with a unique batch or identification number, dated, and signed when issued. In continuous production, the product code together with the date and time can serve as the unique identifier until the final number is allocated.

Documentation of completion of each significant step in the batch production records (batch production and control records) should include the following information:

- Dates and, when appropriate, times
- Identity of major equipment (eg, reactors, driers, mills) used
- Specific identification of each batch, including weights, measures, and batch numbers of raw materials, intermediates, or any reprocessed materials used during manufacturing
- Actual results recorded for critical process parameters
- Any sampling performed
- Signatures of the persons performing and directly supervising or checking each critical step in the operation
- In-process and laboratory test results
- Actual yield at appropriate phases or times
- Description of packaging and label for intermediate or API
- Representative label of API or intermediate if made commercially available
- Any deviation noted, its evaluation, investigation conducted (if appropriate) or reference to that investigation if stored separately
- Results of release testing

Written procedures should be established and followed for investigating critical deviations or the failure of a batch of intermediate or API to meet specifications. The investigation should be extended to other batches that may have been associated with the specific failure or deviation.

■ Finished Dosage Forms (Drug Product)

This section discusses the next step in drug production: the manufacture of the finished dosage form. When we use the term *finished dosage form*, we are speaking of the final drug product that is provided to patients as medication. The drug product contains the API and excipients. Excipients can be subdivided depending on the function they play in the finished dosage such as lubricants, fillers, binders.

Drug products come in a variety of different finished dosage forms including tablets, capsules, topical creams and ointments, topical aerosols, inhaled aerosols, solutions, suspensions, and parenteral preparations. This large variety of different dosage forms provides healthcare professionals more pharmacotherapy options in the armamentarium

TABLE 4-1	Example Batch Formula		
Batch Formula: Good Drug Tablets 50 mg			
Components	Reference to Quality Standards	Amount per Tablet (mg)	Amount per Batch (1,000,000 Tablets) [kg]
Drug Substance	In-house standard	50.0	50
Excipient X	NF, Ph. Eur.	105.0	105
Excipient Y	USP, Ph. Eur.	40.0	40
Excipient Z	NF, Ph. Eur.	8.0	8
Purified water[1]	USP, Ph. Eur.	—	56
Theoretical end weight		203.0	203

[1]Purified water may be added during the granulation step. Water is removed during processing.

against illness. For example, aerosolized albuterol allows for effective drug delivery directly into the lungs of patients with asthma, which is superior to oral administration of albuterol. Without the additional dosage form of albuterol meter-dosed inhalers, the management of asthma would be a challenge for healthcare professionals.

The manufacturing of the drug product starts with the *batch formula*. The batch formula includes a list of all of the components of the final dosage form and their amounts on a per-batch basis. Processing agents (such as purified water) that do not remain in the final drug product should be described in the batch formula.

The amount (ie, weight or measure) of each component should be listed. Any overage in the API (or drug substance) should be explained and justified. For compendial components, the appropriate compendium should be cited. Further explanation of compendial components is addressed later in the chapter. An example of a batch formula is provided in TABLE 4-1.

■ Description of the Manufacturing Process and Process Controls

A flow diagram provides an overview of the entire manufacturing process including packaging and final quality assurance (QA) release. The flow diagram will include the following:

- Where materials enter the process
- Each manufacturing step with identification of critical steps including in-process controls
- The type of equipment being used

An example of a flow diagram is provided in FIGURE 4-1. We continue to use our example of Good Drug tablets. It is important to note that the flow diagram will appear quite different depending on the type of dosage form being described. For example, if Good Drug was a sterile parenteral product, the flow diagram would appear quite different, but it would still depict the main items described previously. Additionally, in an actual flow diagram used for a regulatory submission, the flow diagram contains more specific information such as the actual mixing time or air temperature used for the drying step.

The diagram in Figure 4-1 visually depicts the manufacturing process. For the purposes of our example, we assume the Good Drug tablets undergo wet granulation, a process widely used in the manufacture of tablets. The center column of boxes displays the actual steps of the manufacturing process with the type of equipment utilized during the step.

On the right side of the figure, the in-process controls are displayed. These are tests that are conducted at critical steps in the manufacturing process. The results of these tests are documented on the batch record. Release testing, which is identified in the lower left corner of the diagram, is where a representative sample of the drug product is collected and tested according to release specifications. Specifications are a list of tests and their associated acceptance criteria to which the drug product must conform. This step is discussed in more detail later in the section titled "Control of Drug Product."

The last step of the process is the QA review prior to the final release of the drug product. During this step, the QA department reviews the batch documentation. If satisfactory, the batch is released.

The narrative description of the manufacturing process, which accompanies the flow diagram, provides a detailed analysis of the manufacturing process including quantities of excipients and reagents used, identification of the critical steps and process controls, the type and size of manufacturing equipment used, and the operating conditions such as temperature, pressure, pH, and mixing time.

■ Control of Excipients

Before we discuss how excipients are controlled, it is important to reiterate their function in the final drug product. Often people think of excipients as "inactive" ingredients. Although to some extent this is true, excipients play a crucial role in the drug product. Excipients affect stability, enhance drug absorption, and aid in the manufacture of drug products. Some examples of the role of excipients are presented in TABLE 4-2.

Excipients can be divided into four distinct regulatory categories: compendial nonnovel excipients, noncompendial nonnovel excipients, novel excipients, and excipients of human or animal origin.

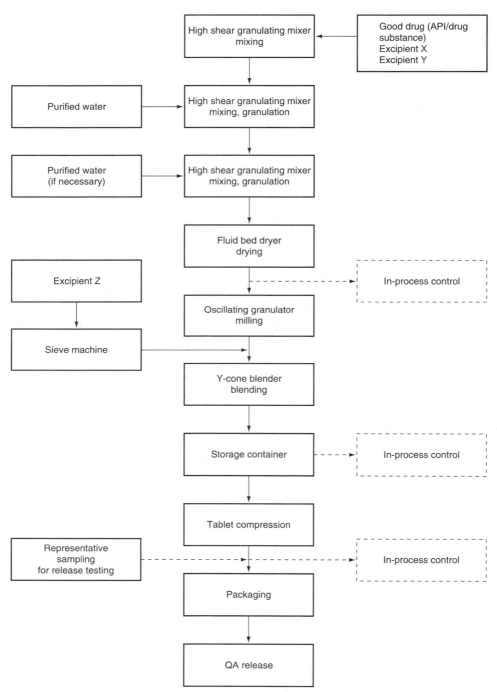

FIGURE 4-1 Example of flow diagram.

TABLE 4-2	Excipients and Function	
Stability	**Drug Absorption**	**Manufacturing**
Antioxidants	Disintegrants	Lubricants
Chelating agents	Drug release modifiers	Glidants
Preservatives	Film formers	Flow and compaction enhancers
Buffers	Encapsulating agents	Suspending agents
pH modifiers	Penetration enhancers	Solubilizing agents
Inert gases	Wetting agents	Propellants
		Bulking agents
		Binders
		Diluents
		Tonicity adjusting agents

As was previously presented, specifications are a list of tests and associated acceptance criteria. A specification for each excipient used in the manufacture of the drug product (ie, listed in the batch formula) should be provided regardless of whether or not the excipient appears in the finished drug product.

The issue of whether the manufacturer needs to provide the analytical procedures, validation, and justification for the specifications for a given excipient depends on the categorization of the excipient (compendial, novel, etc.). Let us revisit our example of Good Drug tablets. Excipients X, Y, Z, listed in Table 4-1, are compendial nonnovel excipients. They are classified as compendial because they are described in an official monograph (United States Pharmacopeia, for example). This means an official monograph exists that describes the specifications for this particular excipient. Therefore, the manufacturer does not need to provide the justification for this specification. For noncompendial excipients, detailed information on the analytical procedures, validation, and justification is necessary.

The determination of whether an excipient is novel or nonnovel depends on whether the excipient has been used previously by another drug product in an approved marketing application. Nonnovel excipients require additional information as described for noncompendial excipients. Additionally, they may require some toxicologic data supporting their safety.

Excipients made from human or animal origin require additional supporting information. This is largely related to concerns over transmissible spongiform encephalopathy (TSE) such as bovine spongiform encephalopathy (BSE). For these cases, the country of origin where the animal and excipient was derived is critical to assessing the risk potential.

■ Control of Drug Product

Specifications for the drug product are critical quality standards that are proposed and justified by the manufacturer and approved by regulatory agencies as conditions of drug approval.

The type specification necessary for a drug product depends on the individual dosage form. For example, the specifications necessary for solid oral dosage form differ from those of sterile parenteral drug product. More information regarding this topic is discussed under the description of the individual drug products given later in this chapter. However, the following tests are applicable to all chemical entity drug products:

- *Description*: A qualitative statement about the appearance of the drug product.
- *Identification testing:* Generally, two identification tests are used. High-performance liquid chromatography (HPLC) is commonly used. Some other methods used include infrared spectroscopy (IR), near-infrared spectroscopy (NIR), thin layer chromatography (TLC), and X-ray powder diffraction.
- *Assay*: A stability-indicating method should be used. HPLC in an example of a common assay.
- *Impurities*: As described under Assay, the method should be stability-indicating, and HPLC is commonly used.

There are additional tests for biologic drug products, such as those presented earlier, that are generally applicable to all biologic drug products. They include purity, potency, and quantity (protein mass).

Release specifications are those tests that are completed at the end of the manufacturing process prior to final release of the drug product. Upon completion of the testing, a certificate of analysis is issued.

In our example of Good Drug 50-mg tablets, a representative sample of tablets would be collected throughout the tabletting run for release testing. This testing would be based on a release specification sheet. TABLE 4-3 provides an example of a release specification sheet.

The in-process testing that occurred with Good Drug 50-mg tablets is not described in the release specification sheet, but would be described in the certificate of analysis. The analytical tests used as specifications for the drug product require appropriate validation and justification. The validation work provides information of the key attributes of the analytical test such as specificity, linearity, range, accuracy, and precision:

- Specificity is the ability to assess unequivocally the analyte in the presence of components that may be expected to be present such as impurities and degradants. In general, the test's identification, assay, and impurities must have sufficient speci-

TABLE 4-3	Sample Release Specification Sheet	
Release Specifications: Good Drug Tablets (50 mg)		
Test	Acceptance Criteria	Method Number
Description	White to off white, round, beveled tablet; debossed with "GD 250" on one side and plain on the other	—
Identification test no. 1	HPLC; the retention time of the major peak in the chromatogram of the assay preparation corresponds to that in the chromatogram of the standard preparation obtained as specified in the assay	SP101
Identification test no. 2	Near-Infrared spectroscopy (NIR)	SP102
Dissolution	NLT 80% (Q) of the labeled amount is dissolved in 30 minutes	SP103
Uniformity of dosage units	According to current USP	SP104
Assay	90.0% to 110.0% of the labeled amount	SP101
Impurities	Degredant A: NMT 0.1%	SP101
	Degredant B: NMT 0.1%	
	Any other degredant: NMT 0.1%	
	Total degradation products: NMT 0.5%	

ficity that they will be able to discern samples with the reference material from those that do not or be able to distinguish between two closely related structural compounds. In the cases where a single test cannot provide such specificity, the combination with another test should be able to provide the necessary specificity.

- Linearity refers to the ability within a given range to obtain results that are directly proportional to the concentration amount of the analyte in the sample:

  ○ *Range:* The range describes the ability to achieve an acceptable degree of linearity, accuracy, and precision within a specified range of the analytical test. Some suggested ranges are the following: assay, 80–120% of the test concentration of the drug product.

  ○ *Impurity:* From the reporting level of the impurity to 120% of the specification. For potentially toxic impurities, the detection limit should be able to detect the level at which the impurities need to be controlled.

  ○ *Dissolution:* Dissolution should be ±20% over the specified range.

  ○ *Content uniformity:* Content uniformity should cover a minimum of 70–130% of the test concentration.

- Accuracy is the trueness of the measurement, how close of an agreement exists between the value that is accepted as true and the value found.
- Precision of an analytical procedure expresses the degree of agreement between a series of measurements. It is considered at three levels: repeatability, intermediate precision, and reproducibility.

Two other important pieces of methodology for validation are detection limit and quantitation limit.

■ Container Closure Systems

Packaging, as shown in Figure 4-1, is one of the last steps in the manufacturing process. The primary role of packaging is to provide containment and protection to the drug product, but it also plays a role in product identification and, in some cases, patient compliance.

Packaging can be divided into two categories: primary and secondary packaging. Primary packaging is that which directly interacts with the drug product and therefore is more important from a manufacturing perspective than secondary packaging, which does not directly interact with the drug product.

The choice of primary packaging depends on the type of dosage form and the specific attributes of the drug product. Before a package system is chosen for a drug product, the manufacturer must ask several questions:

1. Which packaging material would be most appropriate for the drug product?
2. Will the packaging provide adequate protection against environmental concerns such as light and moisture?
3. Will the package affect stability and shelf life?
4. Will the packaging enhance the effect of the medication? Will it affect degradation and impurities?

These questions are important because some dosage forms, such as liquid preparations, have more interaction with the primary packaging than solid oral dosage forms do. The route of administration is also important; the packaging for injectables plays an integral part in the drug product's stability, sterility, and potency. For this reason, injectables and inhalation products are examples of dosage forms that are of high concern to regulatory agencies. The various dosage forms, routes of administration, and degrees of interaction are presented in TABLE 4-4.

An individual drug product's attributes also play a role in selection of primary packaging. To illustrate this, let's look at our example of Good Drug tablets. Solid oral dosage forms are the lowest concern of any of the routes of administration and have the lowest interaction with packaging material. Let us assume that Good Drug tablets are sensitive to moisture and that moisture accelerates the degradation of the

TABLE 4-4	Dosage Forms of Concern to Regulatory Agencies		
Degree of Concern With Route of Administration	Potential for Packaging/Drug Product Interaction		
	High	Medium	Low
Highest	Inhalation aerosols Parenterals	Sterile powders for injection	
High	Opthalmic solutions Nasal aerosols Transdermal patches		
Low	Topical Solutions Oral Solutions	Topical powders	Oral tablets and capsules

drug product. If this were the case, we would select packaging that would afford Good Drug tablets sufficient protection against moisture including the use of desiccants in the primary packaging. Additional examples of environmental factors that could lead to degradation of drug products include light, temperature, and microbial contamination. Some drug products may have direct incompatibilities with the primary packaging material. For example, the API may bind to the packing material or a component of the packaging material may leach into the drug product itself.

Primary packaging material should not leach harmful substances into the final dosage form; leachables in the final drug product raises concerns over safety. In the case of select dosage forms such as sterile products (parenteral and ophthalmics) and inhalation solutions, this situation is more worrisome. In these cases, additional testing is required. Specifically, an extraction study to evaluate which substances may enter the dosage form and toxicologic testing on any substance that is found during the extraction study should be performed.

Secondary packaging is less critical than primary packaging because it does not directly contact the drug product. Therefore, the amount of data required to support secondary packaging is modest. Secondary packaging generally consists of outer packaging over the primary container. For example, a cardboard box containing primary packaging of glass prefilled syringes or a plastic high-density polyethylene (HDPE) bottle filled with oral tablets. If the secondary packaging does afford protection to the drug product, then more detailed data are required.

Ultimately, the packaging must address the following needs for the final drug product:

- Compatibility with the formulation of the drug product
- Protection from environmental factors (light, moisture, etc.)
- Manufacturing capabilities (machine operation, tooling, etc.)
- Commercial considerations (enhanced patient compliance, child-resistant packaging, etc.)

■ Stability

The purpose of stability testing is to provide evidence on how the quality of the drug product varies over time under the influence of environmental factors such as temperature, humidity, and light. This evidence will provide the shelf life of the drug product under specified storage conditions.

The design of the stability program is based on experience with the API, both its physical chemical characteristics and prior completed stability studies on the API. Data on at least three primary batches of the drug product should be provided in marketing applications. These batches should be the same formulation and packaging that will be used commercially.

Stability studies should include testing the drug product according to its specifications to discern any changes that occur over the storage time. For Good Drug tablets, we need to test the drug product according to the specifications listed in Table 4-2 over time at specified intervals to assess the changes in the drug product.

Long-term testing should cover a minimum of 12 months duration on at least three primary batches at the time of submission and should be continued for a period of time sufficient to cover the proposed shelf life.

The general scheme for stability data for drugs is provided in TABLE 4-5: Table 4-5A is for drugs intended to be stored at room temperature, Table 4-5B is for refrigerated drugs, and Table 4-5C is for drugs that are to be stored under freezing conditions.

The schemes presented are general and several factors may affect extent of the data required at submission such as whether the packaging is permeable to moisture, whether a significant change in the drug product was observed during the stability study, and the number of drug product strengths and container closure systems being evaluated.

A stability protocol with a well-planned study design is the key to a successful stability program. In addition to the chemical, physical, and microbiological attributes of the drug product that need to be considered in planning a stability study, several statistical and regulatory perspectives also need to be taken into account.

TABLE 4-5A	Room Temperature	
Study	Storage Conditions	Minimum Time Period Covered by Data at Submission
Long-term	25°C ± 2°C/60% RH ± 5% RH or 30°C ± 2°C/65% RH ± 5% RH	12 months
Intermediate	30°C ± 2°C/65% RH ± 5% RH	6 months
Accelerated	40°C ± 2°C/75% RH ± 5% RH	6 months

TABLE4-5B	Refrigerated Conditions	
Study	Storage Conditions	Minimum Time Period Covered by Data at Submission
Long-term	5°C ± 3°C	12 months
Accelerated	25°C ± 2°C/60% RH ± 5% RH	6 months

TABLE 4-5C	Freezing Conditions	
Study	Storage Conditions	Minimum Time Period Covered by Data at Submission
Long-term	−20°C ± 5°C	12 months

■ Individual Dosage Forms

In this section, we discuss some of the individual manufacturing processes and specifications associated with different dosage forms.

Solid Oral Dosage Forms

Solid oral dosage forms, such as tablets and capsules, are the most common form of drug product and account for more than 70% of pharmaceutical products produced. Tablets and capsules contain the API and excipients. The excipients play a variety roles including as fillers, disintegrants, binders, and lubricants.

The API and excipients are mixed using blenders or tumblers prior to the compression process. The two most common manufacturing methods for tablets are direct compression and granulation.

In direct compression, the API is blended generally with one or more excipients and directly compressed into the tablet. In this process, excipients (binders) often act as fillers and impart compressibility to the powder blend. The cohesive properties of binders may reduce friability of the tablets. Direct compression is a relatively simple process and is considered economical from a manufacturing perspective. It is also associated with less degradation issues for materials sensitive to heat or moisture. However, to utilize direct compression the powder needs to have good compressibility and flowability. This is seldom the case though, and generally these attributes need to be imparted to powder by methods of granulation.

Granulation is widely used because of its versatility. Its main objective is to improve the flow properties and compression characteristics of the mix, increase particle strength, and prevent segregation of the constituents. However, these gains must be weighed against the fact that granulation requires multiple-unit processes, such as wet massing, drying, and screening, which are costly in terms of the time, space, and equipment required, and they add complexity because each unit process brings its own set of complications.

There are two main methods of granulation: wet granulation and dry granulation. Wet granulation uses fluid to help form granules and is the most widely used granulation method. Dry granulation is a mechanical process in which granules are formed via pressure. It is generally utilized when the formulation is sensitive to moisture or cannot tolerate the drying process used in wet granulation.

Melt granulation, another form of granulation, is when the excipients are melted and then granulated with the API. Capsules can be further subdivided into either hard or soft capsules, with hard capsules being more common. Soft capsules or "softgels" are generally made of gelatin film that contains liquid solution.

Hard capsules share many of the manufacturing processes of tablets with the final step of tabletting or capsule filling being the major distinction. One advantage of hard capsules over tablets is that they may be easier to formulate because there is no need for the formulation to account for variables related to tablet compaction. The main disadvantage of capsules is that the machinery associated with filling the capsules is considerably slower than tabletting machines are.

The soft capsules share some of the same advantages of hard capsules. Liquid capsule formulations often provide, greater flexibility than those of tablets. However, the process of manufacturing soft capsules is relatively expensive and time-consuming.

The following specifications/tests may be applicable to solid oral dosage forms.

- Dissolution
- Disintegration
- Hardness/friability

■ Parenterals

Parenteral medications come in a variety of different dosage formulations and are available for several routes of administration, with intravenous (IV), intramuscular (IM), and subcutaneous (SC) being the most common.

These different routes of administration along with more broad-based concerns with parenterals (such as sterility and pyrogens) make the formulation and manufacturing of these products a complicated proposition. For example, any preparation intended for IV administration needs to be isotonic with the intravascular space to avoid inflammation of the blood vessel walls.

Parenteral drug products fall into several categories:

- *Solutions.* The most common formulation of parenteral formulations. Solutions are often manufactured by dissolving the API and excipients and adjusting the pH as necessary.
- *Suspensions.* Suspensions consist of the API suspended in an aqueous vehicle. These are often manufactured by asepetically combining a sterile solution vehicle with a powder.
- *Dry powders.* When the drug product is too unstable to prepare in a solution or suspension, it may be manufactured as a dry powder to be later reconstituted. In this process, the drug product solution is freeze-dried in a process called lyophilization. This is an expensive and complicated process but is the only alternative for some drug product formulations. Other methods are used for solid/dry powders such as spray drying, but they are less common than lyophilization.
- *Emulsions.* Emulsion formulations are less common than the other formulations presented. These are oil-in-water or water-in-oil preparations made stable through an emulsifying agent.
- *Protein formulations.* Most protein formulations fall into one of the previous categories (solutions or dry powders), but they present special challenges because of the nature of their delicate formulation that warrant special attention. Many factors can adversely affect the protein in these preparations, so additional procedures are often applied to the formulation and manufacturing process to ensure a quality product.

Excipients play an important role in parenteral products; they provide many of the attributes (stability, sterility, and tonicity) that make administration possible. Some examples of the excipients used are provided in the TABLE 4-6.

TABLE 4-6	Role of Excipients in Parenteral Products
Excipient Role	Examples
Tonicity-adjusting agents	NaCl, mannitol
Antioxidants	Ascorbic acid
Bacteriostatic preservatives	Benzyl alcholol, benzalkonium chloride
pH adjusters	HCl, NaOH
Buffering agents	Phosphates, citrates
Chelating agents	ETDA

The manufacturing process of a parenteral is dependent on the formulation; the process for parenteral solutions is quite different from dry powders undergoing lyophilization.

However, some manufacturing steps are common to all parenteral products. All parenteral products have their packaging components (vials, ampules, rubber stoppers, etc.) sterilized prior to filling. All equipment must be of the best available grade of stainless steel. The filling area of the manufacturing site is always aseptic with numerous quality control measures such as HEPA-filtered laminar-flow within in the aseptic area.

The sterilization process is particularly important in the manufacture of parenteral drug products and warrants additional attention. *Sterilization* can be defined as a process that removes and kills all microorganisms through a chemical agent or physical process. However, when pharmaceutical products are manufactured, there is no absolute certainty that all the units will be sterile. The common methods of sterilization are the following:

- *Moist heat.* Moist heat sterilization is a process in which steam and pressure are used to sterilize via an autoclave. This process is effective, relatively quick, and inexpensive. However, the drug product must be stable to moisture and heat.
- *Dry heat.* Dry heat sterilization utilizes a drying oven with heated filtered air. The air is distributed throughout the chamber by convection via a blower system. This process is often used to sterilize the glassware used in parenteral manufacture.
- *Filtration.* This process utilizes filters ranging from 0.1 µm to 0.22 µm to filter bacteria. This process is desirable for heat-labile drug products.
- *Ethylene oxide.* This sterilization process uses ethylene oxide gas to sterilize and is employed when the temperatures used in moist and dry heat sterilization procedures are unacceptable. Ethylene oxide is highly flammable, mutagenic, and leaves the possibility of toxic residues in treated materials. This process is generally used only with medical devices.
- *Ionizing radiation.* This process is generally used on medical devices. One advantage over the use of ethylene oxide is the lack of any potential toxic residue from ionizing radiation.

The choice of which sterilization process to use depends on the capacity of the formulation and the ability of the package to resist the treatment applied. For instance, a liquid formulation may be sterilized by using autoclaving (moist heat) or filtration, whereas medical devices are treated using ethylene oxide. The majority of sterile drugs are manufactured by aseptic processing because terminal sterilization degrades the chemical stability of a given formulation and damages the container/closure system.

Although we did not discuss biologics and biotechnology engineered products in specific detail in this chapter, most differences as compared to chemical entities are related to the manufacture of the API, and those differences can be profound. However, in most cases, these drug products are parenteral products and are manufactured in similar manners as chemical entity drug products. For example, etanercept, which is a dimerized protein molecule, has its API produced via recombinant technology. The finished dosage form is manufactured as a sterile, lyophilized powder formulated with excipients (mannitol, etc.) in a similar manner as presented in this section.

The following tests/specifications are generally applicable to sterile parenteral dosage forms:

- pH
- Sterility
- Endotoxins/pyrogens
- Particulate matter
- Antimicrobial preservative
- Extractables
- Functionality testing of delivery system (if a syringe or device is used to aid in the delivery of the injection)

The packaging of parenteral products is a critical part of the drug product because it may have direct effects on the sterility, stability, potency, and toxicity. As was described earlier in the section titled "Container Closure Systems," particular attention must be paid to the choice of packaging for parenteral solutions. In general, glass containers are the best. The United States Pharmacopeia (USP) classifies glass containers as type I, II, or III. We do not discuss the details of each classification, but type I is superior to the others and is often the grade of glass used in parenteral products.

■ Ophthalmic Drug Products

Ophthalmic drug products are unique in that they allow the pharmacologic agent to be placed in the direct target of concern. These preparations have additional challenges such as the need to bypass physiologic barriers in the eye such as the cornea.

Not unlike parenteral drug products, the formulation and final drug product intended for ocular delivery must be sterile. The sterilization procedures for ocular products are the same as those used for parenterals described previously.

An additional concern in the manufacture of ocular drug products is the assessment of ocular irritation. This may affect the concentration of the API and type of excipients used in the manufacturing process. For example, many antimicrobial preservatives cause irritation to the eye.

Ocular dosage forms come in several formulations, as described here:

- *Solutions*. Like parenteral products, solutions are the majority of the ocular preparations available. These formulations are generally desirable from a large-scale manufacturing perspective because of the relative simplicity of formulation.

However, great care must be taken with the pH, solubility, tonicity, and viscosity (aid in drug delivery by keeping the drug in the eye longer).

- *Suspensions.* The manufacture of suspensions is more complicated than manufacturing solutions. This is because of a variety of reasons including variables such as particle size of the API, rate of sedimentation, the resuspendability of the API, and choice of solubilizing and suspending agents utilized.
- *Ocular ointments.* These drug products can provide excellent drug delivery to the eye. However, because of complications of use, such as blurred vision, their application is generally limited to nighttime use only. In the manufacture of ocular ointments, the API is often sterilized by dry heat, ethylene oxide, or ionizing radiation. Then, the sterilized API is added aseptically to a petroleum-based vehicle.
- *Gels and gel-forming solutions.* These ocular drug products utilize mucoadhesive polymers that bind to tissue in the eye. This helps overcome the main disadvantage of ocular solutions: a relatively short residence time in the eye. In the case of the gel-forming solutions, these products have gelling systems that cause the solution to gel upon contact with enzymes found in the eye.

Ocular agents have additional specification/tests required for release. In general, these tests are similar to those presented for parenteral drug products.

The manufacturing equipment should be of the best grade stainless steel, and all filling areas must be aseptic environments like that described previously for parenteral products. The packaging for ocular drug products is generally plastic dropper bottles.

One unique item that is associated with ocular products is the use of color-coded caps to identify medication types. The color scheme is provided in TABLE 4-7.

■ Metered Dose and Dry Powder Drug Products

Aerosolized solutions and powders allow for organ-targeted therapy; they allow for the drug product to be administered directly into the lungs of respiratory-compromised patients.

Metered dose and dry powder drug products are some of the most complicated drug products to manufacture because of the complexity of the issues that surround these

TABLE 4-7	Color Schemes for Ocular Medications
Drug Class	Cap Color
Beta-blocker	Yellow or blue
Non-steroids	Grey
Anti-infectives	Brown or Tan
Carbonic anydrase inhibitors	Orange

dosage forms. Respiratory drug products have the smallest particle sizes of all drug products, and the composition of the formulation is crucial in defining physical stability and performance.

Additional concern is related to the delivery device for these products because almost all inhalation products use some form of device for drug delivery. Excipients often comprise a significant portion of the formulation and have a substantial effect on the safety, quality, stability, performance, and effectiveness of these drug products. The manufacturing process and formulation concerns are too complicated to address fully in this chapter, but some specifications that are applicable to metered dose and dry powder inhalers are as follows:

- Microbial limits
- Moisture content
- Net content weight
- Dose content uniformity
- Dose content uniformity throughout container life
- Particle size distribution
- Spray pattern and plume geometry
- Leak rate
- Leachables
- Pressure testing

Similar to the situation with parenteral products, the primary packaging is a critical parameter for these drug products. One issue unique to metered dose and dry powder inhalable products is that design and performance of the inhaler can directly affect the efficacy of the drug product. Because these formulations are a "high to highest" concern based on route of administration and potential interaction with the primary packaging (see Table 4-4), additional attention must be paid to leachables, and extraction studies are necessary.

■ Topical Drug Products

Topical drug therapy is that which is applied directly to the skin. This in itself presents some challenges because one of the main functions of the skin is to maintain a barrier against foreign substances entering the body. The rationale for topical therapy is either to apply a drug product directly to the skin to produce some effect on the skin itself or to achieve some systemic effect via administration of the drug on the skin (ie, transdermal therapy).

Transdermal therapy is often used when the drug product cannot be administered orally because of decreased potency or chemical stability in the gastrointestinal tract (ie, testosterone replacement therapy) or to achieve a superior pharmacokinetic/

pharmacodynamic profile (ie, transdermal selegiline). Topical therapy can be divided into several dosage forms including creams, ointments, pastes, and gels.

Although these dosage forms have differences in vehicles, they are basically manufactured in a similar manner. In the fusion method, the vehicle is heated to the liquid state and the API and excipients are added as the formulation dictates. The mixture is then cooled and homogenized as necessary.

Transdermal drug products deliver medication systemically via various patch technologies. These drug products are somewhat more complex to manufacture because their efficacy and performance are correlated to the patch technology (size of patch, location on body of administration, duration of contact, etc.).

Topical products can be associated with irritation and skin sensitivity. This sensitivity may develop from the API and/or one of the excipients used in the formulation. Some specifications that are applicable to topical products include the following:

- Homogeneity
- Particle size distribution
- pH
- Visual appearance, color
- Texture and viscosity
- Release and bioavailability (transdermal patches)

■ Suggested Reading

Ali Y, Lehmussaari K. Industrial perspective in ocular drug delivery. *Adv Drug Delivery Rev*. 2006;11:1259–1267.

Avis K. *Pharmaceutical Dosage Forms: Parenteral Medications*. Drugs and the Pharmaceutical Sciences. New York, NY: Marcel Dekker; 1992.

Banker G, Rhodes C. *Modern Phamaceutics*. 4th ed. Drugs and the Pharmaceutical Sciences. New York, NY: Marcel Dekker; 2002.

Berger C, Donne, P, Winderman H. Use of substances of animal origin in pharmaceutics and compliance with TSE-risk guideline—a market survey. *Biologicals*. 2005;33:1–7.

Burgess D. *Injectable Dispersed Systems: Formulation, Processing, and Performance*. Drugs and the Pharmaceutical Sciences. Boca Raton, Fla: Taylor and Francis; 2005.

DiFeo T. Drug product development: a technical review of chemistry, manufacturing, and controls information for the support of pharmaceutical compound licensing activities. *Drug Dev Ind Pharmacy*. 2003;29:939–958.

Food and Drug Administration. *Guidance for Industry: Container Closure Systems for Packaging Human Drugs and Biologics*. Washington, DC: US Department of Health and Human Services; May 1999.

International Conference on Harmonisation. *Guidance for Industry: Q3B(R2) Impurities in New Drug Products*. Rockville, Md: ICH; July 2006.

International Conference on Harmonisation. *Guidance for Industry: Q2B Validation of Analytical Procedures*: Methodology. Rockville, Md: ICH; 1996.

International Conference on Harmonisation. *Guidance for Industry: Q1A(R2) Stability Testing of New Drug Substances*. Rockville, Md: ICH; November 2003.

International Conference on Harmonisation. *Guidance for Industry: Q2B Validation of Analytical Procedures: Methodology*. Rockville, Md: ICH; 1996.

International Conference on Harmonisation. *Guidance for Industry: Q3B(R2) Impurities in New Drug Products*. Rockville, Md: ICH; July 2006.

International Conference on Harmonisation. *Guidance for Industry: Q6A Specifications: Test Procedures and Acceptance Criteria for New Drug Substances and Drug Products: Chemical Substances*. Rockville, Md: ICH; 2000.

International Conference on Harmonisation. *Guidance for Industry: Q6A Specifications: Test Procedures and Acceptance Criteria for New Drug Substances and Drug Products: Chemical Substances*. Rockville, Md: ICH; 2000.

International Conference on Harmonisation. *Guidance for Industry: Q6B Specifications: Test Procedures and Acceptance Criteria for Biotechnological/Biological Products*. Rockville, Md: ICH; August 1999.

Lin T, Chen C. Overview of stability study designs. *J Biopharm Stat*. 2003;13:337–354.

Mitchell R, Marzolini NL, Hancock SA, Harridance AM, Elder DP. The use of surface analysis techniques to determine the route of manufacture of tablet dosage forms. *Drug Dev Ind Pharmacy*. 2006;32:252–261.

Pifferi G, Santoro P, Pedrani M. Quality and functionality of excipients. *Il Farmaco*. 1999;54:1–14.

Shekunov B, et al. Particle size analysis in pharmaceutics: principles, methods, and applications. *Pharm Res*. 2007; 24:203–227.

Zhang G, Law D. Phase transformation considerations during process development and manufacture of solid oral dosage forms. *Adv Drug Delivery Rev*. 2004;56:371–390.

Ethics in Clinical Research

Michael McGraw and Adam George

Clinical research involving human volunteers is conducted to establish generalizable knowledge to understand and support human health and wellness. It has produced many advances in medicine but continues to present ethical questions that must be considered. Clinical research has fallen under intense scrutiny as a result of serious events that have occurred over the years. This chapter describes the ethical principles and guidelines that influence the current and future conduct of clinical research and provide a historical perspective of the clinical research landscape.

■ Clinical Research Versus Clinical Practice

It is important to distinguish between clinical research and clinical practice. Clinical research is unlike clinical practice because the objectives are very different. The intention of clinical research is to conduct an investigation of human biology, health, or disease to benefit society as a whole. It utilizes elements of the scientific method whereby a hypothesis is developed and tested and conclusions are drawn from the results of those tests.[1] Clinical research does not always benefit the individual who is participating and should not be considered an approach to treatment. Instead, the purpose of clinical research is to generate data that may enhance general medical knowledge. The objective of clinical practice, on the other hand, is to treat an individual patient's medical condition with the confidence that the treatment has a reasonable expectation of success and direct benefit to the patient. However, clinical research can give patients access to high-quality health care and cutting-edge therapies, but this is not the intended purpose of research.

■ Ethics and Clinical Research

Ethics are standards that describe how human beings should live and behave in society. One of the many ethical debates that surround clinical research is the question of the "good of society" versus the "good of the individual." It is necessary to conduct clinical research to advance medical care and promote public health, but it is important to respect the rights and humanity of an individual person. Given this information, the question becomes whether it is ethical to jeopardize the safety of an individual knowing that society will benefit from the knowledge gained by the individual's participation in clinical research. Historical events have brought such questions to the forefront. These events have perpetuated the composition of various documents that have become the ethical foundations that guide the conduct of clinical research as we know it today.

■ Ethical Foundations

The foundations for ethics in clinical research lie within the confines of specific documents discussed below.

Nuremberg Code

To understand the ethical issues influencing the conduct of clinical research, it is essential to understand the basic foundations. The Nuremberg Code (TABLE 5-1) merges Hippocratic ethics and protection of human volunteers into 10 concise principles. This document was developed after World War II in response to the experiments that took place in the concentration camps of Nazi Germany. During this time, medical doctors conducted clinical research without the consent of the patients. Furthermore, these experiments were conducted without any rational background and yielded results with no benefit to society.[2–4]

The first principle of the Nuremberg Code stresses that voluntary consent of human volunteers is essential for participation in clinical research trials. Subjects must have the capacity to give consent and the ability to exercise free choice without outside influence or coercion. During the informed consent process, all volunteers must be explained the nature, duration, purpose, and all possible risks or hazards involved with participation. The responsibility for attaining and conducting proper informed consent lies in the hands of the individuals conducting the research. It is also important to understand that before a volunteer can be approached regarding participation in research, it is necessary to make sure the research is valuable.[3,4]

The second principle of the Nuremberg Code states that the anticipated results of a research project should be beneficial to society and that the only means of obtaining this knowledge is by conducting the research in humans. In other words, if the same information could be obtained by conducting research in animals or through other methods, then it is unethical to conduct the research in humans. Furthermore, experimental design should be based on the results of animal studies and the rationale of disease history to justify the purpose of conducting the research.[3,4]

TABLE 5-1	The Nuremberg Code

1. The voluntary consent of the human subject is absolutely essential.

   This means that the person involved should have legal capacity to give consent; should be so situated as to be able to exercise free power of choice, without the intervention of any element of force, fraud, deceit, duress, overreaching, or other ulterior form of constraint or coercion; and should have sufficient knowledge and comprehension of the elements of the subject matter involved as to enable him to make an understanding and enlightened decision. This latter element requires that before the acceptance of an affirmative decision by the experimental subject there should be made known to him the nature, duration, and purpose of the experiment; the method and means by which it is to be conducted; all inconveniences and hazards reasonably to be expected; and the effects upon his health or person which may possibly come from his participation in the experiment.

   The duty and responsibility for ascertaining the quality of the consent rests upon each individual who initiates, directs or engages in the experiment. It is personal duty and responsibility which may not be delegated to another with impunity.

2. The experiment should be such as to yield fruitful results for the good of society, unprocurable by other methods or means of study, and not random and unnecessary in nature.

3. The experiment should be so designed and based on the results of animal experimentation and a knowledge of the natural history of the disease or other problem under study that the anticipated results will justify the performance of the experiment.

4. The experiment should be so conducted as to avoid all unnecessary physical and mental suffering and injury.

5. No experiment should be so conducted where there is an a priori reason to believe that death or disabling injury will occur; except, perhaps, in those experiments where the experimental physicians also serve as subjects.

6. The degree of risk to be taken should never exceed that determined by the humanitarian importance of the problem to be solved by the experiment.

7. Proper preparations should be made and adequate facilities provided to protect the experimental subject against even remote possibilities of injury, disability, or death.

8. The experiment should be conducted only by scientifically qualified persons. The highest degree of skill and care should be required through all stages of the experiment of those who conduct or engage in the experiment.

9. During the course of the experiment the human subject should be at liberty to bring the experiment to an end if he has reached the physical or mental state where continuation of the experiment seems to him to be impossible.

10. During the course of the experiment the scientist in charge must be prepared to terminate the experiment at any stage, if he has probable cause to believe, in the exercise of the good faith, superior skill, and careful judgment required of him, that a continuation of the experiment is likely to result in injury, disability, or death to the experimental subject.

Source: The Nuremberg (1949), as printed in Levine R. *Ethics and the Regulation of Research*, 2nd ed. New Haven, Yale University Press, 1986.

Protection of human volunteers is a concept that is described in the remaining principles of the code. These principles state that all research should be conducted to avoid unnecessary physical and mental suffering. It is unjust to conduct any research that the investigator believes will cause death or disabling injury. Also, the risk involved with study participation should not be greater than the benefit of the results. Physician investigators and members of the study staff must take into consideration that all volunteers who participate in clinical research trials will be exposed to potential risks.

For example, patients have blood drawn as standard of care for most disease states. Even though the risks associated with having blood drawn are minimal, they are still present but are outweighed by the benefit of the results in managing their disease state. When conducting a clinical research study, it is easy to forget that blood drawn for the study can expose volunteers to the risks involved with having blood drawn, such as pain, with little or no direct benefit. This may seem like a trivial scenario. However, it is possible that a volunteer could develop a serious bacterial infection from a study blood draw that was not essential to prove a study endpoint. No matter how insignificant the risks may seem, it is always important for everyone involved in the conduct of clinical research to protect the health and safety of all human volunteers. To do this, it may even be necessary to let volunteers discontinue their participation in a study that is providing them with direct benefit.[3,4]

Giving volunteers the ability to terminate their participation in a research study is another concept derived from the Nuremberg Code. There may come a time when volunteers feel that they are no longer physically or mentally willing or able to participate in the research. As a physician investigator, this decision maybe difficult to accept particularly if the research is clearly benefiting the person's condition. However, the volunteer's decision must be respected without efforts to persuade the person to continue.[3,4]

Every day clinical investigators and all members of the study staff are required to make difficult impartial ethical decisions. During the course of any research project, investigators must, in good faith, be prepared to stop a study if they believe continuation will result in injury, disability, or death to participants. This decision must be made regardless of the potential benefits to society. When posed with an ethical dilemma such as this, it is essential for researchers to use the principles, outlined in documents such as the Nuremberg Code, as a guide.[3,4]

Declaration of Helsinki

The Declaration of Helsinki was developed by the World Medical Association (WMA) and is a statement of ethical principles to provide guidance to physicians and other participants in medical research involving human volunteers.[5] The Declaration stresses, in detail, the same ethical concepts of the Nuremberg Code but also identifies other principles. The uniqueness of the Declaration is that, unlike the other foundation documents, it is periodically updated by the WMA to address the ever evolving ethical issues in clinical research.

Similar to other foundation documents, the Declaration addresses the principle of protection of human volunteers. The WMA recognizes that "medical progress is based on research which ultimately must rest in part on experimentation of involving human volunteers."[6] It states that the purpose of medical research involving human volunteers is to improve prophylactic, diagnostic, and therapeutic procedures. To do so, it is necessary to continuously challenge the effectiveness of these procedures through research. In analyzing this principle, it is evident that there will always be a need to conduct research trials with the intention of discovering new, more safe and effective standards of care. It is important to remember that the well-being of the patient is the primary concern. The Declaration states that the duty of physicians is to promote and safeguard the health of the people and binds them with the words, "The health of my patient will be my first consideration."[6] This principle is continued by the statement that it is the duty of the physician in medical research to protect the life, health, privacy, and dignity of the human volunteer.

The Declaration identifies that some research populations are vulnerable and require special protection. It is necessary to recognize the needs of volunteer populations that are economically and medically disadvantaged. Consideration must also be given to vulnerable populations such as those who cannot give or refuse to give consent for themselves, those who volunteer by giving consent under duress, and those for whom research is combined with care. In the setting where research is combined with care, it is the physician's responsibility to inform volunteers which aspects are related to research and which are related to patient care.[6]

In the Nuremberg Code, it is stated that research should be designed and based on previous experiment results and pertinent background information: The Declaration takes this a step further to say that the design and performance of each clinical trial should be clearly formulated in an experimental protocol. To ensure that research proposals are ethical, the Declaration affirms that they must be submitted for consideration, comment, and guidance for approval to an ethical review committee. Often these committees are called institutional review boards (IRBs) or independent ethics committees.[6] The topic of IRBs is covered in greater detail later in this chapter.

Also addressed in the Declaration are the principles of voluntary participation and informed consent. The basic concepts stressed by the WMA are very similar to those presented in the Nuremberg Code. The Declaration takes these a step further to include that precautions must be made to not only safeguard the patient but to respect the privacy and confidentiality of the patient's information. To conform to this concept it is common practice in research that volunteers are identified by randomly generated numbers. Beginning the moment the patient signs the informed consent all study-related documents and laboratory materials are identified with this number and not the volunteer's name.[6]

Since its conception, updates to the Declaration occur to provide ethical guidance on newly developing issues. In the modern era, we are fortunate to have a drug or multiple drugs to treat almost every disease. In research, it is common to test a new drug against placebo. In the case of a drug study, *placebo* is a tablet or capsule made to look like the comparator drug but that does not contain any medication. These have also been referred to as sugar pills. This was done in the past because in most cases other treatment options were not available for comparison against a new medication. An amendment to the Declaration addresses the ethical issue behind placebo controlled studies. To summarize this amendment the benefits, risks, burdens, and effectiveness of a new drug should be tested against the best current medication used to treat the target disease state. This concept seems plausible, but there are many different opinions and arguments that surround this topic. The rationale and ethical dilemmas surrounding placebo research are discussed in greater detail later in this chapter.[6]

For example, a drug company wants to discover whether a new compound is carcinogenic. Experiments have yet to be conducted in animals for this purpose, but to speed up the development process the drug company would like to conduct the initial experiment in humans. Being that this is a new compound and its efficacy at treating any disease state has yet to be proven, it is not ethical to conduct this research in human volunteers. It is possible that more information or a definitive answer can be discovered by first conducting research in animals.

Belmont Report

The Belmont Report, drafted by the National Commission for the Protection of Human Subjects, identifies and summarizes the basic ethical principles in biomedical and behavioral research. The three basic ethical principles outlined in the report are respect for persons, beneficence, and justice.[7]

Respect for persons recognizes that individuals should be treated as autonomous agents and that persons with diminished autonomy are entitled to protection. This principle is the basis for human volunteer informed consent and respects that autonomous individuals are able to make decisions about personal objectives and act under the direction of such decisions. Informed consent of human volunteers is a process that explains the potential risks and benefits involved with participation in clinical research. In this process, clinical researchers are obligated to prove potential research volunteers with all the information necessary to make an educated informed decision. It is essential that individuals with disabilities that may affect their capacity to make an informed decision are protected from the potential risks of clinical research. Sometimes it is necessary to exclude individuals from participation in clinical research because they are not able to make rationale informed decisions or because they may be coerced into participation.[7]

An ethical debate that continues in the research community is whether or not to allow prisoners to participate in clinical research. Based on the concept of respect for persons we must recognize that these individuals are able to act autonomously and should be given the same opportunity to participate in research. However, it is possible that these volunteers may be coerced into participating in exchange for shortened prison terms or special treatment. The same issue can also emerge with employees of research institutions. Should employees of research facilities be excluded from participating in studies conducted by that the facility? If so, are we denying them the opportunity to participate in possible beneficial research? In making important ethical decisions it is important to keep the best interests of the research volunteers in mind.[7]

Beneficence is another basic principle outlined in the Belmont Report and is expressed by two rules: do not harm, and maximize potential benefit and minimize possible harm. It is not possible to know all the risks involved in conducting clinical research, but we must not intentionally harm volunteers to benefit the greater good. The answers to questions posed by certain studies may be of great benefit to society, but obtaining these answers may require conducting a study that intentionally harms or puts volunteers at considerable risk. Even though the results of this research are important, it is not always ethical to intentionally harm even a small group of volunteers.[7]

The risk versus benefits must always be weighed when considering conducting a clinical research study. In most cases studies provide potential benefit to participants while subjecting them to minimal risk. Other studies may not have potential benefit to volunteers directly involved with the study but may provide a great benefit to society while subjecting volunteering participants to minimal risk. It is the job of both the research community and investigators to make every effort to reduce the risk involved in conducting clinical research. We are able to offer research volunteers the ability to participate in potentially beneficial research without unjustly jeopardizing their overall health and well-being.[7]

Identifying potential volunteers for clinical research trials requires careful selection of individuals that are able and willing to participate, without denying individuals the potential benefit of participation. In the Belmont Report, the concept of justice states that research must justly distribute the potential benefit and burden involved with recruiting study participants. One assumption is that "equals must be treated equally." The report suggests some widely accepted formulations on which to base the distribution of benefits and burdens. These formulations are as follows: to each person an equal share, to each person according to individual need, to each person according to individual effort, to each person according to societal contribution, and to each person according to merit.[7] It is important to understand these implications to trust that researchers are not taking advantage of groups of people such as the poor, chronically ill, and uneducated.

■ Rules and Regulations

The previous section discusses ethical foundations that researchers use as guidelines to conduct ethical clinical research. However, these documents act only as guidelines. Rules and regulations regarding clinical research have been developed by the United

States, Europe, and the International Conference on Harmonisation (ICH). Each agency has its own set of rules and regulations that must be followed. For the United States, these are outlined in the Code of Federal Regulations. In Europe, rules and regulations regarding clinical research are outlined in the European Union Clinical Trials Directive. ICH is responsible for creating international guidelines for conducting clinical research trials.[8-10]

Code of Federal Regulations

The Code of Federal Regulations (CFR) is the codification of the general and permanent rules published in the *Federal Register* by the executive departments and agencies of the federal government. The CFR is divided into 50 titles. Title 21 of the code outlines the rules and regulations for food and drugs governed by the US Food and Drug Administration (FDA). In Title 21, there are three sections that discuss the ethical conduct of clinical research: Part 50, Part 54, and Part 56. Title 45 CFR Part 46 was first adopted in 1981 to regulate research funded by the US Department of Health and Human Services (DHHS; formerly the Department of Health, Education, and Welfare). In 1991, these regulations were expanded and became known as the Common Rule. The Common Rule applies to all research funded by federal agencies. These regulations were also codified in Title 21 CFR Parts 50 and 56, and guidelines from the World Health Organization (WHO), which were incorporated into the ICH Guidelines for Good Clinical Practices. These regulations specify the composition and responsibilities of an institutional review board (IRB) or an independent ethics committee (IEC), the criteria for reviewing and approving research protocols, and the elements of informed consent, described further later.[1,11] This section discusses Part 50 and Part 54. CFR Part 56 defines the function and operation of IRBs and is discussed later in this chapter.[12]

European Union Clinical Trials Directive

Developed by the European Parliament and the Council of the European Union, the European Union Clinical Trials Directive outlines the rules and regulations for the conduct of clinical research in the countries that comprise the European Union. The directive is divided into 24 articles of which Articles 3 through 12 pertain to clinical research. This document is very similar to the US CFR, so it is appropriate that these be discussed in tandem.[9]

The Nuremberg Code and Declaration of Helsinki introduced the principle of informed consent and explained its ethical purpose. The main intent of CFR Part 50 and Article 3 of the directive is the protection of the rights and safety of human volunteers involved in clinical research. These documents recognize the significance of this principle and state that human volunteers may not participate in research without voluntary informed consent. The elements of informed consent are outlined in both documents and are discussed later in this chapter.[8,9]

Many clinical research studies are sponsored or funded by the government or private industry. Investigators may have ties to these sources by means of stocks, bonds, or part-time employment. These ties can potentially confound research, especially if the investigator can benefit financially or personally from the results of the study. Part 54 of the CFR addresses the issue of financial disclosure by clinical investigators. It is mandated that a list of clinical investigators who conducted the research must be submitted to the FDA for review. Included is a description of the financial ties, if any, the investigator or any member of their immediate family may have to the research. The clinical trials directive differs from the CFR on this topic and does not mandate that investigators disclose personal financial ties to the research. However, Article 6 explains that the amounts and arrangements for rewarding or compensating investigators along with agreements between the sponsor and the site must be disclosed to an ethics committee.[8,9]

International Conference on Harmonisation

The ICH was created with the goal of harmonizing regulations from the three major players in drug development: western Europe, Japan, and the United States. Regulatory bodies from these countries meet periodically to construct guidelines for the development of investigational compounds. The intention is that these guidelines will be globally accepted and streamline the drug approval process. Section E6 of the ICH guidelines describes the expectations and requirements of all participants in the ethical conduct of clinical trials.[10,13]

■ Protection of Human Subjects

The National Commission for the Protection of Human Subjects of Biomedical and Behavioral Research stated that the three ethical principles found in the Belmont Report (respect for persons, beneficence, and justice) shape "the basis on which specific rules could be formulated, criticized, and interpreted."[1] These three principles, along with the standards set by the Nuremberg Code and Declaration of Helsinki, are the framework for legislation and guidelines promulgated by government agencies and organizations such as the US Department of Health and Human Services (DHHS), the World Health Organization (WHO), and the International Conference on Harmonisation (ICH). The legislation and guidelines developed by these organizations and government agencies were designed to protect the welfare and safety of human volunteers and to ensure the integrity of clinical trial data. The introduction of the ICH guidelines state that "compliance with this standard provides public assurance that the rights, safety, and well-being of trial volunteers are protected, consistent with the principles that have their origin in the Declaration of Helsinki, and that the clinical trial data are credible."[14]

Institutional Review Boards and Independent Ethics Committees

Institutional review boards (IRBs) and independent ethics committees (IECs) are a critical element of the system designed to protect individual volunteers as well as public health by critically appraising the scientific and ethical content of clinical research studies. It is necessary that research is evaluated by an IRB or IEC to determine that the rights, safety, and well-being of volunteers are taken into consideration and that the research is valuable according to ICH guidelines. These committees have to carefully assess research protocols with the essential scientific knowledge and evaluate the endpoints of new studies and the methods used.[15]

Title 45 CFR Part 46 details the composition of an IRB (TABLE 5-2) as well as the criteria for evaluating a research protocol (TABLE 5-3). It is imperative that an IRB is properly constituted to ensure that research protocols are evaluated with the necessary scientific rigor. For example, if an IRB or IEC is evaluating research protocols that involve children, then the IRB should have at least one member whose specialty is pediatrics. On the other hand, the IRB or IEC must also consist of members whose main focus is not scientific in nature. Instead, some members must provide the perspective of a lay person. This person is often a member of the clergy or another local community representative.

The main responsibility of an IRB or IEC is to evaluate the level of risk to the research volunteer versus the possibility of benefit to the volunteer or society as a whole. This can be a difficult task given the intricacy of some research protocols and the complexity of some innovative therapies. This evaluation is conducted by scrutinizing the protocol procedures and the risks and benefits outlined in the informed consent form in addition to the expertise of the individual committee members. An IRB or IEC meets periodically to discuss these issues and determine whether or not the research should be conducted.[11]

There are different types of review committees and systems for review throughout the world. The United States uses a system involving both local and central commercial IRBs. Local IRBs are often affiliated with a college, university, or hospital. A local IRB evaluates research conducted at its affiliated institution. Central or commercial IRBs in the United States evaluate research at multiple institutions and frequently operate on a for-profit basis. They have the same responsibilities as a local IRB but are not necessarily affiliated with the institution whose research is under evaluation.[11]

The European Union utilizes a national system of ethics committees to evaluate the conduct of research. All research involving human volunteers is evaluated at a national level to determine whether a particular research protocol should be conducted. The standards set for these national ethics committees are outlined in the EU Clinical Trials Directive and are similar to the CFR and the ICH guidelines.[9]

TABLE 5-2	IRB Membership

45 CFR 46.107

(a) Each IRB shall have at least five members, with varying backgrounds to promote complete and adequate review of research activities commonly conducted by the institution. The IRB shall be sufficiently qualified through the experience and expertise of its members, and the diversity of the members, including consideration of race, gender, and cultural backgrounds and sensitivity to such issues as community attitudes, to promote respect for its advice and counsel in safeguarding the rights and welfare of human volunteers. In addition to possessing the professional competence necessary to review specific research activities, the IRB shall be able to ascertain the acceptability of proposed research in terms of institutional commitments and regulations, applicable law, and standards of professional conduct and practice. The IRB shall therefore include persons knowledgeable in these areas. If an IRB regularly reviews research that involves a vulnerable category of volunteers, such as children, prisoners, pregnant women, or handicapped or mentally disabled persons, consideration shall be given to the inclusion of one or more individuals who are knowledgeable about and experienced in working with these volunteers.

(b) Every nondiscriminatory effort will be made to ensure that no IRB consists entirely of men or entirely of women, including the institution's consideration of qualified persons of both sexes, so long as no selection is made to the IRB on the basis of gender. No IRB may consist entirely of members of one profession.

(c) Each IRB shall include at least one member whose primary concerns are in scientific areas and at least one member whose primary concerns are in nonscientific areas.

(d) Each IRB shall include at least one member who is not otherwise affiliated with the institution and who is not part of the immediate family of a person who is affiliated with the institution.

(e) No IRB may have a member participate in the IRB's initial or continuing review of any project in which the member has a conflicting interest, except to provide information requested by the IRB.

(f) An IRB may, in its discretion, invite individuals with competence in special areas to assist in the review of issues which require expertise beyond or in addition to that available on the IRB. These individuals may not vote with the IRB.

Source: Title 45, United States Code of Federal Regulations Part 46.

Informed Consent

Informed consent is the process by which persons decide whether or not they want to volunteer to participate in a research study. Consent is an ongoing process and may be withdrawn by the volunteer at any time during the study. This process is documented by asking a volunteer to sign an informed consent form, but informed consent is more than just the document. The Belmont Report discusses three aspects of informed consent: information, comprehension, and voluntariness.[7]

TABLE 5-3	Criteria for IRB Approval of Research

45 CFR 46.111

(a) In order to approve research covered by this policy the IRB shall determine that all of the following requirements are satisfied:

 (1) Risks to volunteers are minimized: (i) By using procedures which are consistent with sound research design and which do not unnecessarily expose volunteers to risk, and (ii) whenever appropriate, by using procedures already being performed on the volunteers for diagnostic or treatment purposes.

 (2) Risks to volunteers are reasonable in relation to anticipated benefits, if any, to volunteers, and the importance of the knowledge that may reasonably be expected to result. In evaluating risks and benefits, the IRB should consider only those risks and benefits that may result from the research (as distinguished from risks and benefits of therapies volunteers would receive even if not participating in the research). The IRB should not consider possible long-range effects of applying knowledge gained in the research (for example, the possible effects of the research on public policy) as among those research risks that fall within the purview of its responsibility.

 (3) Selection of volunteers is equitable. In making this assessment the IRB should take into account the purposes of the research and the setting in which the research will be conducted and should be particularly cognizant of the special problems of research involving vulnerable populations, such as children, prisoners, pregnant women, mentally disabled persons, or economically or educationally disadvantaged persons.

 (4) Informed consent will be sought from each prospective volunteer or the volunteer's legally authorized representative.

 (5) Informed consent will be appropriately documented.

 (6) When appropriate, the research plan makes adequate provision for monitoring the data collected to ensure the safety of volunteers.

 (7) When appropriate, there are adequate provisions to protect the privacy of volunteers and to maintain the confidentiality of data.

(b) When some or all of the volunteers are likely to be vulnerable to coercion or undue influence, such as children, prisoners, pregnant women, mentally disabled persons, or economically or educationally disadvantaged persons, additional safeguards have been included in the study to protect the rights and welfare of these volunteers.

Source: Title 45, United States Code of Federal Regulations Part 46.

The information provided to human volunteers should include the research procedures, purpose, risks, and anticipated benefits, including what a reasonable volunteer would want to know before giving consent. The information must be in lay language that the volunteers can understand, and attempts should be made to ensure that it is understood, especially when risks are involved.[7]

The volunteers should have the legal capacity and the ability to understand or comprehend the information and risks involved so that they can make an informed decision. Some participants, such as children, are not legally competent to make decisions of consent for themselves, so others must make the decision for them. This is usually the parent or guardian, but the child also must assent to the procedure. However, the age at which a child is capable of giving assent is determined by the IEC or IRB. Comprehension also may be diminished in persons with mental retardation or emotional disability. These persons should be allowed to assent or not, but a third party should be chosen to act in their best interest.[7]

The third aspect of informed consent, voluntariness, means that the human volunteer freely, without threat or undue inducement, has decided to participate in the study. There should not be any element of deceit, constraint, or coercion. Voluntariness is also reduced when the research offers financial or other inducements that the potential participants would find hard to refuse.[7,16]

It is the responsibility of the IRB or IEC to determine whether the informed consent process will be conducted according to these principles. The CFR and ICH guidelines provide a list of required elements of informed consent that account for the principles expressed in the foundation documents. The required elements of informed consent can be found in 21 CFR Part 50 and in the ICH guidelines (TABLE 5-4).

There are many issues that can undermine proper informed consent. One of these issues is the concept of *therapeutic misconception*. The therapeutic misconception is defined as a mistaken belief of human volunteers that treatment and research have the same primary goal. However, the primary goal of research is not to treat the individual patient, but to provide generalizable knowledge to benefit society. It is important that researchers stress this concept to human volunteers and that the distinction between research and treatment is clearly understood.[17]

The CFR and ICH guidelines also ensure that care is taken to protect vulnerable populations. Vulnerable populations are defined as persons who may have a diminished capability of providing informed consent because they do not meet all three criteria established by the Belmont Report.[7]

Children, prisoners, pregnant women, and persons with any form of cognitive impairment are all examples of vulnerable populations.[18-27] Research in vulnerable populations is a complicated issue. It is important to protect these populations from the risks of participating in clinical research, but it may also be harmful if vulnerable populations do not participate in research. Therapies may be unavailable to these populations because they have not been studied appropriately.

For example, children are often treated with medications that may not have been studied in a pediatric population. The safety and efficacy of these therapies may not be established in this population, but there may be no alternative treatments available. The Best Pharmaceuticals for Children Act was passed by the US Congress in 1997 to provide incentives to the pharmaceutical industry to study new and marketed drugs in a pediatric population. The incentive to conduct these pediatric studies is 6 months of market exclusivity.[28] Therefore, pharmaceutical companies have conducted more studies in children in recent years.

Conducting research in prisoners has been a controversial issue over the years. The principle of justice states that prisoners should have an equal opportunity to participate

TABLE 5-4	Basic Elements of Informed Consent

45 CFR 46.116, 21 CFR 50

Each volunteer shall be provided with a description of the following:

(1) A statement that the study involves research, an explanation of the purposes of the research and the expected duration of the subject's participation, a description of the procedures to be followed, and identification of any procedures which are experimental.

(2) A description of any reasonably foreseeable risks or discomforts to the subject.

(3) A description of any benefits to the subject or to others which may reasonably be expected from the research.

(4) A disclosure of appropriate alternative procedures or courses of treatment, if any, that might be advantageous to the subject.

(5) A statement describing the extent, if any, to which confidentiality of records identifying the subject will be maintained.

(6) For research involving more than minimal risk, an explanation as to whether any compensation and an explanation as to whether any medical treatments are available if injury occurs and, if so, what they consist of, or where further information may be obtained.

(7) An explanation of whom to contact for answers to pertinent questions about the research and research subjects' rights, and whom to contact in the event of a research-related injury to the subject.

(8) A statement that participation is voluntary, refusal to participate will involve no penalty or loss of benefits to which the subject is otherwise entitled, and the subject may discontinue participation at any time without penalty or loss of benefits to which the subject is otherwise entitled.

Source: Title 21, United States Code of Federal Regulations Part 50; Title 45, United States Code of Federal Regulations Part 46.

in research. However, their circumstances make them a vulnerable population subject to coercion and undue influence. For centuries prisoners have been used, often unscrupulously, as subjects of research. Today, most prisons do not allow inmates to volunteer for clinical research studies.[22]

Title 45 Part 46 also provides criteria for conducting research in pregnant women and fetuses (TABLE 5-5). All of these criteria must be met to legally include pregnant women in a research study. Inclusion of pregnant women in research is often avoided for the most part even though many pregnant women receive medications and treatments during pregnancy that may not have been studied.[24]

Respecting autonomy and the right to self-determination in patients with cognitive impairment are complicated by difficulties associated with ensuring understanding and voluntariness in the informed consent process. Protecting patients with cognitive impairment from harm may be complex because it is difficult to determine the ability of these patients to comprehend the research at hand.[25–27]

TABLE 5-5	Research Involving Pregnant Women or Fetuses

45 CFR 46.204

Pregnant women or fetuses may be involved in research if all of the following conditions are met:

(a) Where scientifically appropriate, preclinical studies that included studies with pregnant animals and clinical studies that included studies with nonpregnant women have been conducted and provided data for the assessment of potential risks to pregnant women and fetuses.

(b) The risk to the fetus is caused solely by interventions or procedures that hold out the prospect of direct benefit for the woman or the fetus; or if there is no such prospect of benefit, the risk to the fetus is not greater than minimal, and the purpose of the research is the development of important biomedical knowledge that cannot be obtained by any other means.

(c) Any risk is the least possible risk for the achievement of the objectives of the research.

(d) If the research holds out the prospect of direct benefit to the pregnant woman, the prospect of a direct benefit both to the pregnant woman and the fetus, or no prospect of benefit for the woman nor the fetus when the risk to the fetus is not greater than minimal and the purpose of the research is the development of important biomedical knowledge that cannot be obtained by any other means, then the pregnant woman's consent is obtained in accord with the informed consent provisions.

(e) If the research holds out the prospect of direct benefit solely to the fetus, then the consent of the pregnant woman and the father is obtained in accord with the informed consent provisions, except that the father's consent need not be obtained if he is unable to consent because of unavailability, incompetence, or temporary incapacity or the pregnancy resulted from rape or incest.

(f) Each individual who provides consent is fully informed regarding the reasonably foreseeable impact of the research on the fetus or neonate.

(g) For children who are pregnant, assent and permission are obtained in accord with the provisions 45 CFR 46.

(h) No inducements, monetary or otherwise, will be offered to terminate a pregnancy.

(i) Individuals who are engaged in the research will have no part in any decisions as to the timing, method, or procedures that are used to terminate a pregnancy.

(j) Individuals who are engaged in the research will have no part in the determination of the viability of a neonate.

Source: Title 45, United States Code of Federal Regulations Part 46.

■ Ethical Research Methodologies

Randomized clinical trials and placebo controlled clinical trials are the most widely accepted designs used in clinical research. The ethics of these two research methodologies are discussed next.

Randomized Clinical Trials

Randomized clinical trials remain the gold standard for demonstrating the safety and efficacy of new therapies. Clinical trials are often randomized, blinded, and evaluated with a formal statistical analysis. Randomization means that the therapeutic intervention is assigned by chance. This concept differs from normal clinical practice because the researcher does not decide the best therapy for the individual. A randomized clinical trial typically compares two or more therapies to confirm the superiority of one therapy over the other.[1] Sometimes it is difficult for human volunteers to understand the notion of randomization. This is often explained using common terminology such as "flipping a coin" or "rolling the dice."

Placebo Controlled Trials

The Declaration of Helsinki states that placebo controlled trials should be avoided if alternative comparators are available.[6] However, some regulatory agencies require placebo controlled studies for marketing approval, if feasible. Comparing an experimental new therapy to a placebo allows the investigator to establish efficacy in an efficient and rigorous manner.[1] Placebo controlled trials are warranted when there is no standard treatment, when new evidence has raised doubts about the effectiveness of a standard treatment, or when investigating therapies in groups who historically do not respond to standard treatments.[29] A placebo control should not be used if no treatment or treatment with placebo would result in death, disability, or permanent morbidity.[1]

■ Summary

Ethical principles of clinical research are in place to protect the safety, welfare, and well-being of human volunteers and to protect the integrity of clinical trial data. The principles found in the Nuremberg Code, the Declaration of Helsinki, and the Belmont Report were developed in response to historical events in which the rights and welfare of human subjects were not respected. These documents now provide the framework for the regulations and guidelines that govern the conduct of research throughout the world. The development of innovative therapies and the mapping of the human genome have opened the door to new ethical issues in the years to come, but the foundations of research ethics presented in this chapter should be applied universally to these issues. In the end, the ethical treatment of human volunteers is in the hands of the researchers conducting the investigations.

■ References

1.   Grady C. Ethical principles in clinical research. In: Gallin J, ed. *Principles and Practice of Clinical Research*. San Diego, Calif: Academic Press; 2002.

2. Carrese JA, Sugarman J. The inescapable relevance of bioethics for practicing clinician. *Chest*. 2006; 130(6):1864–1872.

3. Shuster E. Fifty years later: the significance of the Nuremberg Code. *NEJM*. 1997;337(20):1436–1440.

4. The Nuremberg Code (1949). In: Levine R, ed. *Ethics and the Regulation of Research*. 2nd ed. New Haven, Conn: Yale University Press; 1986.

5. Carlson R, Robert V, et al. The revision of the Declaration of Helsinki: past, present and future. *Brit J Clin Pharm*. 2004;57(6):695–713.

6. World Medical Assembly. Declaration of Helsinki (1996). *JAMA*. 1997;277(11):925–926. Available at: http://www.wma.net. Accessed December 2, 2008.

7. National Commission for the Protection of Human Subjects of Biomedical and Behavioral Research. *The Belmont Report: Ethical Principles and Guidelines for the Protection of Human Subjects of Research*. Washington, DC: US Government Printing Office; 1979.

8. Title 21. United States Code of Federal Regulations Part 50.

9. Council/20/EC. Implementation of good clinical practice in the conduct of clinical trials on medicinal products for human use. *Off J Euro Communities*. 2001;No L121/34.

10. ICH Global Cooperation Group. *ICH Information Brochure*. May 2001. Available at: http://www.ich.org/LOB/media/MEDIA410.pdf. Accessed April 4, 2007.

11. Title 45, United States Code of Federal Regulations Part 46.

12. GPO Access. Code of Federal Regulations: about. Available at: http://www.gpoaccess.gov/cfr/about.html. Accessed April 1, 2007.

13. International Conference on Harmonisation of Technical Requirements for Registration of Pharmaceuticals for Human Use. Synopsis of ICH guidelines and topics. May 2004. Available at: http://www.ich.org/LOB/media/MEDIA407.pdf. Accessed April 4, 2007.

14. International Conference on Harmonisation of Technical Requirements for Registration of Pharmaceuticals for Human Use. Home page. Available at: http://www.ich.org/cache/compo/276-254-1.html. Accessed April 4, 2007.

15. Garattini S, Bertele V, Li Bassi L. How can research ethics committees protect patients better? *BMJ*. 2003;326:1199–1201.

16. Morgan GA, Harmon RJ, Gliner JA. Ethical problems and principles in human research. *J Am Acad Child Adolesc Psychiatry*. 2001;40(10):1231–1233.

17. Dresser R. The ubiquity and utility of the therapeutic misconception. *Soc Philosophy Policy*. 2002;19(2):271–294.

18. National Institutes of Health. NIH policy and guidelines on the inclusion of children as participants in research involving human subjects. March 6, 1998. Available at: http://grants.nih.gov/grants/guide/notice-files/not98-024.html. Accessed December 2, 2008.

19. Hampton T. Experts ponder pediatric research ethics. *JAMA*. 2005;294(17):2148–2151.

20. Barfielda RC, Church C. Informed consent in pediatric clinical trials. *Curr Opin Pediatrics*. 2005;17:20–24.

21. Ecoffey C, Dalens B. Informed consent for children. *Curr Opin Anaesthesiology*. 2003;16:205–208.

22. Arboleda-Florez J. The ethics of biomedical research on prisoners. *Curr Opin Psychiatry*. 2005;18:514–517.

23. Gostin LO. Biomedical research involving prisoners: ethical values and legal regulation. *JAMA*. 2007;297(7):737–740.

24. McCullough LB, Coverdale JH, Chervenak FA. A comprehensive ethical framework for responsibly designing and conducting pharmacologic research that involves pregnant women. *Am J Obstet Gynecol*. 2005;193:901–907.

25. Roberts LW. Informed consent and the capacity for voluntarism. *Am J Psychiatry*. 2002;159:705–712.

26. Stocking CB, Hougham GW, Baron AR, Sachs GA. Are the rules for research with subjects with dementia changing? *Neurology*. 2003;61:1649–1651.

27. Sevick MA, McConnell T, Muender M. Conducting research related to treatment of Alzheimer's disease. *J Gerontol Nurs*. 2003;February:6–12.

28. Best Pharmaceuticals for Children Act. Public Law 107-109. January 4, 2002. Available at: http://www.fda.gov/opacom/laws/pharmkids/contents.html. Accessed April 4, 2007.

29. Freedman B. Placebo controlled trials and the logic of clinical purpose. *IRB: Rev Human Subjects Res*. 1990;12(6):1–5.

Clinical Research

Steven P. Gelone

■ What Is Clinical Research?

In 1999, the American Medical Association and the American Association of Medical Colleges (AAMC) Task Force on Clinical Research convened a clinical research summit. The output of this summit was a national call to action that included a working definition for clinical research that states that clinical research is

> *a component of medical and health research intended to produce knowledge essential for understanding human diseases, preventing and treating illness, and promoting health. Clinical research embraces a continuum of studies involving interaction with patients, diagnostic clinical materials or data, or populations, in any of these categories: disease mechanisms; translational research; clinical knowledge; detection; diagnosis and natural history of disease; therapeutic interventions including clinical trials; prevention and health promotion; behavioral research; health services research; epidemiology; and community-based and managed care research.*

■ Historical Perspective on Clinical Research

The beginnings of clinical research date back to the Old Testament in the Book of Daniel (Daniel 1:11–16) in the Bible, where a comparative protocol of diet and health is documented and to Hippocrates (460–370 BC), considered to be the father of modern medicine, who exhibited the strict discipline required of a clinical investigator. The first modern clinical trials were conducted in the 1700s to address the growing problem of scurvy in the British Navy, and in the late 1800s Robert Koch established "Koch's postulates" to prove that an infectious agent causes disease. The 20th century brought with it amazing advances in the medical sciences, the establishment of medical colleges in Europe and the Untied States, and the discovery of such drugs as penicillin and insulin. In 1925 Abraham Flexner, a noted medical educator, wrote, "Research can no more be divorced from medical education than can medical education be divorced from research."

Like many advances, progress in clinical research also brought with it troubling events including human experimentation by the Nazis and the Tuskegee syphilis experiments in African American men that lasted more than 30 years. These events lead to the enactment of several key measures to ensure ethical clinical research, including the Nuremberg Code (1949), the Harris Kefauver amendment to the Food and Drug Act in 1962, the Declaration of Helsinki in 1964, and the Belmont Report in 1979. Implicit in the conduct of all clinical research are ethical principles and integrity that are discussed in greater detail in Chapter 5 of this text. The remainder of this chapter focuses on clinical research involving drug products intended for use in humans.

■ Why Is Clinical Research Needed?

Given the uncertain nature of diseases and the potentially large variation that exists in biological systems and measures, it is extremely difficult to determine whether a new treatment or intervention makes a difference on a patient's outcome on the basis of uncontrolled observation. In addition, a true risk versus benefit analysis cannot be conducted outside the context of a controlled situation. Although the controls that are sometimes employed in clinical research may not exactly mimic clinical practice, they do provide a standardized manner in which to evaluate the safety and effectiveness of interventions to treat or prevent disease. The types of evaluations of medicines or interventions are outlined in TABLE 6-1.

■ The Phases of Drug Development

The development of drug products is generally divided into four phases. Phase 1 studies are exploratory clinical research designed to evaluate the safety of new medicines

TABLE 6-1	Types of Evaluations of Medicines
Safety	
Efficacy	
Pharmacokinetic/pharmacodynamic	
Mechanism of action	
General population	
Clinical methodology	
Clinical pharmacology	
Post marketing	

to determine whether further investigation is appropriate. Phase 1 studies involve the first administration of a new therapy to humans (the so-called first-in-man studies) and are often conducted on normal, healthy subjects. In addition to evaluating safety, phase 1 studies are commonly designed to describe the clinical pharmacology of a new drug. They may evaluate single versus multiple dose exposure, establish a maximum tolerated dose (MTD), describe drug–drug or drug–food interactions, or evaluate the pharmacokinetics of a drug in special patient populations such as those with renal insufficiency. Phase 1 investigations are conducted throughout the development life cycle of a drug, the earliest of which evaluate safety and pharmacokinetics, whereas drug–drug interaction studies and special patient population studies may be conducted later in the development cycle.

Phase 2 studies are the first attempt to evaluate the safety and efficacy of a drug in patients with the disease to be diagnosed, treated, or prevented. The overall objectives for phase 2 evaluations are to acquire information on dose-response relationship, estimate the incidence of adverse reactions, and provide additional insight into the pathophysiology of disease and the potential impact of new therapy. Some have divided phase 2 studies into phase 2a, which are small pilot studies, and phase 2b, which are larger studies and may be considered a pivotal trial (key studies used for submission to regulatory authorities). Regardless of whether phase 2a or 2b, this phase of clinical research often evaluates dose-response or different patient types (eg, young versus old or different ethnicity).

Phase 3 studies are considered the definitive evaluation of a new therapy to determine the safety and efficacy of new medicines in patients with the disease to be diagnosed, treated, or prevented. These clinical investigations most commonly compare a new therapy to the standard of practice at the time and involve large numbers of patients, including special patient populations. Phase 3 studies are often called "pivotal" or "registration trials" (also called phase 3a studies) because they are the clinical research backbone of a New Drug Application (NDA) or biologics license application (BLA) to the Food and Drug Administration (FDA) and will ultimately provide the basis for labeling of a new medicine. Phase 3b studies are clinical trials conducted after the submission of an NDA or BLA and may supplement earlier studies and add new information to the labeling of a medicine.

Phase 4 studies are trials conducted after a medicine has been approved and marketed. These studies monitor the use of a new therapy in clinical practice and are designed to gather additional information on the impact of a new therapy on the treatment of disease, the rate of use of a new therapy, and a more robust estimate of the incidence of adverse events of a new therapy. Phase 4 trials are sometimes referred to as postmarketing surveillance studies and may be required by a regulatory authority as a condition of approval of a new product. Phase 4 research can be observational in nature and is often not as well controlled as investigations in phases 1 through 3. A summary of the phases of the drug development life cycle is presented in FIGURE 6-1.

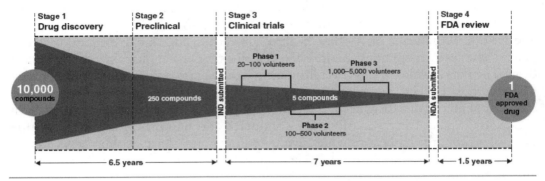

Source: Pharmaceutical Research and Manufacturers of America.

FIGURE 6-1 Drug development life cycle.

Where Clinical Research Begins

All clinical research begins with an unanswered question and the development of a concise and specific primary objective. The objective is the springboard for all of the analysis to occur from the data generated from the clinical research study. Although one can theoretically change the primary objective of a clinical research study after initiation, this usually results in major problems with analysis and interpretation of the data obtained as well as the acceptability of the data by the medical community. As such, it is critical that prior to initiating a clinical research study one invests the time upfront to explore and develop a primary objective that will allow for the most robust analysis to occur.

Critical Concepts in Clinical Research

The two fundamental aspects of all clinical research are whether the results are valid and generalizable. The most compelling evidence in research is the ability to replicate the outcome of an investigation. Because not all studies undergo replicate analysis, one should critically evaluate the study design and analysis utilized as a surrogate marker of the validity of a study. If one concludes that a study result is valid, it is equally important to consider whether the findings of the study are applicable to multiple clinical practice settings. Again, replication of a study is very helpful in this assessment but often is not conducted.

In the absence of a replicate study, one should evaluate the inclusion and exclusion criteria utilized in the clinical study to assess the generalizability of the results. Researchers from the McMaster University have developed a series of questions that are useful in interpreting the results of clinical research studies:

Are the results of the study valid?

- Primary guides:

  - Was the assignment of patients to treatments randomized?
  - Were all patients who entered the study properly accounted for at its conclusion?
  - Was follow-up complete?
  - Were patients analyzed in the groups to which they were randomized?

- Secondary guides:

  - Were patients, clinicians, and study personnel blinded to treatment?
  - Were the groups similar at the start of the trial?
  - Aside from experimental intervention, were the groups treated equally?

What were the results?

- How large was the treatment effect?
- How precise was the treatment effect (confidence intervals)?
- Will the results help me caring for my patients?
- Does my patient fulfill the enrollment criteria for the trial? If not, how close is the patient to the enrollment criteria?
- Does my patient fit the features of a subgroup analysis in the trial report? If so, are the results of the subgroup analysis in the trial valid?
- Were all the clinically important outcomes considered?
- Are the likely treatment benefits worth the potential harm and costs?

■ Approaches to the Design of Clinical Research Studies

As noted previously, the design of a clinical study is critical to the analysis, interpretation, validity, and generalizability of clinical research. Although an in-depth review of statistical approaches to clinical trial design and all of the permutations with which a clinical research study can take on are beyond the scope of this text, the following represents an overview of the approaches to clinical research design.

Clinical research design can be divided into one of a couple of broad categories: retrospective versus prospective studies, and those involving a single group versus multiple groups. In short, retrospective studies evaluate events that occurred in the past and as such are limited by the data that were collected. As a result, retrospective studies are unable to definitively answer research questions. Although these limitations are a reality, retrospective studies are easier to conduct, usually require less resources and time than prospective studies do, and are very useful for hypothesis generating. Prospective studies evaluate events in the present time and forward. As such, these studies' greatest strengths are the ability to control bias more effectively and have more robust data collection than retrospective studies. A timeline for clinical studies is presented in FIGURE 6-2.

In single-group studies, all subjects are treated with the same intervention or medicine. In multiple-group studies, subjects in each group are treated with different interventions and the results are compared between groups. The major study designs employed for two groups of subjects are cross-sectional and longitudinal trials. Cross-sectional studies are usually short-term trials (weeks) in which a cross-section of the patient population is evaluated and data obtained from each group are compared. Most safety and efficacy studies conducted are cross-sectional trials. Longitudinal trials are typically longer in duration (months), and patients' data are generally compared with the patients' baseline data to identify any changes. Many epidemiological studies and phase 4 studies are longitudinal trials.

The two most commonly utilized designs comparing two groups of subjects are the parallel and crossover designs. In the parallel design, subjects are randomized into one of two groups and typically receive one of two potential treatments as assigned for the entire duration of the study. These studies are applicable to most experimental situations. In crossover studies, subjects receive both treatments being compared. To effectively utilize a crossover design, subjects should have a stable, chronic condition during both treatment periods and a similar baseline condition at the start of each treatment. Examples of diseases for which a crossover-designed study may be con-

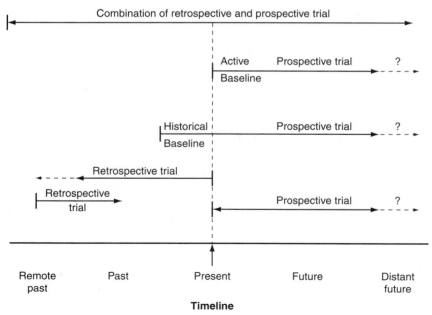

FIGURE 6-2 Timeline of retrospective and prospective studies.

ducted include migraines, epilepsy, and glaucoma. For the same sample size, the parallel design is less sensitive in detecting differences between the two groups. The analysis of crossover studies is more greatly affected by patient dropouts and missing data.

Two other designs comparing two groups of subjects are matched pairs and historical control studies. Neither is as robust as parallel or crossover studies. Matched pair design is a type of parallel design in which subjects who are identical with regard to relevant factors are identified. One subject within each matched pair receives one treatment, while the other receives the other treatment. The obvious limitations of this design are the difficulty in identifying well-matched pairs and that all relevant factors to match pairs may not be known.

In historical control trials, all subjects receive the same treatment and the control group is composed of a similar group of subjects who were previously treated, often by different investigators. The advantage of historical controlled trials is that enrollment may be easier, but this must be counterbalanced by the fact that it is very difficult to have an adequately controlled historical group with all the relevant information required.

Phase 4 study designs can be divided into five broad categories, including descriptive studies, cross-sectional studies, case-control studies, cohort studies, and controlled clinical research studies.

Descriptive studies provide information on the pattern of disease occurrence in populations. The data used in descriptive studies is often collected passively to describe rare events or generate hypotheses. Cross-sectional studies involve data from a random sampling of a target population and data are classified based upon exposure and observed outcomes. This type of study can provide the prevalence of an event and as such is a snapshot in time. Case-controlled studies are retrospective research in which the cases have the disease in question and the controls do not. Each case is matched based on relevant factors to a control subject, which is often difficult. Case-controlled studies can evaluate multiple exposures and uncommon diseases, and are logistically easy. A cohort study follows forward in time a group of subjects who have been exposed to an event or intervention. The outcomes in the cohort are then compared retrospectively with a control group that was not exposed to the event or intervention. Cohort studies can evaluate multiple outcomes and uncommon exposures. Last, controlled clinical trial designs have been presented previously and are the most convincing clinical research design.

■ Bias in Clinical Research

Bias are errors that enter into a clinical research study that distort the data collected. Bias may be introduced by anyone involved with the design, conduct, or analysis of clinical research. Because the introduction of various forms of bias into a clinical research study may significantly affect the validity and generalizability of a study, one of the primary goals in designing a clinical research study is to eliminate or minimize

TABLE 6-2	Types of Bias in Clinical Research
Type of Bias	Description
Selection bias	Occurs during recruitment and selection of potential subjects
Information bias	Information collected directly from subjects can be biased based on beliefs or values
Observer bias	Clinical investigator objectivity for measuring outcomes varies greatly
Interviewer bias	The expectation of the interviewer may influence how information is collected

the introduction of bias. As described earlier, some clinical research designs inherently introduce bias (eg, case-control or retrospective designs), but the best way to avoid bias is to identify its potential during the design of a clinical research study. The types of bias to be considered in clinical research are summarized in TABLE 6-2.

The main methods used to control bias in clinical research include blinding, randomization, and when possible the administration of placebo to the control population in the study. Blinding is a method used to keep the identity of the treatment used in a group unknown. Groups that can be blinded include patients, investigators, data review committees, ancillary personnel, statisticians, and monitors. With regard to blinding, clinical research studies can be described as outlined in TABLE 6-3.

TABLE 6-3	Types of Blinding in Clinical Research
Type of Blinding	Description
Open-label	No blinding is used. Both patient and investigator know the identity of the treatment being used. Least rigorous design.
Single-blind	Patient is unaware of the treatment being used.
Double-blind	Neither the patient nor the investigator is aware of what treatment is being used.
Full-double-blind	The patient and anyone that interacts with the patient group is unaware of the treatment being used.
Full-triple-blind	The patient, the investigator, and anyone that interacts with the patient or investigator are unaware of the treatment being used.
Full-clinical-trial-blind	The patient, and anyone that interacts with the patient or the data are unaware of the treatment being used.

TABLE 6-4	Randomization Methods
Method	Description
Simple randomization	Uses a predetermined code to assign patients to one of two or more treatments
Block randomization	A block size is chosen and the number of patients assigned to each treatment is proportional (eg 1:1, 2:1, 3:1)
Systematic randomization	Patients are assigned to receive treatment based on a random order in the first block, whose pattern is repeated in subsequent blocks or by a sequential assignment to treatment

Randomization is a process by which patients in a clinical research study are randomly assigned to receive one of the potential treatments using a predetermined randomization code. Randomization decreases the effect of interjecting an investigator's bias(es), allows for breaking a blind on one patient while keeping it on the remaining subjects, and permits statistical testing conducted on resulting data in a valid manner. Examples of randomization methods are provided in TABLE 6-4.

■ Challenges in Conducting Clinical Research

After a clinical research idea is developed more fully into a study protocol, one must consider the complexity and various moving parts that are critical to the efficient conduct of a clinical research study. The two major groups include a coordinating group and a support group. These groups can be further subdivided into their functional units, all of which are critical to the successful completion of a clinical research study.

The overall roles of the functional groups are to provide intellectual and scientific leadership for the study (eg, investigators, medical directors), selection and management of investigational sites (eg, clinical operations, study managers, research associates), data gathering and analysis (eg, data management, programming, biostatisticians), and infrastructure support (eg, finance, human resources, information technology). It is only with the collaboration of all of these functional groups that one can efficiently conduct clinical research that is scientifically and ethically sound.

■ The Interpretation and Integration of Clinical Research Into Clinical Practice

The ultimate goal of conducting clinical research is to improve patient care. To this end, the results of clinical research must be integrated into clinical practice. The interpretation

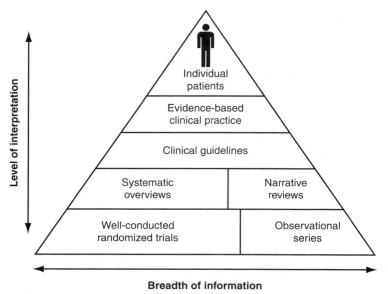

FIGURE 6-3 Methods to integrate results into clinical practice.

of the results of clinical research studies is therefore a critically important part of the process and must be undertaken with great care. In an effort to adequately synthesize empirical information, a variety of methods are currently used to aid clinicians in effectively integrating clinical research study results into clinical practice (FIGURE 6-3).

In particular, national and international societies and other organizations, most notably the Centers for Disease Control and Prevention, the Cochrane Collaborative Group, and the World Health Organization, regularly prepare evidenced-based guidelines derived from the available clinical research results to aid clinical decision making and improve patient care.

Ultimately, for the results from a clinical research study to influence medical practice they need to be published in a peer-reviewed journal, be interpreted by clinicians as positive, and must be generalizable to the clinician's specific patient population. It is worth noting that many well-designed trials results have had little effect on medical practice and many poorly designed studies have had a major influence. In the end, it is the responsibility of each clinician to make his or her own assessment of new clinical research data. Critical evaluation of such studies requires one to pose questions related to the endpoints, methodology, and data obtained from the study. Only after answers to these questions are generated and an understanding of the strengths and limitations of a study is obtained can a clinician proceed to integrate the results into clinical practice.

■ What Does the Future Hold for Clinical Research and What Opportunities Exist for Allied Health Professionals?

The clinical research summit conducted by the AAMC in 1999 identified several issues that are critical to the conduct of clinical research, including: (1) a general lack of understanding by the general public of what clinical research is and what its potential value is to patient care; (2) a lack of data on funding for clinical research and productivity; (3) a lack of interest and funding in some types of clinical research; (4) a lack of sufficiently trained clinical researchers; (5) an insufficient emphasis on incorporating clinical research into clinical practice; (6) inadequate coordination among research centers and disciplines; (7) significant impact of fiscal concerns at academic centers that may negatively affect clinical research; and (8) the lack of a comprehensive clinical research agenda.

Subsequently, the AAMC published a follow-up report in 2006 directed at addressing many of the issues identified, in particular recommending that all future physicians receive as part of their education and training instruction in the basic principles of clinical research. In the author's opinion, it would be beneficial if this goal were extended to all future healthcare professionals.

A variety of training programs (both certificate and degree conferring) are currently available that provide an in-depth exposure to the various aspects of clinical research. As identified by the AAMC report in 2006, there is a shortage of well-trained clinical research professionals. Opportunities for allied health professionals in the field of clinical research are numerous and exist in academia, foundations, government, and industry. The 21st century has brought with it incredible advancement in the medical sciences. These advancements have been the by-product of basic science and clinical research efforts. Patient care will continue to improve only through the combined efforts of educational institutions and well-trained translational and clinical researchers, skilled in research design and interpretation.

■ Suggested Reading

Association of American Medical Colleges. Clinical Research: A National Call to Action. November 1999. Washington, DC.

Association of American Medical Colleges. Promoting Translational and Clinical Science: The Critical Role of Medical Schools and Teaching Hospitals. May 2006. Washington, DC.

Association of American Medical Colleges. Task Force on Clinical Research. November 1999. Washington, DC.

Fletcher AJ, et al. *Principles and Practice of Pharmaceutical Medicine*. West Sussex, UK: John Wiley; 2002.

Gallin JI. *Principles and Practice of Clinical Research*. San Diego, Calif: Academic Press; 2002.

Kelley WN. *Careers in Clinical Research: Obstacles and Opportunities*. Washington, DC: Committee on Addressing Career Paths for Clinical Research, Institute of Medicine, National Academy Press; 1994.

Spilker B. *Guide to Clinical Trials*. Philadelphia, PA: Lippincott Williams & Wilkins; 2000.

United States Government Accountability Office. *New Drug Development: Science, Business, Regulatory, and Intellectual Property Issues Cited as Hampering Drug Development Efforts*. Washington, DC: US GAO; November 2006.

Regulatory Affairs

Kristie Stephens

Regulatory affairs (RA) is a vital part of any pharmaceutical company. Employees in the RA department act as liaisons between their company and health authorities, such as the US Food and Drug Administration (FDA). They prepare correspondence in all forms, written and verbal, in support of Investigational New Drug applications, which notify the FDA of a company's intention to begin clinical trials on a new drug product, and New Drug Applications (NDAs) or Abbreviated New Drug Applications (ANDAs), which are mechanisms for receiving marketing approval in the United States. RA employees are the link between regulatory bodies and the company. It is an area of the company that is made up of responsible, well-trained employees who have pharmaceutical experience and the people skills necessary to handle stressful situations and communicate efficiently and effectively with different types of personalities. This chapter provides an overview of the RA department of a pharmaceutical company and the documents the group prepares to receive marketing authorization in the United States.

It is critical for personnel working in RA to be well versed in laws, regulations, guidances, and Manual of Policies and Procedures (MaPPs; FDA's standard operating procedures) the FDA issues to help companies understand their expectations. These documents can be found on the FDA website at www.fda.gov. The most fundamental law that must be followed is the Federal Food, Drug, and Cosmetic Act. This act provides the basis for all legal requirements governing the pharmaceutical industry. In the hierarchy of law, the act is at the top, followed by the regulations found in the Title 21 Code of Federal Regulations (CFR) guidances issued by the FDA, and MaPPs. The act is the statute passed by Congress that is binding for everyone. Regulations interpret the law and provide guidance on what needs to be performed to comply with the law. Guidances provide nonbinding opinions on how the FDA feels the tasks designated by the law can be accomplished.

The FDA is a very transparent organization; it makes many of its documents and decisions available to the public. The Freedom of Information Act (FOIA) allows anyone to request and receive documentation of interest. In many cases, proprietary information will be redacted from the document, but the nonproprietary material is available to garner information about most topics. Warning letters, inspection reports, and summary basis of approvals are examples of documents available through Freedom of Information (FOI). Information on FOI can be found on the FDA website. Because communication is available in the public domain, it is vital for an RA professional to have a thorough knowledge of FDA rules and regulations and of company policies and procedures because any person (especially competitors) can access the information and utilize it. RA is one of the primary groups in a company that prepares documentation to be submitted to the FDA, so potentially their communications will be available to the public. It is important that communication is prepared in compliance with all governing rules because it will be accessible to anyone requesting it.

■ International Conference on Harmonisation

In April of 1990, three entities met to discuss harmonizing certain technical aspects of the pharmaceutical industry.[1] The entities—Japan, United States, and the European Union—worked diligently to harmonize important tasks performed during the drug development process. The countries formed a group, called International Conference on Harmonisation (ICH), which meets regularly to discuss various topics and develop guidance documents for industry and regulatory agencies to utilize when preparing or reviewing documents pertaining to drug development and marketing approval. The ICH is a joint venture involving regulatory authorities and industry to streamline the drug development process globally. More information on ICH can be found at www.ich.org.

Topics covered by ICH are broken down into four categories: Quality (Q), Safety (S), Efficacy (E), and Multidisciplinary (M). The Quality category focuses on the chemical and quality assurance aspects of the industry. An example of a quality topic is the ICH guidance document *Q2, Validation of Analytical Procedures: Text and Methodology*.[2] This guidance document provides a framework for companies that are validating analytical methods. It includes specific parameters that must be included in the validation plan. The Safety category provides guidance on nonclinical (animal and in vitro) testing and expectations. For example, *S1A, Guideline on the Need for Carcinogenicity Studies of Pharmaceuticals*,[3] provides industry with a guideline on when carcinogenicity studies are required. The Efficacy category focuses on human clinical trials and provides guidance on conducting various aspects of a clinical program to demonstrate efficacy in humans. For example, the guidance document *E6, Good Clinical Practice: Consolidated Guideline*,[4] describes the responsibilities and expectations of those conducting clinical trials. The Multidisciplinary category contains those extra topics that do not fit into one of the other areas. For example, the guidance document *M4, The Common Technical Document*,[5] provides a harmonized application format for NDAs. The Common Technical Document (CTD) is discussed later in this chapter.

The ICH is so important to RA personnel because the FDA is following these guidances more and more and requesting that industry follow the recommendations made in these guidances. It is vital to know how to access these documents so that a company can stay current with the FDA's expectations and submit paperwork that meets the FDA's current standards. To learn more about ICH and to read ICH guidance documents, please refer to their website at www.ich.org.

■ The Investigational New Drug Application

At the conclusion of a positive preclinical drug development program, a company will begin preparing to conduct clinical trials on humans. According to the Federal Food, Drug, and Cosmetic Act, no person may introduce an unapproved drug product into interstate commerce (Section 505(a)). This means that no unapproved drug may be shipped from state to state. The Investigational New Drug (IND) application is a formal mechanism to apply for an exemption of this law so that clinical trials may be conducted. Clinical trials are most often conducted by many investigators at many different sites across the United States or globally, so an exemption is necessary to ship the drug across state lines. The contents of the IND provide scientific data to justify the exemption and to allow a drug to be administered to humans. Title 21 Code of Federal Regulations Section 312 (21 CFR 312), describes the legal requirements for using investigational products in humans, including the documentation required to be submitted in an IND prior to beginning clinical trials.

RA personnel in a pharmaceutical company will compile the IND for submission to the FDA. The FDA is looking at the safety aspects of the drug, based on preclinical animal and in vitro studies. Safety is of the utmost concern for the FDA and they want to ensure that the investigational product is safe for human use.

There are different types of IND applications. The one described in this chapter is a commercial IND, with the purpose of filing ultimately being marketing of the proposed drug product. There are also INDs for other aspects of drug research. Physicians and academics may need INDs for noncommercial purposes, such as for emergency use.[6] A physician may request to use an unapproved drug product in a medical emergency where no other treatment options are available. The sponsor of the drug product submits the IND at the physician's request.

The IND is composed of 10 sections. The regulatory requirements for an IND may be found in 21 CFR 312.23. The FDA has also issued guidance documents for the format and content of an IND application, including *Guidance for Industry: Content and Format of Investigational New Drug Applications for Phase 1 Studies of Drugs, Including Well-Characterized, Therapeutic, Biotechnology-Derived Products*, and these can be found on the FDA website at www.fda.gov/cder/guidance/clin2.pdf.

The first section of the IND is FDA Form 1571.[7] This form is provided on the FDA website (www.fda.gov/opacom/morechoices/fdaforms/FDA-1571.pdf). FDA

Form 1571 provides basic information about the contents of the submission, including the name, address, and telephone number of the sponsor (the company responsible for all clinical work); the date of the submission; the name of the drug; IND number if previously assigned; proposed indications covered by the IND submission; the phase of clinical testing to be conducted (phase 1, 2, 3, etc.); the submission type (initial IND, response to clinical hold, amendment, etc.); and checkboxes for the contents included in the submission. There is also a section for describing the investigators and a section asking for information about contract research organizations (CROs) (if applicable). A responsible employee of the sponsor company must sign the form stipulating that the sponsor will wait 30 days prior to initiating clinical studies, that they will have an institutional review board (IRB) review and approve all studies, and that the conduct of the trials will be in accordance with all regulatory requirements.

The second section of the IND is a comprehensive table of contents that details the contents of the submission.[8]

The third section of the IND is an introductory statement.[9] This statement provides an overview of the drug, the development program, and the proposed uses of the drug. The introductory statement should discuss the name of the drug and the active ingredients, the drug's pharmacological class, the structural formula, the formulation of the drug product, the proposed route of administration (eg, oral, by injection), broad objectives for the study and the planned duration of the trial, a summary of any previous human experience, a reference to any other INDs covering the drug, a description of any investigational or marketing experience in other countries, and an explanation if the drug was withdrawn from investigating or marketing and the reason for action.[10]

The fourth section, the General Investigational Plan, is a brief description of the overall plan for the clinical program for the upcoming year. The plan should include rationale for the study, indications to be studied, the general approach for evaluating the drug, the kinds of trials that are to be conducted in the year, the estimated number of patients to be given the drug, and the risks expected based on toxicologic data in animals or prior human studies.[11]

The fifth item in an IND is the Investigator's Brochure (IB). This is a very important document because it provides clinical investigators with information on the new drug and describes the product's attributes. It is similar to the package insert for an approved drug product. Included in the IB is a description of the drug substance, formulation of the drug product, the chemical structure, the known pharmacologic effects, the known toxicologic effects, pharmacokinetics and biological action, effects in humans including a summary of previous human safety and efficacy findings, and a description of possible risks and side effects.[12] ICH has issued a guidance document, *E6, Guideline for Good Clinical Practice* (Section 7), which describes the contents and format of an IB.[13]

The next section contains clinical study protocols for each of the proposed studies. Full protocols must be submitted. A protocol contains the following information:

a statement of the objectives and purpose of the study, investigator information (including IRB information), patient information (including inclusion/exclusion criteria and the expected number of patients participating in the study), the study design (including the controls to be used and the methods used to minimize bias), the dose of the drug to be administered (including duration of dosing), observations and measurements to be made, and clinical and laboratory procedures designed to monitor drug effect and minimize risk.[14]

The seventh section of an IND is the chemistry, manufacturing, and controls information. This section provides information on both the drug substance and the drug product, including the composition, the manufacturing procedure, and the testing controls for both the drug substance and drug product.[15] The purpose of this section of an IND is to ensure the investigational product's identity, strength, quality, and purity. Because this drug will be used in humans, this section must demonstrate the drug's quality. Information provided in this section for the drug substance and drug product include physical, chemical, or biological characteristics; manufacturer information; method of manufacture; information on excipients (inactive ingredients in drug product); packaging information; specifications and analytical methods used to ensure quality, purity, strength, and identity; and product stability based on stability studies.[16] There is also a description of the placebo used in clinical trials and its manufacturing, testing, and composition.[17] Any labeling corresponding to the drug is also included in this section.[18] An environmental analysis may also be required for this section based on 21 CFR 25.40.[19] Most products qualify for a waiver of this analysis, called a Claim for Categorical Exclusion (21 CFR 25.30 or 25.31), and that waiver request is included in Section 7.

The eighth item in an IND is the pharmacology/toxicology study information. This section demonstrates the safety of the drug based on animal and in vitro studies. The sponsor of the application must demonstrate that the data generated during these studies clearly shows that it is safe to continue the drug development program and begin administering in humans.[20] Information on the people conducting the research must be defined, including identification and qualifications.[20] The studies performed during preclinical development will show the pharmacologic aspects of the drug, including its mechanism of action, drug disposition, and interactions with other drugs.[21] Toxicologic information is also provided, including full study reports for all preclinical studies conducted.[22] A statement must also be included in this section certifying that all testing was conducted in accordance with Good Laboratory Practices (GLPs; 21 CFR 58).[23]

Section 9 contains information on previous human experience. Information should be provided for any previous human experience including previous clinical trials, marketing in other countries, and any published information on the investigational drug.[24] If the drug has been withdrawn from the market for safety or efficacy reasons in the United States or another country, this information must be included in section 9.[25]

The last section of an IND contains any additional information necessary for the FDA to review the application. This information may include drug dependence and abuse potential of the proposed drug, meeting minutes from previous FDA/sponsor meetings, references to previously submitted information, and certification that any foreign language translations are accurate and complete.[26]

The purpose of an IND is to demonstrate to the FDA that there will not be an unreasonable risk to humans if they take the drug, so a sponsor must include enough information to clearly show that humans will not be unnecessarily exposed to risk. When the IND is compiled, the RA department will submit three copies, one original and two copies, of the document to the FDA.[27]

When the IND application is received by the FDA, the agency has 30 days to review the contents. An acknowledgment letter is sent to the sponsor when the IND is received by the FDA. There is a passive approval process: if a company does not hear any feedback from the FDA 30 days after the agency receives the application, the company may begin clinical trials. It is prudent for the sponsor company to call the FDA and make certain that the IND was adequate and that it is safe to begin trials. If the FDA finds that there is a problem with the documentation presented in the IND, they will place the product on clinical hold until the problem is rectified. *Clinical hold* means that a company may not administer the drug to humans.

During clinical trials, there are several occasions when an RA employee will need to send additional documentation to the FDA. IND applications are updated regularly. When a submission is made to an active IND, it is called an amendment to the IND. Amendments may include protocol amendments, safety reports, annual reports, and information amendments. An employee will be required to submit these amendments at various time intervals during the life cycle of the IND. Protocol amendments (as described in 21 CFR 312.30) are submitted any time there is a change to an existing protocol; for example, a change to the dosage form for capsules to tablets must be reported to the FDA. Any change that may affect safety or efficacy of the product must be reported. When there is a change in investigators or a new investigator or site is added to the study, it must also be reported in a protocol amendment. For all protocol amendments, IRB approval is obtained before instituting the change.

Information amendments (as described in 21 CFR 312.31) are submitted when new vital information becomes available that is not ordinarily included in a protocol amendment and that must be reported prior to the next annual report, for example, if new toxicology animal data are available.

IND safety reports (as described in 21 CFR 312.32) are submitted to notify the FDA of adverse events encountered during the course of a clinical trial. It is important for the sponsor company to notify all clinical investigators of the adverse event because many studies are conducted by several different investigators at different sites. It is imperative for a sponsor to review all safety information received in a timely manner to determine its impact on the clinical trials being conducted. Serious adverse events are life-threatening or result in death, hospitalization, persistent or significant incapacity, or birth defects and other congenital anomalies.[28] An unexpected adverse event is any adverse event that was not described in any plan or protocol based on data generated during nonclinical studies, the specificity or severity of which is not consistent with the expectations, and the risk information is not included in the general investigational plan or elsewhere in the IND application.[28] For unexpected fatal or life-threatening adverse events, the FDA must be notified via telephone or fax within 7 days of the initial notification to the sponsor.[29] For serious adverse events that are unexpected and associated with the drug, a written report must be submitted to the FDA within 15 calendar days of the first report to the sponsor.[30] Also, any finding from nonclinical testing on animals that suggests a significant risk for human subjects, including reports of mutagenicity or carcinogenicity, should be reported in a written report.[31] The written reports should contain information on the patient, the adverse event, the causal relationship to the drug (the possibility that the drug caused the adverse event cannot be ruled out), and previous reports for similar adverse events along with any other information that is available. Written safety reports must continue to be submitted to the FDA as the company attains information until the file is closed on the adverse event (including follow-up reports about the 7-day or 15-day reports). The FDA has a form for adverse events, Form 3500A (also called the MedWatch Form), that is submitted with safety reports. This form can be found on the FDA website at www.fda.gov/medwatch/SAFETY/3500.pdf. The FDA may request safety reports at a different frequency and will notify the sponsor of its intentions.[32]

Each year, a brief report of the progress of the studies covering the previous year is submitted, called the annual report (as described in 21 CFR 312.33). The annual report should be submitted within 60 days of the anniversary date of when the IND went into effect. Each annual report should include individual study information (a brief description of the status of ongoing and completed studies), summary information (a summary of clinical/nonclinical information, summary of adverse events, a summary of all IND safety reports for the year, summary of information learned about dose response, bioavailability, information from controlled trials, a list of ongoing and completed nonclinical studies with any findings, and a summary of manufacturing/microbiological changes), the general investigational plan for the upcoming year, IB revisions, any modifications to protocols or foreign developments, and a log of outstanding business with the FDA.

A compliant IND program is necessary for a successful drug development program, so it is imperative for a sponsor and the RA employees who prepare documentation for submission to the FDA to be diligent when preparing paperwork and ensure that all information is relayed to the FDA in a timely fashion. The FDA is available to industry for questions and concerns and its expertise should be utilized when necessary.

■ Meetings With the FDA

The Food and Drug Administration Modernization Act of 1997 (FDAMA) contains a section concerning the FDA meeting with a sponsor for the purpose of discussing aspects of development, such as coming to agreement about the size and scope of clinical trials that form the basis of the efficacy claims for an investigational product.[33] The Prescription Drug User Fee Act (PDUFA) of 1992 allows the FDA to collect user fees from sponsor companies so that they can attain the resources necessary to review and act on new marketing applications in a specified amount of time. With the passage of PDUFA, the FDA is bound to very specific time frames, and time allotted for meetings must be controlled and the meeting process must be streamlined to ensure maintaining certain time frames. The FDA can no longer spend large quantities of time meeting with the sponsors/applicants because its resources are limited and it is held accountable to the times specified in PDUFA.

The FDA has issued a guidance document describing the meeting process titled *Guidance for Industry, Formal Meetings with Sponsors and Applicants for PDUFA Products.*[33] According to this guidance, there are types of meetings requested by a company, Type A, Type B, and Type C. Type A meetings are for serious issues that have an impact on the critical path of the drug program, such as clinical hold or refuse to file situations. These meetings are generally granted within 30 days of receipt of the meeting request because of the serious nature of the problem. Type B meetings are conducted at various points in a drug development process, for example, a pre-IND meeting, an end of phase 2 meeting, and a pre-NDA meeting. These are generally scheduled within 60 days of the request. Type C meetings are for miscellaneous topics, such as labeling or to ask advice from the FDA and are generally scheduled within 75 days of request. For each type of meeting, the FDA will issue meeting minutes within 30 days after the meeting.

The FDA does not grant every meeting request that is made. The FDA may determine that the nature of the problem can be discussed in a teleconference and may schedule one instead or the FDA may feel that the problem can be addressed by a written response. It is important for meeting requests to be sufficient in detail for the FDA to determine the necessity of a meeting. It is also important for an employee preparing the request to assess the need for a meeting; it is not wise to request meetings prematurely or when the issue does not warrant the need for a face-to-face meeting.

RA personnel are often intimately involved in meetings with the FDA. There are certain meetings that are important for the development of new drug products.[34] The pre-IND meeting is an opportunity for a company to discuss phase 1 plans for agreement with the FDA and to discuss any other problems or concerns prior to beginning clinical trials. This meeting takes place prior to submitting the IND, before beginning human clinical trials. The end of the phase 2 meeting is also an important meeting. The end of phase 2 is usually a critical time for a pharmaceutical company because it represents the time when a decision is made to continue conducting very large, expensive phase 3 trials. At this time, a company evaluates all the data it has collected so far to decide whether there is an adequate benefit to risk ratio to continue. The FDA meeting at this time is a great opportunity to get FDA feedback and discuss whether its interpretation of the data matches that of the sponsor company. It is also a great opportunity to discuss the pivotal trials to be conducted in phase 3 and adequate clinical endpoints.

The pre-NDA meeting is conducted at the end of all clinical testing and is an opportunity for a company to discuss whether the data generated during the trials supports the efficacy claims. It is also a good time to discuss technical aspects of the NDA submission to ensure that the FDA agrees with the company's strategies.

A fourth type of meeting that may be conducted is a meeting to discuss labeling. This meeting generally takes place after submission of the NDA. This meeting is set up to discuss the proposed labeling submitted in an NDA so that the FDA and the company can come to an agreement on the contents of the labeling.

It is important to mention that generic drug products are not required at this time to pay PDUDA fees, so all aspects of the generic program should be discussed with the Office of Generic Drugs.

■ The New Drug Application

At the culmination of the drug development program, the RA group will begin preparing a New Drug Application (NDA) for submission to the FDA. An NDA is submitted to request permission to market the new drug product. It is a very large, complex document that includes all results of all studies performed to support the safety and efficacy claims made for the drug. Compilation and submission of the NDA represents many years of work performed by many different employees of the company. It is a very significant achievement for a company.

The regulatory requirements for an NDA can be found in 21 CFR 314. The NDA must include all safety and efficacy information determined by the many studies conducted on the investigational drug, as well as proposed labeling for the new drug product, and all chemistry, manufacturing, and controls (CMC) information to demonstrate that the drug can be consistently produced meeting all specifications. There are now different formats for submission of an NDA, including the standard paper format described in 21 CFR 314 as well as an electronic version of the NDA and the Common Technical Document (CTD) format (which is discussed later in the chapter). The contents of the application remain the same for any format selected; it is the order of the contents within the document that changes. This chapter discusses the NDA format detailed in 21 CFR 314.50, but it is important to keep in mind that there are FDA guidance documents for the electronic version of a submission and the Common Technical Document (CTD) if a company chooses to submit an application in these formats. The main goal of a company should be to prepare a well-organized, thorough document that is easily navigated so that an FDA reviewer can find information quickly and easily.

There are many different elements submitted in an NDA. The first item submitted is a cover letter, which gives the applicant the opportunity to briefly discuss the new drug and point out any areas of significance.

The second item submitted in the application is FDA Form 356h, which can be found on the FDA website at www.fda.gov/opacom/morechoices/fdaforms/FDA-356h.pdf. This form identifies the name and address of the applicant, date of application, the application number (if previously assigned), drug information (name, dosage form, route of administration, and strength), identification numbers for INDs or Drug Master Files referenced in the application, proposed indication for use, the type of application (original application, resubmission, etc.), the drug type (Rx or over-the-counter [OTC]), and the signature of the responsible person at the applicant company.[35] Form 356h also contains checkboxes for the contents of the attached submission.[36]

The third section of an NDA is a comprehensive index, which identifies contents by both volume number (the application is quite large and will have several volumes) and page number.[37]

The next documentation submitted is the labeling.[38] Most original applications will contain four copies of draft labeling. Final printed labeling (FPL) is generally submitted after the FDA has reviewed the draft labeling and made any necessary changes to the text. When it is time to submit FPL, 12 copies are sent to the FDA. Labeling consists of all labeling for the drug, including the package insert, the container label, the carton label, and so forth. The package insert also must be submitted electronically and will be discussed later in the chapter.[39]

The next section, the summary, is submitted to provide a general overview of the data. It should be written at the same level as a document for publication in a scientific journal.[40] This section contains annotated labeling, which is the proposed package insert text and references to every statement made and where the justification for the claim can be found in the application.[41] For example, if the package insert states that the drug product will clear acne, the annotated labeling must direct the reviewer to the data that demonstrate that the drug product does indeed clear acne. No claims may be made in a package insert that are not justified by the data contained in the application. The summary section also discusses the drug's pharmacologic class, any previous marketing history for the drug, a summary of the technical sections, including chemistry, manufacturing, and controls data, nonclinical pharmacology and toxicology data, human pharmacokinetics and bioavailability data, microbiology (if necessary), clinical data with statistical results, and a conclusion of the benefit to risk for the proposed drug and any postmarketing studies or surveillance that may be conducted (eg, a risk management plan).[42]

The next sections contain the technical information of the application. The technical aspects of the application provide the data and information necessary to allow FDA reviewers to make an informed decision on the drug product.

The first technical section is the Chemistry section, containing information on chemistry, manufacturing, and controls (CMC).[43] The composition, manufacture, and specifications for the drug substance and drug product are detailed in this section. These sections are critical to ensure the quality, strength, identity, and purity of the drug product being marketed to the public.

The CMC sections contain information concerning the manufacturing, packaging, composition, specifications, and analytical testing of the drug (drug substance and drug product), including batch records, stability data for expiration dating, in-process controls, methods of testing, container/closure systems, excipients, and so forth.[44] It is critical to establish that a reproducible method of manufacture, packaging, and testing is available for the drug substance and drug product. The CMC section of an NDA contains the Environmental Impact Assessment or a request for a waiver of this assessment.[45] Environmental impact is required only under extraordinary circumstances; most drugs will receive a categorical exclusion (waiver) from providing this information. A field copy certification is also included in this section, certifying that a true copy of the technical sections of the application have been sent to the company's district field office.[46]

The second technical section is Nonclinical Pharmacology and Toxicology. This section contains all animal and in vitro studies. The nonclinical studies are performed in animals and in vitro to demonstrate pharmacologic actions, potential adverse events, toxicologic effects shown when the drug is taken as it is intended, and the absorption, distribution, metabolism, and excretion of the drug product.[47] Reproductive and developmental effects of the drug are also assessed during nonclinical testing.[48] Some of the studies included in this section of the application are acute, subacute, and chronic toxicity; reproductive toxicity; and carcinogenicity (if required). When conducting nonclinical studies, Good Laboratory Practices (GLPs) must be adhered to throughout testing. A statement is included in this section certifying that studies were conducted in accordance with GLPs.[49]

The third technical section of an NDA is Human Pharmacokinetics (PK) and Bioavailability. This section contains the studies conducted in humans or a request for a waiver of certain bioavailability studies. A description of each study conducted in humans to demonstrate PK and/or bioavailability must be included with a discussion of the analytical methods and statistical methods used to assess the samples.[50] Rationale for establishing the analytical methods, specifications, and acceptance criteria must be included for the methods used during testing, including data for each drug product.[51] The formulation(s) of the drug product used during the studies should be included. IRB approval for the studies or the reason why IRB approval was not required for each study is also included in the section.[49] A summary of the studies should be included in the section, summarizing the PK and metabolism of the active ingredient and the bioavailability/bioequivalence of the drug product based on the conducted studies.[52]

The next technical section, Microbiology, is only required for anti-infective drugs. The biochemical basis of action on microbial physiology, the antimicrobial spectra of the drug, any known mechanism of resistance for the drug, and clinical microbial laboratory methods needed for effective use must be included in the application.[53]

The fifth technical section, Clinical Data, is one of the most important sections of an NDA. It contains the human data, which provide the proof of safety and efficacy for the claims made in the application for the proposed drug product. This section describes each of the clinical studies performed, including a comparison to the acquired animal data.[54] This section also contains information on each controlled clinical study performed to support the proposed indication, including the protocol and the statistical analyses used to assess the study.[55] A discussion of each uncontrolled study is also part of this section including a summary of the results and an explanation of why the study was uncontrolled.[56] There should also be information on any other data relevant to the drug's safety and efficacy.[57] There is an ICH guidance for the format and content of clinical study reports, ICH *E3, Structure and Content of Clinical Study Reports*,[58] that guides the author on how to compile report information.

In the clinical data section of an NDA, the applicant must include an integrated summary of safety (ISS),[59] an integrated summary of effectiveness data (ISE),[60] and an integrated summary of risks and benefits.[61] The ISS provides details of all studies containing safety information, describes the overall extent of exposure of the drug, provides demographics for the subjects studied, and describes adverse experiences seen during the course of the clinical trials. The ISS should contain all pertinent information found while conducting many studies of the drug such as drug–drug interactions. The statistical analyses used to analyze the data should also be discussed.[59] The ISE describes controlled studies showing that the drug has the intended effect and defines the effect of the drug in the controlled studies conducted. The purpose is to pool efficacy data from all pivotal studies and analyze it. The ISE contains an analysis of responses in the overall population as well as subgroup analysis to look for trends in the various subgroups. It is vital because it supports the dosage and administration section of the labeling and identifies dosage modifications resulting from analysis of subgroups and diseases present while taking the drug, such as renal, hepatic, or varying levels of severity of the disease being treated.[60] An integrated summary of the benefits and risks of the drug provides a justification for why the benefits outweigh the risks for the conditions stated in the labeling.[61]

The next item, the Safety Update Report, is not submitted with the original application. It contains any additional safety information generated during the course of the review period. It is submitted to the FDA 4 months after filing the NDA, following the receipt of an approvable letter issued by the FDA, or as per FDA request.[62]

The next section included in an NDA is the Statistical section. This section discusses the statistics used to interpret the data generated during the clinical trials. This section describes the assessment of the drug based on statistics used on the data generated during clinical studies and information provided about the safety of the drug product, including documentation and statistical analyses used to evaluate safety information.[63]

The next section, the Pediatric Use section, describes the studies conducted to evaluate the drug for use in pediatric populations, including a summary of the information that is pertinent to the safety and efficacy and benefits and risks of the drug in pediatrics for the claimed indications (eg, controlled clinical studies).[64] 21 CFR 314.55 describes in detail the expectations of the FDA concerning pediatric assessment of the drug product.

The next section of an NDA contains the case report tabulations (CRTs). CRTs (data sets) are data tables containing information on data from phase 1 studies, effectiveness data from each controlled study, and all safety data. The tabulations must include the data on each patient in each study, except those who are not pertinent to the review of the drug's safety or effectiveness (with FDA permission).[65] Upon request, the FDA will discuss with the applicant those tabulations that may be removed at the pre-NDA meeting.

Case report forms (CRFs) are contained in the next section of the application. CRFs must be included for any deaths or patients who did not complete the study because of adverse experiences.[66] CRFs for patients with severe adverse events may also be included. During application review, the FDA may request additional CRFs, if necessary.

Patent information is also included in the NDA. Patents that claim the drug, the drug product, or the method of use are submitted by the applicant. 21 CFR 314.53 details patent information that should be included in an application. Patents are critical to innovator companies because they delay the introduction of generic competition on the market for as long as possible. Once a generic product becomes available to the public, a large portion of the innovator's sales is lost to this generic competition.

Patent certification for patents that claim the drug is the next section of the application. An applicant must submit certification for each patent issued by the United States Patent and Trademark Office that claims a drug (the drug product or drug substance that is part of the drug product) or that claims an approved use for the drug.[67] For each patent, the patent number should be listed and the applicant should certify to one of the following circumstances: Paragraph I certification—the patents have not been submitted to the FDA; Paragraph II certification—the patents have expired; Paragraph III certification—the applicant will not market the drug until all pertinent patents have expired (certification should include date of expiration); and Paragraph IV certification—the patent is invalid, unenforceable, or will not be infringed by the submission of an application.[68] More information on patent certifications can be found in 21 CFR 314.50 and 21 CFR 314.52.

For certain biologics, an establishment description is required as per 21 CFR 600. This section is not applicable for most products.

The next item in an NDA is the Debarment Certification, which certifies that the applicant did not and will not use the services of a debarred person in any capacity for this drug product. A list of debarred people can be found on the FDA website.

In addition to a Debarment Certification, an applicant must also provide a Field Copy Certification, which certifies that a true copy of the CMC section, the summary section, and the FDA Form 356h of the application have been sent to the FDA District Office of the applicant.[69] All applications are sent to the Center for Drug Evaluation and Research (CDER) or Center for Biologics Evaluation and Research (CBER), but a copy must be sent to the district office because this office is the one that will conduct a prior approval inspection of the facility and operations to ensure that all regulatory areas conform to GMP regulations (Good Manufacturing Practices; 21 CFR 210 and 211).

The next item in the application is the User Fee Cover Sheet, FDA Form 3397. This form provides proof that applicants subject to user fees under PDUFA have sent payment for application review and it can be found on the FDA website at www.fda.gov/oc/pdufa/coversheet.html.

Financial information is the next item in an application.[70] Financial information must be submitted for each clinical investigator used for clinical studies, in accordance with 21 CFR 54. FDA Form 3454[71] is submitted when an applicant certifies that there were no financial interests and arrangements with the clinical investigator. FDA Form 3455[72] is submitted to disclose any financial arrangements for each clinical investigator associated with the clinical study conducted.

The last section is titled Other. This section contains any information not covered in the other sections, including references to previously submitted information and a statement that accurate and complete English translations are provided of any foreign language documents.[73]

For generic drug products, an Abbreviated New Drug Application (ANDA) is submitted because generic companies do not perform the extensive nonclinical and clinical testing the innovator companies do on the drug. Generics rely on the data generated by the innovator companies. Regulations governing the format and content of ANDAs can be found in 21 CFR 314.94. Generic drugs cannot be introduced to the market until all patent protection and/or marketing exclusivity has expired on the innovator product, unless a patent Paragraph IV certification has been submitted and the innovator either does not contest the claim (no lawsuit is filed) or the generic company successfully shows that the patent either is not infringed or is not valid for its drug product (determined via ruling in court). It performs bioequivalence testing, which demonstrates that the generic drug product works the same way in the body as the innovator drug. Generic manufacturers utilize the *Approved Drug Products with Therapeutic Equivalence Evaluations* book (commonly referred to as the Orange Book), found at http://www.fda.gov/cder/orange/default.htm, to determine which drug product is the reference listed drug (RLD) for their proposed product. The RLD is the drug that generics conduct bioequivalence testing against to demonstrate that their drug is equivalent. A large part of an ANDA application is the CMC section, which describes the chemistry, manufacturing, and controls used to manufacture and test the drug substance and drug product. Bioequivalence study data are also submitted in an application. Labeling submitted for a generic drug must be equivalent to the RLD labeling, excluding any proprietary names or patented/exclusive claims. Generic companies do not pay user fees under PDUFA for the review of their ANDA submissions. Applications are reviewed by the Office of Generic Drugs, a part of CDER.

■ The Common Technical Document

The Common Technical Document (CTD) is an application format that is becoming more widely used globally. It is an ICH initiative whose goal is to develop a harmonized marketing application format. Prior to the CTD, companies that submit applications globally had to essentially assemble the same information in many different formats, taking a tremendous amount of time to prepare applications for different health authorities around the world. Each health authority required information in different places within an application. In an effort to harmonize the process of assembling applications, the ICH developed a modular format, called the CTD. There is a specific guidance document that details the format of a CTD titled *M4: Organization of the CTD*.[5] The CTD is not a global dossier; specific content will be different for different countries based on individual regulations. For example, the United States requires FDA Form 356h to be submitted with an application, whereas other ICH regions, including the European Union (EU), Japan, and Canada, do not. The CTD format is now required for the EU, Japan, and Canada. The FDA is encouraging applicants to submit in CTD format, but it is not required at this time.

The CTD is composed of five modules. Module 1 contains all the required regional information for each country. For example, for a US submission to the FDA, Module 1 contains all FDA forms required in an application (eg, Forms 356h, 3397, 3454, 3455), all certifications (patent, debarment, field copy), and any other regional documents. Labeling is also submitted in Module 1 because labeling requirements differ for each country.

Module 2 contains all the overviews and summaries. There is a Quality Overall Summary, a Nonclinical Overview, a Clinical Overview, a Nonclinical Summary, and a Clinical Summary. Overviews are brief documents written to present the overall findings and results of the drug development program. The applicant can discuss and interpret findings in this section. Overviews are approximately 30 pages in length. Summaries are detailed, factual documents that summarize the information contained in the application. Summaries contain facts only; there is no interpretation of the facts in these documents.

Module 3 contains the quality components of the application. The quality section is essentially the CMC information of an NDA. ICH has a guidance document for the contents of this module titled *M4Q, Quality*.[74] This guidance also discusses the necessary contents of the Quality Overall Summary contained in Module 2.

Module 4 contains all the nonclinical documents of the application. The ICH guidance document that discusses the contents of the module is *M4S, Safety*.[75] This guidance also provides information on the contents of the nonclinical summary and overview.

All clinical data are found in Module 5. The ICH guidance document *M4E, Efficacy*[76] describes what is required for this module. The clinical summary and overview are also discussed in this guidance. The Integrated Summary of Safety and Integrated Summary of Efficacy are regionally specific to the United States and are not required when using CTD format. The information included in these reports can be incorporated into the clinical summary and overview.

■ Electronic Documents

In recent years, the FDA has been encouraging companies to begin submitting documents in electronic format. There are guidances covering the submission of applications in eNDA (electronic New Drug Application) format and eCTD (electronic Common Technical Document) format on its website. Electronic submissions allow multiple reviewers to look at an application at the same time, without having to make multiple copies of the same documents. Paper copies comprise many, many volumes for one complete application. Multiple copies of the application take up a large amount of space at the FDA and the documents must be stored.

Electronic submissions consist of as little as one CD or disk being submitted containing all the necessary documentation. It is much easier to handle, and it allows access to reviewers. At this time, only the content of labeling is required to be submitted electronically, but the FDA is strongly encouraging companies to submit entire applications electronically to facilitate a faster review period. Companies may submit applications in eNDA or eCTD format at this time. The FDA is focusing more and more on the eCTD format. There is a wealth of information available on the FDA website covering this format.

■ Communication During the Review Period

There are many times during review of an NDA that the FDA will communicate with a company and a company will communicate with the FDA. When an application is first received, the FDA has 60 days to determine whether the submission is acceptable for filing.[77] This determination is made by staff who do a first review of the application to make sure that all necessary documents are present, complete, and in the right sections. If there are problems with the application, the FDA may refuse to file the application. If there is information missing, the FDA will not accept the filing until the problems are corrected. 21 CFR 314.101 details the filing procedure and refuse to file criteria. When the application is accepted for filing, the application is assigned to a project manager, who becomes the first point of contact for the applicant. The application is also assigned an

NDA or ANDA number. This number must be placed on all future correspondence to the FDA because this is how the application is tracked at the FDA.

CDER is divided into several different offices. The Office of New Drugs reviews NDA applications. The Office of New Drugs is divided into different divisions, with each division concentrating on a particular therapeutic class of drugs. For example, the Division of Neurology Products reviews all applications for drugs indicated for neurologic conditions.

After day 60, when the application is accepted for filing, the FDA has 180 days to review the application and make a determination.[78] This is not necessarily 180 days to approve an application; it is just the amount of time the FDA has to complete its first review and notify the applicant of issues or findings made during review. As per *Guidance for Review Staff and Industry, Good Review Management Principles and Practices for PDUFA Products*,[79] the FDA may issue letters to notify the applicant of any potential issues identified during the first review of the application (during the acceptance for filing determination). This letter is issued to alert the applicant of any potential problems so that the applicant can begin to address the issues immediately, thus reducing the time the application remains unapproved. These letters do not affect the mandated time clock set by PDUFA.

During the 180-day review period, the various disciplines review the application to determine its acceptability. The FDA will issue one of three action letters after its primary review: the approval letter, the approvable letter, or the not approvable letter. The approval letter (21 CFR 314.105) is issued when the application submitted provides the necessary information to demonstrate that the drug product is safe and effective for the proposed claims. The applicant may begin to market the drug product on the effective date, the date the approval letter is issued.

The approvable letter (21 CFR 314.110) stipulates that the application is essentially ready to be approved, pending the resolution of certain issues found during review. When an approvable letter is issued, the applicant has 10 days to contact the FDA with either the corrected issues, the company's plan to correct the issues, or the company's intent to withdrawal the application.[80]

A not approvable letter (21 CFR 314.120) notifies the applicant that the application does not contain the necessary information to allow the FDA to approve it. The application contains deficiencies that prohibit the FDA from approving the application. The applicant must respond to the deficiencies and correct any problems before an approval can be granted. When a not approvable letter is issued, the applicant has 10 days to contact the FDA with either the deficiencies answered, the company's plan to correct the issues, or the company's intent to withdraw the application.[81]

At the time of original submission, applicants will usually submit draft labeling for review by the FDA. The FDA will most often have changes to the content submitted. The applicant will communicate with the FDA about the content of the labeling, possibly even holding meetings to discuss differences. The FPL is usually submitted closer to approval of the drug product, when all labeling deficiencies and differences are resolved.

Prior to approval of an application, submissions made to an application are called amendments to the application, as detailed in 21 CFR 314.60. Depending on the severity of the issues, these can be major (eg, new efficacy data) or minor (eg, minor deficiencies found during review) amendments or labeling amendments. All documents sent to the FDA should clearly identify the type of correspondence (eg, minor amendment), the drug product, the NDA or ANDA number, and the company name. An exact copy of the amendment must also be sent to the applicant's field office, with a field copy certification enclosed in the amendment application sent to CDER.[82]

Postapproval Communication

The approval of an application is a positive time for a company and the company may now market its new drug product in the countries where it has received approval. In the life cycle of the drug, it is merely the beginning.

Once an application is approved, the RA group will continue to make submissions to the application. As per 21 CFR 314.80, reporting of adverse drug experiences must continue throughout the lifespan of the drug product. The timing of adverse event reporting is dependent on the type and severity of the adverse event. Serious and unexpected adverse events, as defined in 21 CFR 314.80, must be reported within 15 days of the applicant learning of the event (15-day "alert report").[83] After the initial 15-day alert report, follow-up must be done by the applicant and submitted to the FDA within 15 days of initial notification to them. In this time, the applicant must promptly review the adverse event and document all steps taken to seek information about it. Periodic adverse event reports, those not reported by 15-day alert reports, must be sent each quarter for the first 3 years from the date of approval and annually after the first 3 years.[84] Periodic reports should contain a discussion of the information in the report and a history of actions taken since the last report, such as labeling changes. FDA Form 3500A (Medwatch Form) is utilized for reporting any adverse events.

Once an application is approved, the applicant must submit an annual report each year within 60 days of the anniversary date of approval. This annual report, as per 21 CFR 314.81, details all new information pertaining to the drug product that occurred during the year. Information in an annual report includes a summary of significant new information from the previous year (eg, changes made, intentions of making changes, and initiation of new studies), distribution data (both foreign and domestic), current labeling and a description of changes made to the labeling during the reporting period, CMC changes, nonclinical studies, clinical studies, status reports on ongoing studies, and a log of outstanding regulatory business (eg, unanswered correspondence between the company and the FDA).[85] FDA Form 2252[86] is submitted with the annual report.

Field alerts are another type of postapproval reporting. Field alerts are sent to the FDA when an event has occurred that causes the drug product or its labeling to be mistaken for a different product, when information concerning any contamination; significant chemical, physical, or other change or degradation of a marketed drug product; or any failure of one or more batches of the drug product to meet the analytical specifications approved for it in the application occurs.[87] Field alerts must be sent to the FDA within 3 working days of receipt by the applicant.[88] This quickly notifies the FDA of potential problems with marketed products.

When an applicant wishes to make a change to an approved application, the applicant is oftentimes required to submit a supplement to the FDA, as per 21 CFR 314.70. Only minor changes may be made to a product and reported in an annual report (without review by the FDA). An example of an annual reportable minor change is the removal of an ingredient that only affects the color of the drug product.[89] More significant changes require a supplement, either a Prior Approval supplement (for major changes), a Changes Being Effected in 30 Days supplement (moderate changes), or a Changes Being Effected supplement (moderate changes). When supplements are submitted to the FDA, a field copy must also be sent to the applicant's district office and a field copy certification must be included in the supplemental application.[90]

Major changes are defined as those that have a significant potential to adversely affect the drug product. A prior approval supplement must be submitted to the FDA and be approved before the company can begin marketing product made with the change. An example of a major change requiring a prior approval supplement is changing the manufacturing process from a wet to dry granulation.[91]

A *moderate change* is defined as a change that has a moderate potential to have an adverse effect on the drug product. The FDA has divided moderate changes into two categories: Changes Being Effected in 30 Days (CBE 30) and Changes Being Effected (CBE). CBE 30 supplements are submitted when the FDA requires a supplement be sent 30 days prior to distribution of the drug product manufactured with the change. An example of this type of moderate change is relaxing an acceptance criterion to comply with an official compendium, such as the United States Pharmacopeia–National Formulary (USP–NF).[92] Certain moderate changes can be made and marketing can occur at the same time the FDA receives a supplemental submission, namely, CBE supplements. An example of a Changes Being Effected supplement change is a change in or addition of a desiccant.[91]

Minor changes are those that have a minimal potential to have an adverse effect on the drug product and are reported in an annual report, as per 21 CFR 314.70 (d). 21 CFR 314.70 provides regulatory guidance for submitting supplemental applications to the FDA. The FDA has also issued guidance documents (eg, *Changes to an Approved NDA or ANDA*[91] and *SUPAC [Scale Up and Post Approval Changes]*[93] guidances) to help companies determine the best course of action when making a change. 21 CFR 314.70 and the *Changes to an Approved NDA or ANDA* guidance also discuss labeling changes and submissions required for such changes.

■ Labeling Initiatives

Recently, the FDA made several changes to labeling in an effort to make it more readily accessible to physicians and pharmacists and to make it more understandable. On December 11, 2003,[94] The FDA published regulations requiring that the content of labeling be submitted to them electronically, effective June 8, 2004. The FDA has issued a guidance to describe the submission of electronic labeling titled *Guidance for Industry, Providing Regulatory Submissions in Electronic Format-Content of Labeling.*[95] More recently, they required labeling to be submitted in the form of Structured Product Labeling (SPL), an Extensible Markup Language (XML)–based computer program. Under collaboration with the National Library of Medicine (NLM), approved product information will be sent to the NLM and displayed on their DailyMed website, an online repository that will make the most current medical product information available to the public on the Internet free of charge. This will make package insert labeling available to all those interested in reviewing it. SPL is a big change for the pharmaceutical industry and companies are still diligently working to comply with the new electronic labeling regulations.

In January 2006, the FDA published a final rule (21 CFR 301.56(d) and 201.57) that changed the content and format of labeling for prescription products and biological products. The revision is designed to make the package insert easier for healthcare practitioners to access, read, and understand. The FDA has issued a guidance document to help industry adapt to the new rule titled *Guidance for Industry: Labeling for Human Prescription Drug and Biological Products: Implementing the New Content and Format Requirements.*[96] As detailed in this guidance, new information was added to the content of labeling, including Highlights of Prescribing Information and Table of Contents sections. Highlights contain information that is most commonly referenced and considered most important for doctors. The purpose is to provide easier access to information that practitioners most commonly refer to and view as most important. Some examples of the changes required by the new regulations include new added labeling sections, including Drug Interactions, which contain information formerly included in the Precautions section. The Clinical Studies and Nonclinical Toxicology sections are now required to be included in the package insert. The Warnings section and Precautions sections have been combined into a new section: Warnings and Precautions. These changes will make specific information easier to find.

■ Conclusion

Regulatory affairs is an ever changing and evolving profession. The FDA and ICH are continually issuing new guidances and revising regulations to keep up with developing and advancing technologies. It is essential for an RA professional to stay current by reading various industry documents, reviewing the FDA and other industry websites regularly, and attending various relevant conferences or meetings to learn the most contemporary, favorable way to communicate with the FDA and other regulatory authorities.

This chapter offers an overview of the duties of the RA department of a pharmaceutical company, but does not encompass every function they may have within a company. Each company varies on who is responsible for what, but as detailed in this chapter, RA employees play a vital role in the continuance of existing applications and the submission of NDAs. The RA group is responsible for the life cycle of the drug product and ensuring its continued compliance with all the rules and regulations of the various health authorities.

■ References

1. International Conference on Harmonisation. History and future of ICH. Available at: http://www.ich.org/cache/compo/276-254-1.html. Accessed December 2, 2008.

2. International Conference on Harmonisation. *ICH Harmonised Tripartite Guideline: Validation of Analytical Procedures: Text and Methodology: Q2(R1)*. November 2005. Available at: http://www.ich .org/LOB/media/MEDIA417.pdf. Accessed December 2, 2008.

3. International Conference on Harmonisation. *ICH Harmonised Tripartite Guideline: Guideline on the Need for Carcinogenicity Studies of Pharmaceuticals: S1A*. November 1995. Available at: http://www.ich.org/LOB/media/MEDIA489.pdf. Accessed December 2, 2008.

4. International Conference on Harmonisation. *ICH Harmonised Tripartite Guideline: Guideline for Good Clinical Practice: E6(R1)*. June 1996. Available at: http://www.ich.org/LOB/media/MEDIA482 .pdf. Accessed December 2, 2008.

5. ICH. Home page. Available at: http://www.ich.org/cache/compo/276-254-1.html. Accessed December 2, 2008.

6. 21 CFR 312.36.

7. 21 CFR 312.23(a)(1).

8. 21 CFR 312.23(a)(2).

9. 21 CFR 312.23(a)(3).

10. 21 CFR 312.23 (a)(3)(i) through (iii).

11. 21 CFR 312.23(a)(3)(iv).

12. 21 CFR.23(a)(5)(i) through (v).

13. International Conference on Harmonisation. *ICH Harmonised Tripartite Guideline: Guideline for Good Clinical Practice: E6(R1)*. June 1996. Available at: http://www.ich.org/LOB/media/MEDIA482 .pdf. Accessed December 2, 2008.

14. 21 CFR 312.23(a)(6)(iii)(a) through (g).

15. 21 CFR 312.23(a)(7).

16. 21 CFR 312.23 (a)(7)(iv)(a) through (b).

17. 21 CFR 312.23 (a)(7)(iv)(c).

18. 21 CFR 312.23 (a)(7)(iv)(d).

19. 21 CFR 312.23 (a)(7)(iv)(e).

20. 21 CFR 312.23(a)(8).

21. 21 CFR 312.23(a)(8)(i).

22. 21 CFR 312.23(a)(8)(ii).

23. 21 CFR 312.23(a)(8)(iii).

24. 21 CFR 312.23(a)(9)(i).

25. 21 CFR 312.23(a)(9)(iii).

26. 21 CFR 312.23(a)(10), 21 CFR 312.23(a)(11).

27. 21 CFR 312.23(a)(11)(d).

28. 21 CFR 312.32 (a).

29. 21 CFR 312.32 (c)(2).

30. 21 CFR 312.32 (c)(1)(A).

31. 21 CFR 312.32 (c)(1) (B).

32. 21 CFR 312.32 (c)(3).

33. US Department of Health and Human Services. *Guidance for Industry: Formal Meetings with Sponsors and Applicants for PDUFA Products*. Procedural. February 2000. Available at: http://www.fda.gov/cder/guidance/2125fnl.pdf. Accessed December 2, 2008.

34. 21 CFR 312.47.

35. 21 CFR 314.50 (a)(1), (2), (3), (5).

36. 21 CFR 314.50 (a)(4).

37. 21 CFR 314.50 (b).

38. 21 CFR 314.50 (e)(2)(ii).

39. 21 CFR 314.50 (l)(i).

40. 21 CFR 314.50 (c)(1).

41. 21 CFR 314.50 (c)(2)(i).

42. 21 CFR 314.50 (c)(2)(ii) through (ix).

43. 21 CFR 314.50 (d)(1).

44. 21 CFR 314.50 (d)(1)(i) and (ii).

45. 21 CFR 314.50 (d)(1)(iii).

46. 21 CFR 314.50 (d)(1)(v).

47. 21 CFR 314.50 (d)(2)(i), (ii), (iv).

48. 21 CFR 314.50 (d)(2)(iii).

49. 21 CFR 314.50 (d)(2)(v).

50. 21 CFR 314.50 (d)(3)(i).

51. 21 CFR 314.50 (d)(3)(ii).

52. 21 CFR 314.50 (d)(3)(iii).

53. 21 CFR 314.50 (d)(4)(i) through (iv).

54. 21 CFR 314.50 (d)(5)(i).

55. 21 CFR 314.50 (d)(5)(ii).

56. 21 CFR 314.50 (d)(5)(iii).

57. 21 CFR 314.50 (d)(5)(iv).

58. International Conference on Harmonisation. *ICH Harmonised Tripartite Guideline: Structure and Content of Clinical Study Reports: E3*. November 1995. Available at: http://www.ich.org/LOB/media/MEDIA479.pdf. Accessed December 2, 2008.

59. 21 CFR 314.50 (d)(5)(vi)(a).

60. 21 CFR 314.50 (d)(5)(v).

61. 21 CFR 314.50 (d)(5)(viii).

62. 21 CFR 314.50 (d)(5)(vi)(b).

63. 21 CFR 314.50 (d)(6)(i) and (ii).

64. 21 CFR 314.50 (d)(7).

65. 21 CFR 314.50 (f)(1).

66. 21 CFR 314.50 (f)(2).

67. 21 CFR 314.50 (i)(1)(i).

68. 21 CFR 314.50 (i)(1)(i)(1) through (4).

69. 21 CFR 314.50 (l)(3).

70. 21 CFR 314.50 (k).

71. US Department of Health and Human Services. Certification: Financial Interests and Arrangements of Clinical Investigators, Form FDA 3454 (4/06). Available at: http://www.fda.gov/opacom/morechoices/fdaforms/FDA-3454.pdf. Accessed December 2, 2008.

72. US Department of Health and Human Services. Disclosure: Financial Interests and Arrangements of Clinical Investigators, Form FDA 3455 (4/06). Available at: http://www.fda.gov/opacom/morechoices/fdaforms/FDA-3455.pdf. Accessed December 2, 2008.

73. 21 CFR 314.50 (g)(1) and (2).

74. International Conference on Harmonisation. *ICH Harmonised Tripartite Guideline: The Common Technical Document for the Registration of Pharmaceuticals for Human Use: Quality—M4Q(R1), Quality Overall Summary of Module 2 Module 3: Quality.* September 2002. Available at: http://www.ich.org/LOB/media/MEDIA556.pdf. Accessed December 2, 2008.

75. International Conference on Harmonisation. *ICH Harmonised Tripartite Guideline: The Common Technical Document for the Registration of Pharmaceuticals for Human Use: Safety—M4S (R2), Nonclinical Overview and Nonclinical Summaries of Module 2 Organisation of Module 4.* December 2002. Available at: http://www.ich.org/LOB/media/MEDIA559.pdf. Accessed December 2, 2008.

76. International Conference on Harmonisation. *ICH Harmonised Tripartite Guideline: The Common Technical Document for the Registration of Pharmaceuticals for Human Use: Efficacy—M4E (R1), Clinical Overview and Clinical Summary of Module 2 Module 5: Clinical Study Reports.* September 2002. Available at: http://www.ich.org/LOB/media/MEDIA561.pdf. Accessed December 2, 2008.

77. 21 CFR 314.101 (a)(1).

78. 21 CFR 314.100 (a).

79. US Department of Health and Human Services. *Guidance for Review Staff and Industry: Good Review Management Principles and Practices for PDUFA Products.* Procedural. April 2005. Available at: http://www.fda.gov/cder/guidance/5812fnl.pdf. Accessed December 2, 2008.

80. 21 CFR 314.110 (a).

81. 21 CFR 314.120 (a).

82. 21 CFR 314.60 (c).

83. 21 CFR 314.80 (c)(1).

84. 21 CFR 314.80 (c)(2).

85. 21 CFR 314.81 (b)(2).

86. US Department of Health and Human Services. Transmittal of Annual Reports for Drugs and Biologics for Human Use, 21 CFR 314.81, Form FDA 2252 (6/05). Available at: http://www.fda.gov/ opacom/morechoices/fdaforms/FDA-2252.pdf. Accessed December 2, 2008.

87. 21 CFR 314.81 (b)(1)(i) and (ii).

88. 21 CFR 314.81 (b)(1).

89. 21 CFR 314.70 (d)(2)(i).

90. 21 CFR 314.70 (a)(5).

91. US Department of Health and Human Services. *Guidance for Industry: Changes to an Approved NDA or ANDA*. April 2004. Available at: http://www.fda.gov/cder/guidance/3516fnl.pdf. Accessed December 2, 2008.

92. 21 CFR 314.70 (c)(2)(iii).

93. US Department of Health and Human Services. *Guidance for Industry: Immediate Release Solid Oral Dosage Forms Scale-Up and Postapproval Changes: Chemistry, Manufacturing, and Controls, In Vitro Dissolution Testing, and In Vivo Bioequivalence.* November 1995. Available at: http:// www.fda.gov/cder/guidance/cmc5.pdf. Accessed December 2, 2008.

94. *Federal Register.* 68(238):69009.

95. US Department of Health and Human Services. *Guidance for Industry: Providing Regulatory Submissions in Electronic Format—Content of Labeling.* April 2005. Available at: http://www .fda.gov/cder/guidance/6719fnl.pdf. Accessed December 2, 2008.

96. US Department of Health and Human Services. *Guidance for Industry: Labeling for Human Prescription Drug and Biological Products—Implementing the New Content and Format Requirements.* Draft Guidance. January 2006. Available at: http://www.fda.gov/cder/guidance/6005dft.pdf. Accessed December 2, 2008.

Medical Information

Tanya C. Knight-Klimas

Pharmacists play a large role in the pharmaceutical/biopharmaceutical industry (which will simply be termed the pharmaceutical industry from this point forward) and hold many positions of employment in many different areas of the industry. In this chapter, I focus on the role of the pharmacist in a specific area of pharmacy practice within the pharmaceutical industry, namely, medical information and communications. As such, this chapter discusses the following topics:

- Provision of drug information as a pharmacy specialty
- Role of drug information within the pharmaceutical industry
- Functions of a drug information department in the pharmaceutical industry
- Opportunities available to a student seeking a potential career in drug information in the pharmaceutical industry

But, in an effort to provide you with a glimpse of the potential opportunities for a pharmacist throughout the pharmaceutical company, I briefly discuss the role of the pharmacist across the organization.

■ Role of the Pharmacist in the Pharmaceutical Industry

According to one survey of pharmacists employed by Eli Lilly and Company in 1998, approximately 7% of all company employees in the United States were pharmacists, and these pharmacists were employed in many areas of the company, including discovery, manufacturing, marketing, medical, product development, sales, regulatory, product and program teams, and quality assurance, as well as legal, government affairs, human resources, and corporate affairs (see TABLE 8-1). Most of the pharmacists who held a doctorate pharmacy degree were employed by the sales, regulatory, and medical departments. Within the medical organization, pharmacists held clinical research, health economics, medical writing, and medical information positions.[1]

TABLE 8-1	The Role of the Pharmacist Throughout the Pharmaceutical Industry*
Example Department and Title	General Role/Responsibilities
Commercial/ Marketing *Assistant Vice President*	Establishes the strategic direction for a product, including areas of investment for various customer groups (healthcare professionals, patients, payors); identifies future clinical development strategies for a product in its life cycle; engages in aspects of manufacturing, supply, and distribution.
Performance Management and Operations *Vice President*	Leads professional orientation, education and training activities; supervises personnel who serve as project managers for clinical trials and other projects; manages budgets, head count, office space and equipment; leads process improvement initiatives; ensures major milestones for clinical trials are delivered on time and that study data is up-to-date; provides support for key meetings and activities; oversees technologies (from a business perspective) used in communication with customers.
Development and Clinical Pharmacology *Clinical Scientist* *Senior Director*	Prepares study-related documents (clinical study protocols, clinical study reports, investigational new drug applications); selects potential sites for drug investigation and conducts monitoring visits to these sites; monitors the safety of study participants and monitors safety reports; participates in the review of data and the resolution of data discrepancy; designs and analyzes the pharmacokinetic and pharmacodynamic components of phase 1–3 clinical trials. *"Industry experience is available through internships; consider post-doctoral industry training; consider mid-career switch after clinical practice; consider seeking a masters in business administration (MBA) or a juris doctorate (JD) degree."*
Safety and Epidemiology, and Labeling *Specialist*	Processes and reviews individual case safety reports, conducts follow-up of adverse event reports as necessary to obtain information needed to clarify reports; ensures timely submissions of adverse event reports; completes product labeling (prescribing information) reviews and communicates safety updates in product labeling; generates various safety reports and prepares and/or reviews reports for submission to the FDA.
Manager, Pharmacovogilance Operations *Senior Director, Risk Management*	Directs and manages risk management activities including risk identification, assessment, communication, and the design, implementation, and evaluation of risk minimization activities. Specifically, collaborates with departments to develop risk management plans for drugs in development and reviews and updates plans as needed; collaborates with departments to identify and assess risks of adverse drug reactions for

| TABLE 8-1 | Continued |

Example Department and Title	General Role/Responsibilities
	marketed products; develops risk management plans that may include risk communication, tools and resources to assist healthcare professionals and/or patients; monitors and evaluates the results of risk management interventions by communicating with patient advocacy groups, professional societies, and healthcare delivery systems regarding risk management activities; serves as a liaison with domestic and international drug review agencies to ensure that risk management activities are consistent with expectations. *"This is not an entry level job in the pharmaceutical industry. Risk Management is for seasoned professionals who have a variety of healthcare and pharmaceutical industry experiences."*
Marketing *Senior Director*	Leads activities regarding the development of the brand's positioning, messaging, promotional campaign, and sales representative tools for selling and promotion; develops content and planning for non-personal (non face-to-face) promotion, such as journal advertising and promotional materials sent via mail.
New Business *Director*	Leads efforts regarding the commercialization of compounds in development, which includes defining the target patient population to use the product, identifying product indications, developing the product profile and labeling (prescribing information), determining publication strategy, determining product positioning and marketing messaging, developing the brand name of the product, determining pricing of the product, determining the size of the sales force needed, estimating profit and loss forecasts, lifecycle planning, and evaluating licensing opportunities. *"A position in Commercial New Business/New Products allows a pharmacist the opportunity to leverage their clinical knowledge, apply it to the drug development and commercialization process and ultimately help the company develop successful products that fulfill key unmet medical needs, in addition to maximizing shareholder value."*
Medical Pharmacovigilance *Senior Scientist*	Identifies safety issues through the evaluation of safety data, adverse event reports, the medical literature and regulatory safety databases; communicates pertinent safety information for marketed and investigational products; collaborates with departments regarding post-marketing safety review, post-marketing studies, and provides input regarding safety

(continues)

TABLE 8-1	Continued
Example Department and Title	General Role/Responsibilities
	topics; prepares safety reports; participates in the development of risk management plans.
	"The final determination of whether a particular event is causally related to a product requires clinical judgment and an understanding of the potential mechanism(s) by which the drug may cause the event. As such, the pharmacist's training in pharmacology and applied therapeutics plays a key role in the process."
Regulatory Affairs *Manager* *Associate Director*	Prepares and submits drug applications and other correspondence to regulatory agencies; acts as a liaison with regulatory authorities to facilitate the prompt review and approval of applications; negotiates complex issues with regulatory authorities.
	"In order to effectively communicate with regulatory authorities, the regulatory manager must have a thorough understanding of how a product was developed (nonclinical pharmacology & toxicology studies, clinical trials, post-marketing studies), how it is manufactured (e.g., chemistry and manufacturing) and its mechanism of action and safety profile, all of which require a strong background in the pharmaceutical sciences. Some pharmacy schools offer graduate programs that focus on new drug development, regulatory affairs, and quality assurance."
	"A career in regulatory affairs requires a broad knowledge-base of the drug development process because it is involved in every step."
Labeling *Manager* *Senior Manager*	Supervises activities related to the development, review, approval, and revision of prescribing labels and related documents for company pharmaceuticals marketed worldwide; develops training for staff on document management policies, procedures, and systems; provides assistance in the continuous improvement of the document management process; supervises the translation of labeling and associated documents into other languages; ensures consistency of labeling decisions for all products, and ensures that labeling decisions are in compliance with company labeling policies; investigates the background of requests for labeling changes, evaluating scientific documentation and analyzing the regulatory situation; provides regulatory counsel.

TABLE 8-1	Continued

Example Department and Title	General Role/Responsibilities
	"Some project management experience is essential as there is much cross-functional team coordination. FDA, international labeling regulations and other core labeling guidelines are followed and thus an understanding of this is essential."
	"As a Labeling Manager, one interacts with many departments, including Legal, Safety, Medical Affairs, Marketing, Clinical Research & Development and Regulatory. This provides a unique insight into almost all aspects of the Pharmaceutical industry."
Sales *Pharmaceutical Sales Representatives*	Liaises with healthcare professionals in hospitals, clinics, pharmacies and other healthcare institutions to develop business relationships and sell company products, often specializing in one or a few products in a particular therapy area; travels regionally or nationally to key meetings to promote products and develop business relationships; completes ongoing training about company products, which may include computer-based training, mailed paper training, and live training.
Sales *Area Business Director*	Manages and leads all sales responsibilities for assigned products in a particular geographical region through a sales team; provides cross-functional support for company initiatives through collaboration with other members of the sales organization. *"There are a significant number of pharmacists in sales roles, ranging from first line sales positions, first line sales managers and several directors."* *"Having the qualifications of a pharmacist gives the employee in pharmaceutical sales added credibility."*
Clinical Pharmacology *Assistant Vice President*	Oversees protocol design, data analysis, modeling and interpretation; serves as a liaison between departments to gain an understanding of dose/response relationships, optimizing dosage regimens, and strategically providing the best environment to develop drug compounds; operationally, leads the company to improving the efficiency of data analysis tools and reporting of data. *"For a research career, graduate training is a prerequisite."*

(continues)

TABLE 8-1	Continued
Example Department and Title	General Role/Responsibilities
Clinical Pharmacy *Associate Director*	Provides leadership and strategic direction for the department in terms of planning, scheduling, and tracking global clinical supplies; acts as a liaison for departments and affiliates globally that manufacture, package, label, and ship clinical trial materials to clinical sites; collaborates with various departments to plan, schedule, and track availability of clinical supplies for worldwide use; analyzes needs and determines appropriate allocation of resources to support worldwide clinical trial objectives; develops the annual budget for the department by assessing projects and staffing.

*Not all-inclusive. Table includes information provided by survey respondents about their personal roles within their organization. The responsibilities of an individual may differ depending upon whether they are in an entry-level position, a more experienced position, or a management position. Similarly, job titles, department names, and responsibilities may differ among different pharmaceutical companies. However, most pharmaceutical companies will have equivalent positions with similar responsibilities.

An informal survey of pharmacists in the pharmaceutical industry can also be used to highlight the positions a pharmacist can hold throughout an organization. The information found in Table 8-1 was collected from this informal survey and briefly describes some of the roles of pharmacists in departments across the industry, other than medical information and communications. Eligibility criteria and qualifications of the successful pharmacist candidate for these positions may vary depending on the position and department, as well as the hiring company. Many of these positions have several levels of candidacy, ranging from junior-level positions to management positions.

Although the job descriptions of course vary by position and company, general job characteristics vary widely as well. For instance, the main place of work may be in the laboratory, in the office, on the road (travel), and some may offer flexible home office arrangements. Some positions require local, regional, national, and/or international travel. Although the core responsibilities of each position are unique, many positions have similar features, including participation in training and development, quality improvement initiatives, and committee work, for example.

■ Drug Information as a Pharmacy Specialty

Drug information is popular specialty practice in the field of pharmacy. The following is a summary of the history of drug information and the variety of venues where this specialty is practiced.

History of Drug Information

Although all throughout history persons in a position to deliver health care have probably rendered medicinal information to their patients, and although the pharmacy profession is inherently a profession specializing in knowledge about medications, interest in formal drug information services dates back to 1962, when Senator Hubert Humphrey and others proposed a national drug information clearinghouse to provide a coordinated approach to disseminate data on new drugs and their adverse effects. One year later, $1 million was given to the National Library of Medicine to develop a drug literature program to "systematically collect, organize, and disseminate drug information." The association, now known as the Pharmaceutical Research and Manufacturers of America, supported this initiative by providing librarians who helped index journal articles about medications and information on their therapeutic use, mechanism of action, and chemical composition.[2]

With the development of increasingly complex therapeutic options and the advent of the Internet, namely, Internet sites containing medical and drug information, there has been an exponential growth in available drug information such that the provision of it has become a pharmacy specialty field unto its own, similar to the specialty practice of geriatrics, pediatrics, cardiology, and so forth.[2–9] Thus, although all pharmacists should demonstrate basic drug information competencies, pharmacists who choose to practice in drug information at an advanced level enter into the specialty practice of drug information.

Drug Information Venues

Drug information can be rendered by pharmacists in many practice settings. Academic centers, hospitals, and health systems often have dedicated drug information services in addition to the general provision of information about medications by pharmacists in hospital pharmacies and other dispensing settings. These specialty drug information services are often rendered in a dedicated physical locale called a drug information center. Drug information is also provided by health maintenance organizations, government organizations, community organizations, and in other nontraditional settings.[3]

Most pharmaceutical companies have drug information departments that serve to deliver information about company products. Although there are some basic tenets of drug information in all settings, the full scope of services offered by the pharmaceutical company differs from those offered by nonindustry drug information centers as a result of corporate, legal, and regulatory considerations.[6] Potential services provided by industry and nonindustry drug information departments are listed in TABLE 8-2.

Herein follows a discussion of the role of the pharmacist drug information in the pharmaceutical industry.

TABLE 8-2	Comparison of Drug Information Services in Different Settings	
Item of Comparison	Industry[3,10,11]	Non-Industry[12,13]
Size	1–53 employees based on 1 survey of companies with 1–500 products[12]	4 employees based on 1 survey[12]
	129 calls per day based on 1 survey[12]	11 calls per day based on 1 survey[12]
Service	Drug Information Provision of drug information to unsolicited requests about company products only	Drug Information Provision of drug information on almost any drug-related topic upon request
	Many questions are repeat questions about company products so standard written responses are often developed and maintained to respond to these questions	Questions are broader in scope and encompass questions regarding any medication, including complementary alternative medications so repeat questions are not very common and custom responses are normally provided
	Provision of drug information is bound by corporate, legal and regulatory constraints that the drug information center needs to be keenly aware of	No particular regulatory or legal implications are known
	Questions are answered very specifically; conclusions are not drawn and treatment recommendations for patients are not given	Conclusions can be made; interpretation of the data and treatment recommendations are normally sought and expected
	Promotional Review Review of promotional materials (materials developed by the marketing department to promote product use among healthcare professionals and consumers) by the drug information pharmacist for medical and scientific accuracy	Pharmacy and Therapeutics Committee Work Drug information pharmacists often participate and sometimes lead this committee to review medication profiles and associated literature to determine acceptability for use on the formulary
	Sales Training Drug information pharmacists assist in training field sales representatives on the science	Drug Use Reviews and Evaluations Drug information pharmacists analyze drug use patterns retrospectively and prospectively to

TABLE 8-2	Continued	
Item of Comparison	Industry[3,10,11]	Non-Industry[12,13]
	behind the company products they promote	determine appropriateness of medication use
	Adverse Event Reporting	Participation in Investigational Drug Trials
	Some drug information departments handle adverse event reporting and monitoring, while some companies have dedicated departments to handle adverse events and related risk management activities	Hospital drug information pharmacists collaborate with the pharmaceutical industry in evaluating the conduct of drug trials at that hospital site. The drug information pharmacist or the hospital pharmacist often dispenses study medication, and ensures site compliance with study protocol
	Other	Adverse Event Monitoring
	Other committee work, newsletter development, other medical writing, teaching students and residents	Drug information pharmacists receive retrospective adverse event reports and prospectively institute measures to monitor adverse events
		Other
		Other committee work including the institutional review board, newsletter development, developing continuing education, other medical writing, outcomes research, teaching students and residents

■ Medical Information and Communications Within the Pharmaceutical Industry

Dr. Charles Depew describes *medical communications*, in the context of the pharmaceutical industry, as "a term that encompasses the practice and provision of drug and/or medical information to health care professionals and/or consumers."[10] Names given to departments in the pharmaceutical company that provide drug information include *professional services*, *medical informatics*, *drug information*, *medical communications*, and *medical information*.[11] The healthcare professionals providing these services are often called *healthcare associates*, *medical specialists*, *medical scientists*, and *drug information coordinators* to name a few.[12] In this chapter, the term *medical information and communications* is used to describe this specialty service.

The medical information and communications department is composed of healthcare professionals, usually pharmacists, physicians, and nurses, as well as administrative

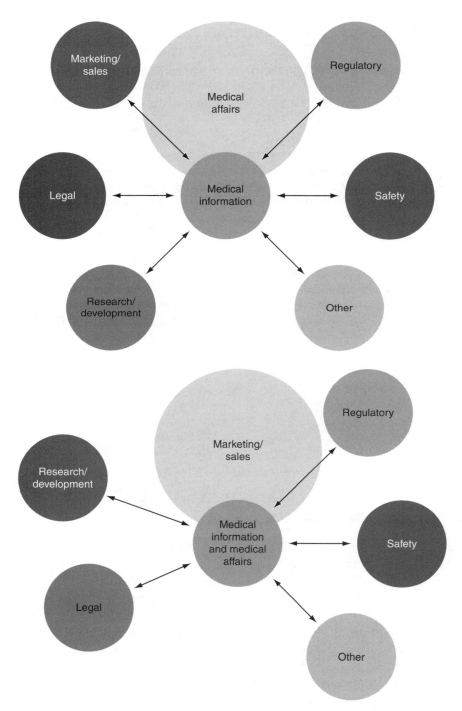

FIGURE 8-1 Medical information and communications within the pharmaceutical organization.[16]

with the larger medical group (often called medical affairs) extensively, often sharing the same or similar policies and procedures. Regardless of where the department resides in the company, the medical information and communications group often interacts regularly with other departments within the organization, such as medical affairs, marketing, sales, legal, regulatory, and safety, among others (FIGURE 8-1). As will be described, the medical information and communications department offers a variety of valued services to other departments, serving as advisors, editors, consultants, and reviewers to many.[13]

■ Functions of a Medical Information and Communications Department

The medical information and communications department of a pharmaceutical company is a valuable department in the organization. It serves largely to support internal (other company departments and employees) and external customers (healthcare professionals and sometimes consumers) by providing needed drug information about company products, although the full breadth and scope of services vary between companies, and many offer a number of services in addition to traditional drug information.[14] Following is a discussion about potential services offered by today's medical information and communications department in the pharmaceutical industry.

Responding to Inquiries for Drug Information

A core function of all medical information and communications departments in the pharmaceutical industry is to respond to inquiries about company products. Based on one survey of 24 pharmaceutical and biopharmaceutical companies in the United States, the number of queries received per product per week ranged from 5 to 183, and the average number of queries handled per staff member ranged from 27 to 196 per week.[12]

However, the pharmaceutical industry is tightly regulated, and the provision of drug information cannot be misconstrued as promotion of a product. Therefore, to maintain compliance with the federal Food and Drug Administration (FDA), medical information and communications departments should only respond to *unsolicited* requests for product information, meaning they should only respond to requests they have no part in originating, and they cannot in any way offer or provide drug information to persons who do not explicitly, wholly, and independently request it. Additionally, drug information provided by the department must be *nonpromotional, data-driven, scientifically balanced* information, meaning the information is not intended to promote the product, must be based on good science using data-intensive sources, and must represent the current thinking of the wealth of the known medical literature, containing known positive and negative information. The FDA also stipulates that the response does not deliberately go beyond the scope of the question and that promotional materials are not included with the response.[15]

Requests for product information may be internal or external. Internal requests originate from personnel within other departments or from affiliates (employees of the parent company located in satellite companies throughout the world). External requests originate from healthcare professionals and consumers. Although all pharmaceutical companies respond to requests for information from healthcare professionals, only some companies, because of additional medical and legal considerations, choose to respond to drug information requests from consumers. For instance, some companies may view the interaction with consumers as an interference with the physician–patient relationship, and some companies are concerned about liability.[12,13,16,17]

Responding to Drug Information Requests from the Healthcare Professional

Questions from healthcare professionals represent the largest source of unsolicited requests for product information, accounting for approximately 60–90% of all queries, according to one survey.[12] Questions from healthcare professionals come into the medical information and communications department via two main routes. First, the sales representatives in the field may submit questions to the department on behalf of a healthcare professional. Questions are often submitted because the sales representative is not authorized to answer certain types of questions because of regulatory constraint. For instance, sales representatives may answer questions about FDA-approved indications, which may be answered by information contained in the prescribing information. However, many questions from healthcare providers are in regard to "off-label" uses of a product (use of a product other than that which is supported by the prescribing information). Sales representatives are unable to answer such questions, and they refer these types of questions to the medical information and communications department.[6] Pharmacists in the medical information and communications department have no regulatory constraint regarding the communication of "off-label" information, as long as the request was unsolicited in nature, the response clearly identifies the information as "off-label" and is scientifically accurate and balanced.[6] The second way in which questions are received by the medical information and communications department is by healthcare professionals who directly call, e-mail, mail, or fax the department with queries.

The Medical Communications Special Interest Section of the Drug Information Association (DIA) identified six activities that together serve as a guide in responding to inquiries from external healthcare professionals. They are as follows:

1. Receiving the inquiry
2. Clarifying and understanding the information needs of the requestor

3. Identifying and evaluating available drug and related medical information
4. Writing the response and having it peer-reviewed
5. Communicating the response to the requestor
6. Checking the requestor's understanding of the response and assessing his or her feedback

Another important activity is to document the interaction in a reliable computer database so that detailed information about the interaction can be retrieved when needed. See FIGURE 8-2.

Common resources the medical information and communications department uses to respond to unsolicited requests for product information include the product prescribing information, peer-reviewed medical literature, and in some instances, unpublished company information. Answers should be based on sound data, should be scientifically balanced, and should not go beyond the scope of the specific question asked, unless a relevant safety issue needs to be highlighted. Personal opinion should be withheld, and treatment recommendations should not be made. Last, a disclaimer should accompany the response stating that the information presented is to assist the healthcare professional in coming to his or her own conclusions, and that the information is not intended to be promotional. An example disclaimer statement is offered by Graves and Baker and reads as follows[6]:

> Company X is providing you with this material as an information service and professional courtesy. It is intended to provide pertinent data that will assist you in forming your own conclusions and making your own decisions. It is not intended to recommend new uses for our products. Company X does not promote the use of any product for any indications, claim, dosage, or route of administration that is not covered in the enclosed package insert.

Standard Written Responses

Because many questions are repeat questions and questions that the company can anticipate (eg, a new study about the safety of a product in a certain patient population may spur renewed interest in the administration of that product in that subpopulation), most pharmaceutical companies develop a database of standard written responses that can be used to answer repeat questions of the like.[6] New standard response letters are written as needed; current ones are reviewed and updated regularly to ensure that they contain all current, relevant information; old ones are retired if they are no longer needed; and all undergo a formal review and approval process based on company policies and procedures.

Medical information and communications departments often own sophisticated databases that store and retrieve these standard responses. Many types of reports can

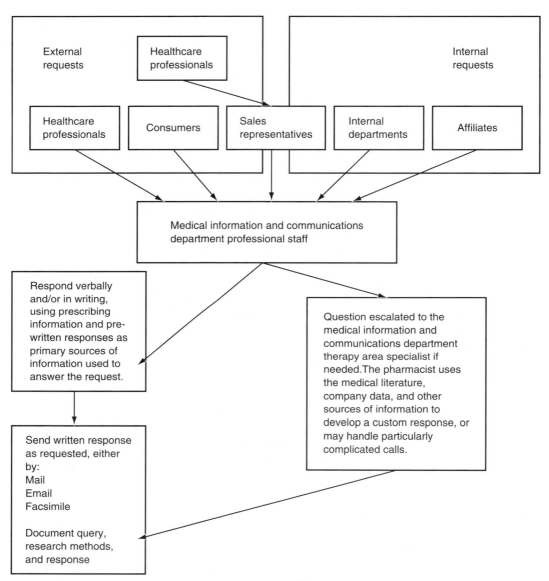

FIGURE 8-2 Example process of handling an inquiry.[21]

be generated by these computer applications so that the department can analyze usage of predeveloped responses, which may assist with documentation and quality improvement initiatives. Many medical information and communications departments have developed standards for the creation of standard written responses, often called a style guide or style manual. These aids are helpful to ensure quality and consistency of written responses.[6] It is important to note that not all questions can be handled by a standard written response. In those instances, a custom response must be developed using the same rigorous search methods and review and approval processes used to develop prewritten responses.

Special Circumstances

Certain types of questions require special thought and consideration owing to their sensitive nature. Questions regarding comparative claims and investigational products are two such types. When answering questions about investigational products, regulatory issues and company policy must be kept top of mind. Comparative claims questions, such as "is your drug better than your competitor's drug" are difficult to handle because only well-conducted randomized, active-controlled trials enrolling an adequate number of subjects and of a sufficient study duration can be used to make superiority claims. Thus, the pharmacist handling the question needs to be very knowledgeable about which studies he or she can use to develop an accurate, complete, scientifically balanced answer. Inadvertently including clinical studies of a lower caliber may lead to an inaccurate portrayal of a product and can lead to repercussions on the pharmaceutical company. The FDA prohibits the promotion of investigational products before they receive FDA approval, and although the medical information and communications department is not involved in product promotion, it needs to avoid any appearance of potential "preapproval promotion," and information sought at this point is often proprietary information.[6]

The provision of medical information for rare disorders and pediatric diseases represents certain challenges as well. Such disorders are often rare, study enrollment is often slow and difficult, and studies are hard to perform. Therefore, manufacturers are less likely to invest resources to manage these diseases. As an incentive to research and develop treatments in these small markets, pharmaceutical companies are given additional market exclusivity for the development of medications used to manage these disorders.

However, because of these same aforementioned challenges, limited information about these medications exists (often as case reports and uncontrolled studies), and medications are often used off-label. Therefore, medical information and communications departments often receive many and varied off-label questions about these medications, and owing to the additional years of market exclusivity, they can anticipate receiving these types of questions for a lengthened period of time. Additionally, because these diseases are rare, with few or no existing treatments available, they are managed by specialists who eagerly await drug availability, study results, and new information. As such, they often request information as soon as the medication is available and before educational materials are reviewed and approved, increasing the request volume for the medical information and communications department.[18]

Responses to other questions require special care as well. These include questions that are by persons who may be misrepresenting their identity or credentials, by persons who may be representing a competitor company, by persons collecting information for a potential lawsuit, and by irate and dissatisfied callers.[13]

Anticipated Changes in Request Volume

Anticipating changes in request volume can help medical information and communications departments prepare for increased request volumes that can strain a department's resources, especially an unprepared one. For instance, an anticipated launch of a new product, new information about a product, or recall of a product, to name a few, may generate an increase in questions that the company may be able to anticipate. In these instances, new standard response letters may be developed, more staff may be dedicated to handle product inquiries, or other measures to manage workload may be used.

In addition to these examples, seasonal patterns may exist. These include an end-of-the-year decrease in inquiry volume as a result of the observance of many holidays; summer declines in inquiry volume resulting from the recess of some health-system activities and committees and an increase in personal vacations taken; an increase in July/August volumes as hospitals employ new residents and fellows who may be less familiar with drug therapy than seasoned professionals are and therefore may be more likely to utilize the services of a medical information and communications department; and last, seasonal variation in the prevalence of certain diseases (such as seasonal allergies and some infectious diseases) that may precipitate an increase in product queries about the medications used to manage them.[19]

Responding to Drug Information Requests from the Consumer

The proportion of questions received by consumers varies greatly and is dependent on company policy (with some companies not responding to consumer questions at all) as well as other factors.[12] There are no FDA regulations that explicitly direct the practice of providing drug information to consumers, but general guidelines have been proposed, and each company will likely have its own policy in place for responding to consumer questions, such as follows[6,16,17]:

- Uncover the consumer's core concern or question.
- Provide only information within the current prescribing information.
- Encourage consumers to discuss drug-related questions with their healthcare providers as well.
- Provide a specific response and ensure that you are answering only the question posed.
- Provide a response that is readily understandable and free of company or medical jargon.
- Do not provide medical advice or counseling.
- Do not provide off-label information. If the consumer is intent on receiving such information, encourage him or her to have a healthcare provider contact the company for that information.

- Assess understanding.
- Communicate sincerely and compassionately.
- Document the interaction.

■ Maximizing Resources to Create Efficiencies in the Provision of Medical Information

Many companies are faced with a high volume of requests for information about their products and are continually trying to determine how to improve efficiency while maintaining or increasing the quality of their responses. Many companies have instituted a same-day standard for responding to requests for product information that can be provided verbally or with a standard written response, whereas more time is allotted for responses that require a custom response.[12,20]

A resourceful company optimizes its use of staff time and technology to better its services. In an effort to respond to inquiries more quickly, while protecting staff time, some companies have instituted a fax-on-demand technology, whereby a requestor dials a fax number, is prompted to order a catalog that contains a list of available documents, and enters his or her own fax number so that within minutes, the catalog is faxed to the requestor. The requestor is then able to view the catalog, call the fax number back, dial in the appropriate catalog number for the document requested, provide his or her own fax number, and then the document is retrieved by a computer at the company and is faxed to the requestor. This fax-on-demand technology is useful for common, repetitive questions the company can anticipate receiving, and because it requires minimal intervention on the part of the pharmacist, it allows the pharmacist to concentrate on more difficult or complex questions that would not be feasible to answer with fax-on-demand. The system also keeps track of callers so that requests can be properly documented. An additional advantage to the system is that it can answer 1500 calls at a time, so it cannot be easily overwhelmed. One important disadvantage is that caller identity cannot easily be verified, making it difficult to control who receives the information.[21] Other technological efficiencies include the use of intranet, extranet, and Internet services, and use of other company-wide or department-wide databases.[22-25] The use of certain company-wide technologies can help to bridge language barriers and time zone differences in global companies with affiliates around the world.[26]

Outsourcing is another method used by medical information and communications departments to handle workload efficiently.[12,27] Outsourcing has been described as the "process of using vendors to perform a function outside of the company."[27] Outsourcing allows a department to focus on certain business goals, while delegating certain functions to a third-party agency. Specific functions that are often outsourced by the medical information and communications department include the handling of drug information requests after business hours for extended coverage time, initial adverse event and product complaint handling, communication of verbal responses to drug information requests, communication of written responses to drug information requests, and development of standard written responses to common, anticipated drug information questions.[5,27,28]

Other ways to create efficiencies include the development of a streamlined review process for standard written responses and other documents requiring approval, cross-referencing centralized literature files, developing new documents in advance of situations that are anticipated and predictable, and using temporary staff or temporarily reassigning staff for needed short-term support.[5]

Handling Adverse Events and Product Complaints

In a medical information and communications department's normal interaction with healthcare professionals and consumers, adverse drug events or product complaints are often "uncovered" in conversation between a company representative and a customer, when it may have not been the intent of the customer to report such an event to the company. In other instances, a healthcare professional or consumer may contact the company specifically to report an adverse event. In either case, adverse events identified by a pharmaceutical company need to followed up on.

Some medical information and communications departments handle adverse event reports and product complaints, whereas other pharmaceutical companies triage these events to other departments dedicated to the handling of them, following proper corporate policy and procedure.[6,29] According to one survey of 24 pharmaceutical companies, 88% stated that their companies had a separate clinical safety group or department.[12] In addition to receiving and processing adverse event information from healthcare providers and consumers, safety departments or related departments vigilantly and proactively audit adverse events and develop short-term and long-term programs to assess and manage adverse events associated with a company product in an effort to minimize known risk associated with the drug.[30]

Participating in Promotional Review

Materials that are developed for promotional use are usually reviewed by several departments, including marketing, editorial, regulatory, legal, and medical, including medical information and communications. The role of medical information and communications is to review promotional materials for medical utility and accuracy.

Examples of promotional items that undergo copy approval or promotional review include journal advertisements, branded (concerning a particular company product) and unbranded (not naming a particular company product but given the content and intent is still considered promotional) websites, and pamphlets sent to healthcare professionals, to name a just a few.

In addition to regular promotional review, medical information and communications often participates in the development of the concept for a potential promotional idea, ensuring that the item would be useful and appropriate for the intended audience (healthcare professional versus consumer).[13] Oftentimes, companies contract with outside vendors to develop certain promotional materials. The medical information and communications department can play a large role in training the outside vendor, by teaching the vendor how to select appropriate medical references to develop the materials, and how to use medical references appropriately. Other company-developed referencing criteria and medical writing standards and styles can be shared with the vendor as well.

Participating in Sales Training Activities

Many medical information and communications departments participate in the training of their sales representatives in several ways.[13] They may participate in the live training of sales representatives, in a traditional classroom setting. In this respect, medical information and communications may deliver lectures to the sales representatives in training, may facilitate questions and answers sessions about company products and the associated disease states they manage, or may engage in role model exercises with the sales representatives in mock detailing to healthcare professionals. Instruction in clinical pharmacology, physiology, and pathophysiology/therapeutics, as well as some biostatistics and literature evaluation can be particularly helpful.

Because the sales force regularly submits requests for product information to the medical information and communications department on behalf of healthcare professionals, medical information can help educate the sales force on company policies and regulatory issues regarding the provision of medical information. Another area of sales training the medical information and communications department can participate in is the development and review of written materials that comprise a curriculum for the sales representatives and that are used to educate them on company products, competitive products, and related disease states.

Launch Preparation

The *launch* of a product is the debut of a product in the marketplace. Pharmaceutical companies may launch a new product, or they may launch a new indication, new route of administration, or new dosage form of an existing product. Oftentimes, new products are developed and approved that are similar chemical entities to other medications. In this instance, the product is not a completely novel product, but rather is one similar to existing products, often called a *line extension*. The launch of a new chemical entity, or a new product launch, requires more resources, whereas less may be required for the launch of a new dosage form, for example.

In any event, as Drs. Werner and Murray have stated, for many departments in the pharmaceutical company, the approval of a product is the culmination of much effort and "signals the end of many years of hard work," but for the medical information and communications department, it "marks the beginning of a new and critical phase of their involvement in the support of a product."[31] When the company is preparing for the launch of a new product in the marketplace (or for an existing product with a new indication, new dosage form, or new route of administration, etc.), tremendous resources (in time, money, and staff) are used. The medical information and communications department plays a critical role in preparing for product launch by both supporting other departments through (well before, during, and after) launch, as well as preparing its own department for launch.

Resource Allocation and Launch Plan Development

The medical information and communications department normally develops a formal launch plan. They first need to determine how many and which persons will be intimately involved in launch preparedness activities so that key individuals can be identified, relied upon, and known by other departments as key contacts.[31] To do so, they need to consider the size of the sales force, the number and sources of possible requests for product information they can anticipate receiving postlaunch, as well as the daily needs of the department independent of product launch. A timeline detailing when key launch activities need to be accomplished should be developed to ensure a successful launch, and involved individuals need to be provided with adequate training and resources.

Support of Other Departments

Well in advance of launch, medical information and communications staff often actively participate in interdisciplinary development teams and marketing teams to provide medical consultation about the investigational product, such as the value the product is expected to have relative to others in the marketplace, proposed life cycle strategies (short-term and long-term strategies to maximize the market potential of a product from its infancy in the marketplace to many years out), potential views that healthcare professionals may have about the product given its profile (risk:benefit ratio), qualities the product must possess to be acceptable to patients and healthcare providers, and so forth.

Some medical information and communications departments have staff that work with regulatory and labeling departments to provide input on proposed prescribing information.[19] Medical information and communications may assist marketing in developing key messages about the product and may participate in advisory board meetings, key workshops, and other events that will assist in the education of healthcare professionals and invited speakers about the investigational product. Medical information and communications will likely review numerous promotional materials that are developed for use after launch.[31] In a survey of medical information and communications departments participating in a myriad of launch activities, including promotional review, the number of hours reported on the promotional review of materials for launch ranged from 150 hours or less to more than 450 hours.[28]

Core Launch Materials

A key role the medical information and communications department has in preparing for product launch is to proactively anticipate and identify the types of requests they will receive from healthcare professionals and consumers about the new product. For example, basic questions about the product's efficacy and safety will undoubtedly be asked, as well as questions about the use of the product in certain patient populations.

If a product is an injectable, an easily anticipated type of question is in regard to product compatibility with other common medications and intravenous solutions, as well as questions regarding storage conditions. Likewise, if it is known that the new product will commonly be used with particular other medications, drug–drug interaction questions can easily be anticipated. A list of such potential high-volume requests for information should be made, and standard written responses developed in advance of launch.

In an industry-wide survey of product launch preparedness methods of pharmaceutical companies, companies reported having developed between 1 and 45 new standard response letters in anticipation of different product launches, although the launch of a new chemical entity may require the development of more standard written letters than the launch of a new route of administration of an existing product does, for example.[28]

Because not all questions can be anticipated, the medical information and communications department can expect to create new written responses postlaunch as actual queries are received by the department and trends in questions are seen. Other core launch documents that may be developed include slide presentations that are to be delivered either internally or externally, dossiers or formulary packets that may be requested by payers planning to review the product for potential formulary inclusion, question and answer documents, and others.[31] It will be necessary for the medical information and communications staff members to collaborate with computer technology departments to ensure that current or new technology can adequately support needed materials. Technology should be reliable, customizable, and user-friendly.

Training

Medical information and communications staff dedicated to the launch of the product is heavily involved in training the sales force on the investigational product and related disease state, as well as information on which types of inquiries are appropriate to submit to the medical information and communications department on behalf of a healthcare professional. This training is akin to that of a full didactic curriculum, with different types of training that are conducted at different time intervals. Medical information and communications is often involved in the development of the sales training syllabus, in the concept of particular training materials, and certainly in the review of all sales training programs.

Live training is often facilitated by medical information and communications in launch workshops, workshops designed to educate and excite the sales force in their new role in selling the new product. Additionally, medical information and communications must train their own department on the product profile, related disease state, and prescribing information specifics; on detailed information about its clinical trials and publications; other core launch materials; and information on standard written responses that will be developed for the product so that staff know when and how best to use them. This is often similarly accomplished by the development of a training curriculum, utilizing different venues and delivery of training, such as classroom training and self-training.[31]

Evaluation and Reassessment

A reassessment of activities postlaunch is effective in determining how better to support the product moving forward and how to better prepare for future launches. One pharmaceutical company surveyed 52 other companies throughout the industry to determine how they prepared for product launches. Of the 14 companies that replied, medical information and communications departments stated they dedicated between 1 and 3 persons to the launch of a product. Although companies stated that they began strategically planning for launch more than 1 year prior to the anticipated launch date, actual launch activities were typically carried out less than 3 months prior to anticipated approval. This may be a result in part of the time-sensitive nature of many of the activities; many tasks cannot be completed until data are available and final documents are approved, for example.

It is also important to note that medical information and communications departments plan for product launches differently. Although some companies dedicate certain individuals to the launch of a product, as launch approaches and passes, some choose to train and involve all team members in support of the product, and some companies, depending on the size of their department, are able to participate in launch activities well in advance of launch, 6 months to 1 year, including the surveying company.[28]

Scientific Meeting Support

Medical information and communications often travels to and actively participates in regional, national, and international professional and scientific meetings. They often sponsor a medical booth or drug information booth to respond to unsolicited requests for product information, similar to the way in which they respond to such questions from their home base.

They also participate in educating the sales force about the different role of the sales force versus that of the medical information and communications department in responding to queries at conventions. They meet with key opinion leaders, learn about competitive products at the meeting, and represent their company at different events.[31]

Other Services of the Medical Information and Communications Department

It is the mission of the medical information and communications department to ensure that company products are being used safely, effectively, appropriately, and optimally. To this end, the medical information and communications department often collaborates with other departments to provide medical and scientific support.[13,14] Medical-marketing relationships exist whereby persons from medical information and communications use their knowledge and clinical expertise to provide medical input to help position company products in the marketplace and to develop a medical education strategy.[32]

Other specialty services include supporting the development of treatment protocols, algorithms, practice guidelines, drug monographs, and other writing pieces; developing special tools (slide kits for presentation, educational platforms, data summaries) that provide support for company products; assisting in the development of dossiers or formulary documents; participating in speakers bureaus, investigator meetings, and advisory board meetings; reviewing company-sponsored continuing education; participating in pharmacoeconomic studies and disease management programs; collaborating with the publication strategy team to optimize their publication plan and to assist in the preparation or review of manuscripts; and participating in patient assistance programs.[13,14] Last, medical information and communications can serve as a consultant to many departments for general medical information.[13,14]

■ Evaluation of Medical Information and Communications Department Services

Medical information and communications department can be evaluated by quality assurance activities and by the use of surveys.

Quality Assurance Activities

Quality assurance has been described as a "formal method that ensures standards are established and maintained, in addition to identifying solutions if standards are not maintained."[12] Medical information and communications departments participate in many informal and formal quality assurance activities. Telephone calls can be monitored to assess the handling of individual information requests. Similarly, computer databases can be tracked to review the appropriateness of written responses to information requests. Regular meetings are often held to discuss complex inquiries to determine how staff could best handle these requests. Standard written responses undergo a formal review and approval process, including peer-review, manager review, and in certain circumstances interdepartmental review.[12]

Using Surveys as a Quality Assurance Measure

Few surveys have been conducted over the years to evaluate services provided by pharmaceutical company medical information and communications departments, either as customer satisfaction surveys or as benchmarking surveys of pharmaceutical companies.[12,33–35] In one survey assessing customer satisfaction with one company's handling of requests for product information, customers (healthcare professionals) ranked accuracy, response time, objectivity, and/or relevance as top characteristics of importance. Overall, healthcare professionals also expressed satisfaction with these characteristics.[35] In another survey conducted to assess the satisfaction of healthcare professionals with another company's handling of requests for product information, 94% of responding healthcare professionals expressed satisfaction with company written response letters, and this satisfaction was shown to have a positive impact on the prescribing of company products.

In a survey of drug information departments providing verbal responses to requests for product information, the following were identified as best practices: using the caller's name in conversation, repeating the question for accurate understanding, asking follow-up questions to elicit further information, summarizing the discussion, and sending written follow-up information in a timely manner.[34]

Participation of the staff in these quality assurance activities can serve to improve the quality and efficiency of work done by the department, as well as potentially reduce legal liability.[36]

■ The Pharmaceutical Industry as a Career

A minority of pharmacists chooses the pharmaceutical industry as an initial career choice following graduation from pharmacy school. Riggins surmises this may be because of an unawareness of job opportunities within the industry and lists several factors that may contribute to this unawareness: (1) lack of formal instruction in pharmacy school curricula, (2) limited interaction of students and pharmacists with employees in the industry other than sales representatives, and (3) limited published literature on career opportunities in the industry.[1]

Pharmacists who leave traditional pharmacy roles to seek careers in the pharmaceutical industry suggest they desired greater job satisfaction, better salary and benefits, more flexible work arrangements, and greater career opportunities as reasons for pursuing a pharmaceutical industry career.[1,37] Riggins conducted a survey of 1,088 pharmacists employed by Eli Lilly and Company in 1998 to evaluate pharmacist employment opportunities and employee satisfaction. According to the survey, approximately 7% of all Eli Lilly and Company employees in the United States were pharmacists. A total of 679 pharmacists responded to the survey, and of these, 85% agreed or strongly agreed that they were satisfied with their current position, and 70% agreed or strongly agreed that they were satisfied with their career progression at the company.[1]

Introduction to the Pharmaceutical Industry in the School of Pharmacy Curriculum

Exposure to the pharmaceutical industry as a career in schools of pharmacy is limited.[1] Some schools have core or elective courses in the curriculum that introduce the student to a variety of traditional and nontraditional pharmacy careers, including that of the pharmaceutical industry. Many schools of pharmacy hold career roundtable discussions whereby they will invite pharmacists who work in different fields of pharmacy to speak with their students. Students are made aware of the different pharmacy careers being represented and can sign up to speak with the career representatives in an informal question and answer forum; pharmacists from different areas of the pharmaceutical industry are often invited to speak with students who would like to learn more about a potential career in the pharmaceutical industry.

For upperclassman, schools of pharmacy hold career fairs whereby potential employers will visit the school and offer information about potential job opportunities; the pharmaceutical industry is often invited to participate and recruit potential candidates.

■ Educational Opportunities for the Student Interested in Industry as a Career

There are a variety of educational opportunities available to students interested in pursuing a career in industry; these include internships, clerkships, residencies, and fellowships. These programs are discussed at length below.

Internships

Student internships are often available in medical information and communications, as well as in other areas of industry. The Drug Information Association (DIA) is a professional, worldwide, nonprofit organization involved in the discovery, development, regulation, surveillance, and marketing of pharmaceuticals. It is a multidisciplinary association that advocates the exchange of information, education and training, networking, leadership, and professional development opportunities in drug information.[9]

Students can search the DIA website for available internships offered by pharmaceutical companies. It is not an all-inclusive site, so internships may exist that are not listed, but it is a helpful start for students seeking such opportunities.

Internships are often completed in the summer (often between the fourth and fifth, or between the fifth and sixth year of the pharmacy curriculum) and are approximately 12 weeks in duration.[9] Whereas some internship curricula are concentrated in medical information and communications, others focus on other areas of industry.

Clerkships

Clerkship rotations, sometimes called externships or experiential rotations, are hands-on practical rotations (usually 4–6 weeks in length) that follow the didactic (classroom) prerequisites in the professional pharmacy curriculum. They became a standard part of the pharmacy curriculum in the 1970s and are a requirement for graduation.[38] Many schools of pharmacy offer drug information clerkships in the pharmaceutical industry setting, either as a required or as an elective rotation. TABLE 8-3 lists example objectives for an industry-based drug information clerkship rotation.

Common exercises and projects that students have the opportunity to complete in an industry-based drug information clerkship (and sometimes in an internship program) include providing verbal and written responses to requests for product information, critically evaluating the medical literature, writing a paper such as a disease state or therapy area "backgrounder" or a standard response letter, developing and delivering an oral presentation, reviewing a promotional item for medical accuracy, preparing a drug monograph, and attending pertinent team or departmental meetings. Other opportunities often exist, including the opportunity to work on special projects that help the department fulfill its mission.[38,39] Often, students have an opportunity to interview or shadow a pharmacist outside of the medical information and communications department to gain an understanding of how the department fits

TABLE 8-3	Objectives of an Industry-Based Drug Information Rotation
Develop a familiarity with drug information resources[41]	
Demonstrate effective probing, gathering, organization, and analysis of drug information[40]	
Strengthen verbal and written communication skills[40,41]	
Improve literature searching and evaluation skills[41]	
Apply didactic knowledge toward problem solving and the development of recommendations[40]	
Develop an appreciation of various roles of pharmacists in industry[40]	
Develop an awareness of corporate organizations, regulatory constraints in the pharmaceutical industry, and the drug development process[40,41]	
Contrast the roles and responsibilities of industry versus institutional drug information centers[40,41]	
Develop professional and interpersonal skills[40]	

into the organization and to gain an understanding of the role of the pharmacist in other departments throughout the industry.

Residencies and Fellowships

Residencies are organized, directed postdoctorate programs that build upon competencies gained from a professional pharmacy curriculum.[7] A survey of pharmacists employed by a major pharmaceutical company in 1998 found that approximately 25% of their PharmDs had completed a residency.[1] These numbers are now likely to be even higher because this survey was completed before pharmacy schools had transitioned to an all–Doctor of Pharmacy curriculum.

Drug information residencies are typically classified as specialty residencies (residencies that concentrate on a focused area of practice) that are traditionally completed in the second postgraduate year and are usually 1 year in length. Although many institutions prefer candidates with prior pharmacy practice residency experience (a postgraduate year-1 residency that strives to enhance general advanced practice competencies), there are other routes for entry into a drug information residency. Some pharmacists apply for a drug information residency following the completion of another type of pharmacy residency, or perhaps after no residency at all if the pharmacist has exceptional work experience that would be deemed equivalent experience. Specific eligibility requirements can be found on the American Society of Health-System Pharmacists (ASHP) website or by contacting the individual program.

The ASHP accredits residency programs. As such, it has developed standards, based upon several guiding principles, that residency programs must meet to maintain accreditation, and it outlines educational goals and objectives for residencies, including drug information residencies. TABLE 8-4 contains a summary of the ASHP goals and objectives of a drug information residency.[40]

The ASHP also has an online residency directory of accredited programs to serve students seeking residency information. The online directory lists more than 20 drug information programs, most of which are hospital, healthcare system, or university/academic center–based, or a combination of such. A few managed care drug information residencies and industry-based drug information residencies are listed on this site as well.[41] Some residencies are dual-track residencies, with a shared focus on two main areas of experience, for example, academic drug information and industry drug information. McCart and colleagues write of a combined industry and academic residency program that offered 6 months of drug information in an academic center and 6 months in an industry setting.[42] Still others are drug information residencies with concentration in a particular setting and a lesser focus in another, such as a drug information residency in an academic center with some focus on industry-based drug information. The provision of drug information in the second setting is accomplished by offering rotations outside of the parent institution in the alternate setting. For example, a drug information residency in an academic center may collaborate with the

TABLE 8-4	Summary of ASHP Educational Goals for Drug Information Residencies

Take responsibility for attaining excellence in drug information practice

Promote activities in pharmacy organizations that relate to drug information

Develop an organized system for staying current in drug information literature

Develop a plan for initiating a drug information service

Develop a quality improvement plan for a drug information service

Develop a plan for documentation of services

Design a drug information storage and retrieval system

Develop and implement drug use policies and procedures

Employ advanced literature analysis skills

Contribute to the biomedical literature

Communicate drug information clearly, verbally and in writing

Use appropriate routes to best communicate the results of work

Provide informational support for investigational drug programs

Assess outcomes literature to determine applicability to population-based decisions

Conduct original research in the practice of drug information

Manage the operation of a drug information center

Maximize efficiency in performing tasks through expert use of technology

Serve as a resource for the lay press in matters related to drug therapy

Demonstrate ethical conduct

Provide instruction to pharmacy trainees

Perform prospective and retrospective financial and clinical outcomes analyses

* Only those applicable for an industry-based drug information program are listed.

Source: American Society of Health-System Pharmacists. Educational Goals and Learning Objectives for Postgraduate Year 2 Drug Information Residencies, www.ashp.org, accessed April 18, 2007.

pharmaceutical industry to provide the drug information resident an opportunity to complete several industry-based rotations.

Features of a drug information residency depend upon the primary practice site. Residency features in industry-based drug information and, in particular, medical communications may include providing drug information to healthcare professionals and consumers, and associated skills such as medical writing and literature evaluation, adverse drug event reporting, management of a drug information service, pharmacoeconomics, and quality assurance, among others. Additional opportunities may be the provision of didactic or experiential teaching of doctor of pharmacy students on internship or clerkship at the pharmaceutical company.

All drug information residents participating in an ASHP-accredited residency must complete a research project, which often culminates with the presentation of the research at a regional meeting. Drug information residents in industry may rotate through other departments in the organization, such as product safety, regulatory, health outcomes, and public relations. The ASHP website lists specific residency features of individual programs.

Last, industry-based fellowships exist. Fellowships are traditionally 2-year, research-based programs, so are usually not in medical information and communications. Examples of pharmacy industry-based fellowships include those in pharmacoeconomics and health outcomes research.

Additional Skills

In addition to the pharmacy-specific knowledge and skills that a pharmacy student should come to develop, certain transferable skills (nonspecific to a pharmacy degree) are highly valued and normally possessed by the successful drug information candidate. They include organization, ingenuity, leadership, collaboration, and effective verbal and written communication skills, to name just a few.[47]

Career Development Opportunities

DIA and ASHP have additional resources for students to network with mentors and to assist in career and professional development. The DIA has an online certificate program in medical communications and has many workshops, training courses, and meetings throughout the year. Although the majority of these are geared toward the working professional, several resources exist to help interested students learn more about the pharmaceutical industry.

■ Evolution of Medical Information and Communications in the Pharmaceutical Industry

The role of medical information and communications within the pharmaceutical industry is currently evolving, and many agree that the practice will continue to evolve and diversify.[6,43,44] Several factors intrinsic and extrinsic to the industry are responsible for this forecast, including an increase in inquiry volume, changes in inquiry sophistication, novel technologies that will assist in inquiry response, globalization efforts, and other factors.[43,44]

Increased Volume and Sophistication of Inquiries

Medical information and communications departments are receiving an increased volume of drug information inquiries. Increasing time constraints placed upon healthcare providers leads to increased queries from busy healthcare professionals. Similarly, an increase in time constraints placed upon healthcare providers when interacting with patients leads to an increase in queries from consumers. An increase in medical information available to the lay public, including that on the Internet (including company-sponsored product-specific and non-product-specific websites), in magazines (including prescription drug prescribing information), in book stores, and on television (direct-to-consumer advertising, nightly news, and even primetime medical dramas), coupled with a society that is increasingly likely to seek self-help, leads to increased consumer queries that are often of a more sophisticated nature.[6,16] The entry of complex, frequently prescribed, life-saving, blockbuster medications into the marketplace leads to an increase in complex inquiries about these products, and as off-label use of medications increases, queries about those products increase in diversity and complexity as well.[19,44]

Novel Technology

The use of an intranet site within a company allows headquarters and field-based personnel to communicate readily, increasing the efficiency of communicating product inquiries from the field to the medical information and communications department. Similarly, the use of fax-on-demand and other voice mail technologies allows for increased efficiencies in responding to product inquiries. For example, some companies have invested in technology that reroutes calls coming in during high-volume instances so that they are redistributed and handled by other personnel, such as an outsourced vendor.[44]

Globalization

Some medical information and communications departments have been steadfast in their commitment to globalize services, striving to partner with affiliate company personnel worldwide on a regular basis to improve communication, quality, and efficiency.[12,14,26,45] Globalization often leads to an increase and diversity of product inquiries because affiliates may seek assistance from headquarters when responding to inquiries regarding products that are made by the parent company but that are not available in the parent country.[43] Headquarter personnel may not be as familiar with these products but will still be expected to support these products.

Additionally, true globalization leads to the partnership between the parent company and affiliates on multiple levels, above and beyond the handling of product inquiries, so additional services may be provided as relationships are better cultivated. For example, shared work, shared resources, sharing of best practices, and other forms of collaboration will occur in a truly globalized department.

Other Factors

In a paper about the changing role of drug information, Curran surmises consolidation of companies, increasing number of co-promotional arrangements and other joint endeavors, outsourcing of drug information responsibilities, and other factors will also result in changes in the size, scope, and function of drug information departments.[44]

■ Summary

Pharmacists play a large role in the pharmaceutical industry, and specifically in medical information and communications. Today's pharmacists practicing in drug information will find themselves looking to tomorrow, as the practice of drug information is constantly growing and evolving. Students interested in a potential career in drug information in the pharmaceutical industry can seek out several career development opportunities, and if they choose to pursue a career in industry drug information, they will find themselves helping to shape the future of drug information.

■ References

1. Riggins JL, Plowman BH. Pharmacist employment and satisfaction trends at Eli Lilly and Company. *Drug Information J*. 2000;34:1223–1229.

2. Knoben JE, Phillips SJ, Snyder JW, Szczur MR. The National Library of Medicine and drug information. Part 2: an evolving future. *Drug Information J*. 2004;38:171–180.

3. Graham AS, Graves DA, Grobman BJ, McCart GM, Tsourounis C. Drug information in industry versus academia: a pharmacy resident's perspective of a sample case. *Drug Information J*. 2000;34:1121–1127.

4. Knoben JE, Phillips SJ, Szczur MR. The National Library of Medicine and drug information. Part 1: present resources. *Drug Information J*. 2004;38:69–81.

5. Curran CF. A progress report: drug information from 1970 to 2000. *Drug Information J*. 2000;34:1355–1363.

6. Graves DA, Baker RP. The core curriculum for medical communications professionals practicing in the pharmaceutical industry. *Drug Information J*. 2000;34:995–1008.

7. American Society of Health-System Pharmacists. Accreditation standard for postgraduate year 1 pharmacy residency programs. Available at: http://www.ashp.org. Accessed April 16, 2007.

8. American Society of Health-System Pharmacists. Accreditation standard for postgraduate year 2 pharmacy residency programs. Available at: http://www.ashp.org. Accessed April 16, 2007.

9. Drug Information Association. Home page. Available at: http://www.diahome.org. Accessed April 16, 2007.

10. Depew CC. Guest editor's note: special series on medical communications. *Drug Information J*. 2000;34:991–993.

11. Salter FJ, Kramer PF, Palmer-Shevlin NL. Pharmaceutical industry medical communications departments: regulatory and legal perils and pitfalls. *Drug Information J*. 2000;34:1009–1015.

12. Hopkins F, Gallagher C, Levine A. Medical affairs and drug information practices within the pharmaceutical industry: results of a benchmarking survey. *Drug Information J*. 1999;33:69–85.

13. Werner AL, Poe TE, Graham JA. Expanding medical communications services to internal customers. *Drug Information J*. 2000;34:1053–1061.

14. Malecha SE, Wiejowski SA, Holt RJ. The applied therapeutic team: an innovative model of drug information in the pharmaceutical industry. *Drug Information J*. 2000;34:1069–1075.

15. Food and Drug Administration. Guidance for industry: industry-supported scientific and educational activities. Part III. *Federal Register*. 1997;62(232):64073–64100.

16. Kline S. Medical-legal considerations regarding the provision of medication-related information to consumers by a pharmaceutical manufacturer. *Drug Information J*. 2000;34:1017–1020.

17. Curran CF, Oh KE. Sources of drug information available to consumers. *Drug Information J*. 2001;35:539–546.

18. Graves DA. Provision of medical information for drugs used in orphan and pediatric disorders. *Drug Information J*. 1999;33:87–90.

19. Curran CF. Planning for variations in level of inquiries received by drug information departments. *Drug Information J*. 2001;35:219–224.

20. Curran CF, Sundar MN, Wesche DR. A same-day standard for responding to drug information requests by a pharmaceutical company. *Drug Information J*. 2003;37:241–249.

21. Gaspic M, Biondi L, Flowers T. Medical information on demand. *Drug Information J*. 1998;32:289–292.

22. Johnson ST, Wordell CJ. Internet utilization among medical information specialists in the pharmaceutical industry and academia. *Drug Information J*. 1998;32:547–554.

23. Agoratus S. Developing a knowledge interface for a document management system. *Drug Information J*. 1999;33:95–99.

24. Yamamoto M, Negi H, Funabashi S, Okada S. Development and utilization of a package insert information retrieval system in the pharmaceutical industry. *Drug Information J*. 1998;32:1109–1117.

25. Curran CF, Buxton MM. Streamlining the information retrieval process in the drug information department. *Drug Information J*. 2001;35:921–933.

26. Riggins JL. Establishing global medical information services: practices and pitfalls. *Drug Information J*. 2000;34:1077–1080.

27. Firth N, Davis LJ, Murray KM, Graves DA. Outsourcing industry medical information services. *Drug Information J*. 2000;34:1105–1113.

28. Donald T, Marsh C, Ashworth L. An assessment of preparation methods and personnel require ments in a medical information department during product launch. *Drug Information J*. 2007;41:241–249.

29. Umrath T, Bess AL. Establishing an adverse event collection team in a pharmaceutical company safety department: impact on report quality and customer satisfaction. *Drug Information J*. 2005;39:81–88.

30. Goldman SA. Auditing safety-related processes and procedures: lessons learned for global compliance and quality. *Drug Information J*. 2006;40:165–175.

31. Werner AL, Murray KM. Preparing for a product launch in a medical communications department. *Drug Information J*. 2000;34:1021–1033.

32. Holt RJ, Finnegan PW, Alexander JC. Making markets and the global medical information imperative: the heat is on! *Drug Information J*. 2001;35:225–230.

33. Shannon ME, Malecha SE, Cha AJ, Moody ML. Evaluation and critical appraisal of a random sample of drug information practice in United States academic and industry medical information centers. *Drug Information J*. 2000;34:1133–1138.

34. Doyle RI, Song KH, Baker RP. An industry-wide evaluation of drug information services. *Drug Information J*. 2000;34:1139–1148.

35. Rawn P. Hoffman-La Roche LTD. Drug information and safety department survey of customer needs and satisfaction. *Drug Information J.* 1999;33:525–539.

36. Fung SM, Martin JS. Quality assurance practice for pharmaceutical industry-based drug information departments: a review and case study. *Drug Information J.* 2004;38:395–405.

37. Riggins JL. Pharmaceutical industry as a career choice. *Am J Health-Syst Pharm.* 2002;59:2097–2098.

38. Fus AF. Drug information clerkships in the pharmaceutical industry. *Drug Information J.* 1998;32:305–311.

39. Riggins JL, Winn JL. Eli Lilly and Company Global Medical Information: pharmacy student clerkships in industry. *Drug Information J.* 1998;32:283–288.

40. American Society of Health-System Pharmacists. Educational goals and learning objectives for postgraduate year 2 drug information residencies. Available at: http://www.ashp.org. Accessed April 18, 2007.

41. American Society of Health-System Pharmacists. Online residency directory. Available at: http://www.ashp.org. Accessed February 19, 2007.

42. McCart GM, Grobman BJ, Tsourounis C, Graves DA. A combined industry and academia residency program. *Drug Information J.* 2000;34:1115–1119.

43. Wolin MJ, Ayers PM, Chan EK. The emerging role of medical affairs within the modern pharmaceutical company. *Drug Information J.* 2001;35:547–555.

44. Curran CF. The evolving role of the United States industry-based drug information departments. *Drug Information J.* 2003;37:439–443.

45. Riggins JL, Ferguson KJ, Miller SI. Globalizing medical information services at Eli Lilly and Company. *Drug Information J.* 1999;33:515–524.

Drug Safety and Pharmacovigilance

Patrick McDonnell

In May 1999, Merck gained approval by the Food and Drug Administration (FDA) to market the drug rofecoxib (Vioxx), a subclass of nonsteroidal anti-inflammatory drugs (NSAIDs) designed to inhibit selectively cyclooxygenase-2 (COX-2). The development of these drugs was based on the hypothesis that the source of inflammation, prostaglandin E_2 and I_2, was mediated by COX-2, and the source of those same prostaglandins that provided protection to the gastric epithelium was mediated by cyclooxygenase-1 (COX-1). By selectively inhibiting only COX-2, patients would have the benefits of therapeutic anti-inflammatory effects, yet still have the cytoprotection of the gastric prostaglandins, reducing the risks of NSAID-induced gastropathy.[1]

On September 30, 2004, Merck withdrew rofecoxib because of an excess risk of myocardial infarctions and stroke. This withdrawal occurred after rofecoxib had been used in more than 80 million patients with annual sales exceeding $2.5 billion, representing the largest prescription drug market in history.[2] In November 2004, Dr. David J. Graham, MD, MPH, Associate Director for Science and Medicine in the FDA's Office of Drug Safety, testified before a congressional committee regarding the rofecoxib withdrawal, stating, "Today, in 2004, you, we, are faced with what may be the single greatest drug safety catastrophe in the history of this country in the history of the world. We are talking about a catastrophe that I strongly believe could have, should have been largely or completely avoided." Graham goes on to state, "In my opinion, the FDA has let the American people down, and, sadly, betrayed a public trust."[3]

These are strong and dramatic statements from one of the leaders in the nation's regulatory body for drug safety. The rofecoxib withdrawal as well as the Institute of Medicine's (IOM) controversial 1999 report *Too Err Is Human: Building a Safer Health System*, which stated that from 44,000 to 98,000 people die each year in hospitals as the result of preventable medication error,[4] have brought the issue of drug safety to the forefront of health care in the early 21st century.

■ History of Drug Safety in the United States

The legislative history of drug safety in the United States has just noted its centennial anniversary with the 1906 Pure Food and Drug Act. This law prohibited interstate commerce of adulterated and misbranded drugs and food. This was the first law that covered *some* safety aspects of drugs, but did not focus on their efficacy. To strengthen against manufacturers of drugs who make false efficacious claims, this law was changed in 1912 to prohibit statements regarding fraudulent drug efficacy claims.

In 1937, a company in the United States manufactured a sulfamonide elixir. This product led to the death of more than 100 people as a result of diethylene glycol toxicity contained in this antibiotic elixir. Because current laws did not require mandated safety testing for drugs, companies were not required to do so. In 1938, the FDA passed a milestone law in the history of drug safety known as the Federal Food, Drug, and Cosmetic Act, which required that safety testing be performed prior to marketing a drug. Proof of this safety mandate was submitted to the FDA in a New Drug Application (NDA). Throughout the next decade additional laws were passed requiring testing for the quality, purity, and strength of drugs.

The next milestone of drug safety was in the early 1960s when an NDA for the drug thalidomide was strongly opposed by Dr. Frances Kelsey at the FDA. Thalidomide was used in Canada and western Europe for the treatment of morning sickness in pregnant women. Women who used thalidomide in early pregnancy were giving birth to children with horrible limb defects known as phocomelia ("seal/flipper limbs" *Greek*). Despite strong pressure to approve thalidomide in the United States, Dr. Kelsey recognized the link of thalidomide and its teratogenic effects and successfully prevented an extenuation of the "thalidomide tragedy" in the United States. Arising from this incident, the Kefauver–Harris amendment became law in 1962 and required drug manufacturers to demonstrate both safety and efficacy to the FDA before the drug would be approved for marketing.

In 1971, the National Drug Experience Reporting System began evolving into the current MedWatch program. This postmarketing surveillance program allows for the reporting of spontaneous adverse drug reactions (ADRs). The program is voluntary for practitioners but is mandatory for pharmaceutical companies, who must report on ADRs they receive. Pharmacoepidemiologists from the FDA continually mine the MedWatch database for potential signals that may suggest a trend of a new or serious adverse drug reaction.

Over the ensuing years, the FDA has had multiple alterations in its structure and function with the Center for Drug Evaluation and Research (CDER) being the subdivision overseeing drug safety and efficacy.

The widely publicized recall of Vioxx in 2004 , as mentioned, is now having all in health care take a second look at current drug safety monitoring and regulations calling for reforms in the FDA's procedures for both pre- and postmarketing drug safety regulation. In response to a growing public concern with health risks posed by approved drugs triggered by the Vioxx withdrawal, the FDA has partnered with the Institute of Medicine (IOM) to conduct an independent assessment of the current system for evaluating and ensuring postmarketing drug safety and to make recommendations to improve risk assessment, surveillance, and the safe use of drugs.[5]

■ Classifications of Adverse Drug Events

Medication errors and the focus of this chapter, adverse drug reactions (ADRs), are just two types of adverse drug events (ADEs). Many feel that an ADE is synonymous with an ADR, so I shall begin with some definitions. To simplify, an ADE is any unfavorable event associated with the use of a drug or drug therapy. The official and accepted definitions used by most are based on the International Conference on Harmonisation (ICH) E2A Guidelines.[6] These definitions are as follows: "Any untoward medical occurrence in a patient or clinical investigation subject administered a pharmaceutical product and which does not necessarily have to have a causal relationship with this treatment"; and "Any unfavorable or unintended sign, symptom, or disease temporally associated with the use of any dose of a medicinal product, whether or not considered related to the medicinal product."

In reference to an ADR there is a defined temporal relationship to the adverse event and the administration of a drug. One of the most common definitions of an ADR is the one used by the World Health Organization (WHO): "any response to a drug that is noxious or unintended, and that occurs at doses normally used in man for the prophylaxis, diagnosis, or therapy of disease."[7] This definition will be elaborated, but in addition to ADRs, this chapter briefly discusses the other forms of ADRs.

Medication errors are another classification of an ADE. Medication errors are defined as "unintended acts (either of commission or omission) resulting in actual or potential harm to a patient, or an act that does not achieve its intended outcome when dealing with drug therapy."[7] Examples of medication errors of commission are generally when something blatant but unintended occurs in drug therapy, that is, a patient is supposed to receive the drug Lamictal (lamotrigine) for seizure control but receives the drug Lamisil (terbinafine) for onychomycosis instead. Or a patient is supposed to receive 1 mg of warfarin and the order is written as "1.0" mg, and this patient is mistakenly given 10 mg of warfarin. The error of commission has occurred, but whether or not it harms the patient shall remain to be seen depending on when the error is discovered along the medication use process system. Medication errors of omission are those that occur when someone fails to detect an important factor in a patient's drug therapy regimen, such as a clinical significant drug interaction or allergy history, failure to detect a disease state contraindication therapy, or the omission of conveying important drug information to prescribers and patients resulting in potential or actual harm.

Two types of ADEs do occur when drug therapy sometimes is "not given" or "not optimally given": *therapeutic failures* and *adverse drug withdrawal events* (ADWEs).[8] In a therapeutic failure, very often suboptimal amounts of drug for some reason or another occur, resulting in a disease state or condition not stabilizing or symptoms becoming worse. For example, certain antibiotics cannot be given at the same time with other drugs that contain minerals because the antibiotic will bind/chelate to these minerals and not be available for absorption, resulting in a treatment failure. Other times, a patient may not fully understand the importance of the drug therapy, especially in chronic disease states, and does not take the drug as prescribed or discontinues therapy altogether. An ADWE occurs when patients on long-term therapies with certain agents experience a withdrawal syndrome when the drug is discontinued, in most cases abruptly. Good examples of ADWEs include rebound hypertension in patients on long-term clonidine use or agitation and/or seizures in patients abruptly discontinuing long-term benzodiazepine therapy.

The last general class of ADEs is an *overdose*, either intentional overdoses or accidental overdoses. How an overdose differs from an ADR is that the doses in these events are not "those that are normally used to treat disease."

You must keep in mind that these definitions are not exclusive of each other and can overlap. Many times some classes of ADEs have a facet of preventability to them and are forms of medication errors. One example[9] is when a patient taking the drug azathioprine for a heart transplant developed the ADR of pancytopenia. The patient was also taking the drug allopurinol for hyperuricemia. There is a well-documented drug interaction between these two agents, and when allopurinol therapy is initiated with concomitant azathioprine therapy, the dose of azathioprine must be decreased by 50–75% to avoid the adverse reaction of bone marrow suppression and resultant pancytopenia. In this case, this interaction was neither detected nor acted upon. The ADR in this case is "pancytopenia" and the medication error in this case was the "omission of detecting a clinical significant drug interaction."

■ Adverse Drug Reactions: Classifications, Severity, Outcomes, and Probability

Returning now to the focus on ADRs, generally two types of ADRs are identified. Type A ADRs are those that are related to the drug's pharmacology and are an extension of these pharmacology effects. They are *A*ugmentations of these effects, such as unintended hypoglycemia from insulin or unintended hypoprothrombinemia with bleeding in a patient on warfarin. Type A ADRs account for about 80% of all ADRs and are dose related. They are, of course, predictable and in many cases potentially preventable. Many times these are referred to as side effects. The term *side effect* often discounts these commonly occurring ADRs and may be a reason that these events are not reported to appropriate bodies that review drug safety. Nonetheless, these events can significantly contribute to a patient's morbidity and mortality and should be viewed as true ADRs.

The other classification of ADRs is type B or *Bizarre-type* reactions. These are reactions that are neither dose related nor related to the drug's pharmacologic effect. Type B reactions may be immunologic or genetically based, or may have some idiosyncratic mechanism of occurrence. Because they are not predictable, they are generally not preventable. They account for approximately 10–20% of ADRs.

Criteria to determine the severity of an ADR are most commonly derived from guidelines and standards from the FDA and the American Society of Health System Pharmacists (ASHP).[10] Severe ADRs are those reactions that are potentially life-threatening, cause permanent damage or even death, or require intensive medical care. ADRs classified as moderate are those that require a change in drug therapy (usually discontinuation of that therapy or dose reduction) and/or initiation of specific treatment to prevent further harm to the patient. Moderate ADRs have symptoms that resolve in more than 24 hours, prolong a hospital length of stay by more than 24 hours, or are the cause of a hospital admission (nonintensive care). Minor ADRs generally have manifestations that resolve in less than 24 hours, do not contribute to a hospital admission, do not prolong a hospital length of stay, or require no therapy or minor intervention for the reaction. Many times the drug therapy is able to be continued during minor reactions.

Although most outcomes from ADRs cause little more than annoyance or inconvenience, the more serious outcomes reported to the FDA were hospitalization (24.1%), threats to life (6.1%), and fatalities (7.1%).[11]

Probability that a reaction is caused by a drug sometimes is difficult to determine. It should be noted that to state emphatically that an adverse event is 100% totally attributed to a drug is more the exception than the rule. Nonetheless it should not deter reporting that event with a temporal relationship to a specific drug therapy. Using clinical judgment alone is often not sufficient enough to make this decision as to whether the drug is the cause because using this method alone has shown poor correlation.[12]

One of the most widely used and validated tools to assess the likelihood that a specific drug is the cause of a specific adverse reaction is the Naranjo algorithm.[13] (See FIGURE 9-1.) This algorithm uses a series of 10 questions with specific numerical values assigned to these assessments to determine an overall score for probability that the event was drug related. A Naranjo score greater than 9 indicates an ADR was definite, scores of 5 to 8 indicate a "probable" event, scores of 1 to 4 indicate "possible" event, and less than 1 indicates a doubtful drug causality. Limitations do exist with this algorithm, and other algorithms exist but do not seem to be as practical or easy to use as the Naranjo algorithm.

Of the three criteria revolving around the regulatory reportability of an individual ADR case (seriousness, expectedness, and causality), causality is often the most difficult to determine when dealing with new drug entities. Generally, in clinical trials

Question	Yes	No	Do Not Know	Score
1. Are there previous conclusive reports on this reaction?	+1	0	0	
2. Did the adverse reaction appear when the drug was administered?	+2	−1	0	
3. Did the adverse reaction improve when the drug was discontinued or a specific antagonist was administered?	+1	0	0	
4. Did the adverse reaction reappear when the drug was readministered?	+2	−1	0	
5. Are there alternate causes (other than the drug) that could solely have caused reaction?	−1	+2	0	
6. Did the reaction reappear when a placebo was given?	−1	+1	0	
7. Was the drug detected in the blood (or other fluids) in a concentration known to be toxic?	+1	0	0	
8. Was the reaction more severe when the dose was increased, or less severe when the dose was decreased?	+1	0	0	
9. Did the patient have a similar reaction to the same or similar drugs in any previous exposure?	+1	0	0	
10. Was the adverse event confirmed by objective evidence?	+1	0	0	
				Total Score

FIGURE 9-1 Naranjo algorithm for determining probability of an ADR.[13]

causality of an ADR with a new drug is determined by the medical research group. Decisions must be made as to whether the event was related or unrelated; there is no gray zone. Unless a case is clearly defined as absolutely unrelated, the causality therefore shall be deemed "related." Those assigned the task of evaluating ADRs must use their experience and introspection in the clinical development of a drug to determine the safety of the agent.

■ Overview of the Scope of the Drug Safety Problem

Adverse drug reactions have been referred to tongue-in-cheek as "America's other drug problem." There really is no drug that is totally safe. What may benefit one patient therapeutically may not be worth the risk of an ADR in another. ADRs occur because of something inherent in the drug, something inherent in the patient, and the combination of these factors.

The costs of ADRs relating to patient morbidity and mortality and, in turn, economics are staggering. The annual cost of drug-related morbidity and mortality in the Unites States has been estimated at more than $136 billion annually.[14,15] Adverse drug reactions occur in all patient settings. Epidemiologic studies indicate that ADRs occur in 5–20% of all hospitalized patients.[16,17] In addition, ADRs can occur in an outpatient setting and can result in hospital admission.[18–22] One recent study (2006) examined just emergency department visits for ADEs and found they accounted for 2.5% of emergency department visits for all unintentional injury and 6.7% of those leading to hospitalizations.[23] As mentioned earlier, causes of these events are inherent in the drug, patient factors, and the combination of these factors. However, what exacerbates both inherent drug and patient factors and increases the risk of an ADR are unsafe practices by healthcare professionals. These include prescribing errors, dispensing errors, administration errors (by self-administration or by nurses in institutionalized patients), and omissions in monitoring. These are considered to be factors involved in preventable ADRs and, because they involve oversights along the medication use process system, are considered to be medication errors of omission. Studies that examine factors relating to preventable ADRs and medication errors of omission report a range of 28–80% of all ADRs being potentially preventable.[24–28]

The Hippocratic Oath "do no harm" is still the credo of medicine, but yet as you can observe, for all the good that drugs do, there still is an overwhelming problem with ADRs. Weighing risks against benefits is one of the most significant factors in determining which patients should get which specific drugs. Trying to identify who will experience an ADR is dependent on many factors. The next sections discuss the inherent factor of the drug and how adverse drug reactions are detected, focusing on new drug entities in the pre- and postmarket periods.

■ ADRs With New Drug Entities: Clinical Trial Sample Size and Postmarketing Surveillance

To gain marketing approval of a drug in the United States and most other countries, a series of clinical trials on patients is required. The scope of these trials is dependent on expected factors inherent to the drug (eg, a novel advanced therapeutic entity, one that may be expected to have toxicities, already approved for other uses and in other formulations), the medical indication being treated (from minor symptomatic relief to life-threatening disease states such as cancer), and the patient-specific population (concurrent comorbid conditions, age, weight, etc.). Following the proper toxicologic and pharmacologic testing in vitro and in animal studies, the drug is then ready to be tested in humans.

A brief review of human clinical trials is as follows. In the United States, the investigator (usually a pharmaceutical company, but sometimes an academic center or individual) submits what is known as an Investigational New Drug (IND) application to the FDA. This contains the protocol for the clinical trial along with introductory data about the drug. The human clinical trials then begin with what is known as the phase 1 portion of the trial.

Phase 1 trials deal with the drug's pharmacokinetics (sometimes referred to as ADME trials, meaning absorption, distribution, metabolism, excretion) and human pharmacology. This phase in primarily designed to find optimal tolerated doses and pathways for metabolism and excretion. Generally, healthy volunteers are selected for these trials and these subjects are generally not the patients for whom the drug therapy is designed for treatment. Safety more than efficacy is the focus of the phase 1 clinical trial. These trials are usually short in duration and patient enrollment is small in number. Serious adverse events are usually rare in this type of trial.

Once a successful phase 1 trial is completed, the phase 2 trial proceeds. Phase 2 trials enroll patients who have the disease for which the particular drug was developed. These trials continue to focus on safety, but efficacy is also observed and measured. One goal of this trial is therefore to find the minimal efficacious doses with the minimal adverse effects. These studies enroll hundreds of patients and may run several weeks to months. The investigators must pay closer attention to serious adverse effects because the *n* for patient enrollment has markedly increased. Any severe or unexpected adverse drug reactions that occur in this phase may be a reason to stop the trial immediately or reevaluate the dose to lessen the likelihood of toxicity. Once this phase of the trial is complete and approved, the trial is ready to progress to phase 3.

Phase 3 trials include hundreds to thousands of the patients with the primary goal of gaining regulatory approval from the FDA to market the drug. Participants in this phase are still those with medical conditions for which the drug was developed. Phase 3 trials are a pivotal portion of the New Drug Application (NDA) dossier submitted to the FDA. These trials are usually double-blinded and multisite, and the new drug being studied is compared to a known and accepted therapy or placebo when applicable and ethical. Phase 3 trials may last several years with a focus still on both efficacy and safety. Again, based on the number of patients enrolled in the trial, serious or unexpected adverse reactions *may* have an increased likelihood of being revealed.

With successful completion of phase 1, 2, and 3 studies, the drug can now be approved. Phase 4 studies are postapproval and postmarketing trials. They may focus on issues such as marketing and pharmacoeconomics, but an extremely important portion of these trials may be specific safety issues. Sometimes these trials can be very large pharmacoepidemiologic studies done in sizeable databases to identify an incidence or patient population at risk for a particular ADR.

It is important to note that all adverse events must be collected in all phases of a clinical trial. Both serious and nonserious adverse drug events should be collected until you can fully understand the safety profile of the drug and attribute relatedness of the ADE to the drug (making it now an ADR). For the most part, the FDA requires only that expected serious adverse events (SAEs), if agreed upon by the FDA and sponsor, and nonserious ADEs be reported at the end of the clinical phase of a trial. Otherwise, SAEs, expected and especially nonexpected, must be collected by the trial's drug safety group and reported within 15 days to the FDA.[29] In the postmarketing surveillance period of a drug, all serious ADEs whether they are expected or not expected are still required to be reported to the FDA as part of the company's NDA for that drug.

Although clinical trials have highly regulated methodology, they do have significant limitations in defining a drug safety profile. Generally, because of the sample size of the trial only frequently occurring ADRs are discovered. For example, if a study enrolls 10,000 patients and not a single patient has a particular serious ADR, you can be only 95% confident that the chance of having a serious ADR in that sample size is less than 1 in 3333. If the threshold for safety is raised to a confidence interval of 99% that a serious ADR would occur with an incidence of 1 in 10,000 patients (or any ADR for that matter), the study would need to have 46,000 people participating.[30]

The 1994 international drug safety standard for a chronically administered drug used long term to treat a non-life-threatening condition recommends that 1500 patients be exposed overall with 600 treated for 6 months and 300 for one year.[31,32] This is considered to be adequate to detect an ADR occurring in 1 of every 300 to 500 patients. These would be deemed the more common ADRs. Even though NDAs contain data on thousands of patients, current drug trials are not large enough for reliable detection of very rare, serious ADRs.

An example of how serious ADRs were not detected until a drug was used in millions in the postmarketing experience is the drug bromfenac, an NSAID that was marketed for acute pain and inflammation. Bromfenac was removed from the market after use in approximately 2.5 million patients because of reports of fatal liver toxicity linked to its use. The incidence of death as a result of hepatotoxicity with bromfenac was below the practical detection limit of most clinical trial protocols. Serious liver damage occurred in approximately 1 in 20,000 patients who used bromfenac for more than 10 days. To reliably detect serious hepatotoxicity in the bromfenac clinical trials, the NDA databases would have had to include 100,000 patients.[31] Even labeling changes[33] to bromfenac's indication (less than 10 days of use) did not eliminate prescribers and patients using this drug longer than 10 days, and given the availability of other analgesics with a much wider safety margin, the FDA believed the risk of hepatotoxicity did not outweigh any benefit as an analgesic/anti-inflammatory agent. Both the FDA and the manufacturer,

TABLE 9-1	Comparison of Patients Exposed to Withdrawn Drugs in Clinical Trials Compared With Actual Use After Approval[31]	
Drug Name	Patients (n) Exposed in Clinical Trials	Approximate Patient (n) Exposed Prior to Withdrawal
Terfenadine	5000	7,500,000
Mibefradil	3400	600,000
Bromfenac	2400	2,500,000
Dexfenfluramine	1200	2,300,000
Fenfluramine	340	6,900,000

Wyeth-Ayerst, did not believe any further labeling warnings would prevent further patient harm and therefore the company withdrew the product.

Therefore, the importance of postmarketing surveillance cannot be stressed enough. An example of how postmarketing surveillance resulted in the identification of serious ADRs in currently marketed drugs occurred during the period of September 1997 through September 1998 when five already marketed prescription drugs were removed from the market because of the identification of unexpected adverse reactions that were not evident in the clinical trials.[31] (See TABLE 9-1.)

The FDA's postmarketing drug safety surveillance program consists of the Adverse Event Reporting System, which gathers and analyzes spontaneous reports from companies as part of the NDA protocols or through spontaneous reports from healthcare workers sent directly to the FDA via the MedWatch program. Serious events are then individually examined with epidemiologic analyses. From the analysis and identification of these serious ADRs, labeling changes or mailings to health professionals may occur, or the drug might even be removed from the market as a result.

■ Current Problems With Drug Safety and the FDA

With the Vioxx withdrawal in 2004, requests for significant changes in drug safety have been proposed. An excellent review article[34] identifies eight major problems with the current system of assessment and assurance of drug safety at the FDA:

1. The design of initial preapproval studies lets uncommon, serious adverse events go undetected.
2. There is a massive underreporting of adverse events to the FDA postmarketing surveillance system which reduces the ability to accurately quantity risk.
3. Manufacturers do not fulfill the majority of their postmarketing surveillance safety study commitments.

4. The FDA lacks the authority to pursue sponsors who violate regulations and ignore their postmarketing safety study commitments.
5. The public increasingly perceives the FDA as being too close to properly regulate the pharmaceutical industry.
6. The safety oversight structure at the FDA is suboptimal.
7. There is a shortage of experts in the area of drug safety and public health at the FDA and in its advisory committees.
8. The drug safety system is inadequate, inappropriately funding, and depends on industry user fees.

■ Proposals for Improvement in Drug Safety

The US Congress, which is ultimately responsible for the performance of the FDA, is urged to do the following[34]:

1. Give the FDA more direct legal authority to pursue violators of their drug safety commitment.
2. For selected drugs authorize the adoption of a conditional drug approval policy.
3. Provide additional resources to support the safety infrastructure of the FDA.
4. Mandate a reorganization of the FDA with the emphasis on improving and strengthening a proactive monitoring program for drug safety.
5. Command a broader representation of drug safety experts and epidemiologists on advisory committees of the FDA.

Currently, several bills are in Congress after the wake of the Vioxx withdrawal and these include the following[34]:

- The Food and Drug Administration Safety Act of 2005 (S 930) would, if passed, give the FDA the authority and independence to implement fully the task of drug safety.
- The Fair Access to Clinical Trials Act of 2005 (S 470), which requires clinical trials be registered and all results, whether positive or negative, for either safety and/or efficacy be posted. Noncompliance would result in monetary penalties.
- The Pharmaceutical Research and Manufacturers Accountability Act of 2005 (HR 879), which would send drug industry CEOs to prison for a minimum of 20 years if they knowingly conceal information regarding serious ADE experiences. CEOs of these companies would be required to attest that all serious adverse drug events have been disclosed. Timelines to complete postmarketing drug safety studies would also be part of this law and would lead to fines up to $5 million for each month that the study goes unfinished.

Conclusion

There is no 100% completely safe drug. Drugs are treated by our bodies as being "foreign" or xenobiotics, so mostly they are treated as potential toxins. Sometimes there is a fine line between efficacy and toxicity, a fine line between risk and benefit. Nonetheless, the countless number of lives saved by drugs cannot be denied; neither can the expected (and sometimes not-so-expected) toxic effects of drugs because it is estimated that deaths from drugs rank among the top 10 causes of death in the United States.[14] It is not only up to the pharmaceutical industry and the FDA to be the caretakers and guardians of drug safety. All in health care have to play a role in being "pharmacovigilantes" either by continued reporting of adverse drug reactions to the FDA or industry; ensuring that the right drug goes to the right patient because one size does not fit all when referring to drugs, dosing, and concurrent disease states; and ensuring patients trust that collectively we shall truly do no harm.

References

1. Fitzgerald GA. Coxibs and cardiovascular disease. *NEJM*. 2005;351:1709–1711.

2. Topol EJ. Failing the public health—rofecoxib, Merck, and the FDA. *NEJM*. 2004; 351:1707–1709.

3. Testimony of David J. Graham, MD, MPH, November 18, 2004. Available at: http://www.finance.senate.gov/hearings/testimony/2004test/111804dgtest.pdf. Accessed December 12, 2008.

4. Kohn LT, Corrigan JM, Donaldson M. *To Err Is Human: Building a Safer Health System*. Washington, DC: Institute of Medicine; 1999.

5. Baciu A, Stratton K, Burke SP, eds. *The Future of Drug Safety: Promoting and Protecting the Health of the Public: Committee on the Assessment of the US Drug Safety*. Washington, DC: National Academy of Sciences; 2007.

6. Center for Drug Evaluation and Research. Adverse event reporting system (AERS). Available at: http://www.fda.gov/cder/aers/default.htm. Accessed December 12, 2008.

7. World Health Organization. *International Drug Monitoring: The Role of the Hospital*. Technical Report Series No. 425. 1969;426:5–24.

8. Leape L. A systems analysis approach to medical error. In: Cohen M, ed. *Medication Error*. Washington, DC: American Pharmaceutical Association; 1999:2.1.

9. McDonnell PJ. $181,000 adverse drug reaction. *Hosp Pharm*. 2004;39(7):648–652.

10. American Society of Health-Systems Pharmacists. ASHP guidelines on adverse drug reaction reporting and monitoring. *Am J Health-Syst Pharm*. 1995;52:417–419.

11. Center for Drug Evaluation and Research. *Annual Adverse Drug Experience Report: 1996*. October 30, 1997. Available at: http://www.fda.gov/CDER/dpe/annrep96/index.htm. Accessed December 12, 2008.

12. Koch-Weser J, Sellers EM, Zacest R. The ambiguity of adverse drug reactions. *Europ J Clin Pharmacol*. 1977;11:75–78.

13. Naranjo CA, Busto U, Sellers EM, et al. A method for determining the probability of adverse drug reactions. *Clin Pharmacol Ther*. 1982:30(2):239–245.

14. Johnson JA, Bootman JL. Drug-related morbidity and mortality: a cost of illness model. *Arch Intern Med.* 1995;155:1949–1956.

15. Talley RB, Laventurier MF. Drug-induced illness. *JAMA.* 1974;229:1043–1048.

16. Colt HG, Shapiro AP. Drug-induced illness as a cause for admissions to a community hospital. *J Am Geriatr Soc.* 1989;37:323–326.

17. Lakshamanan MC, Hershey CO, Breslau D. Hospital admissions caused by iatrogenic disease. *Arch Intern Med.* 1986;146:1931–1934.

18. Dartnell JG, Robert PA, Chohan V. Hospitalisations for adverse events related to drug therapy: incidence, avoidability, and costs. *Med J Aust.* 1996;164:659–662.

19. Caranosos GJ, Stewart RB, Cluff LE. Drug-induced illness leading to hospitalization. *JAMA.* 1974;228:713–717.

20. Miller RR. Hospital admissions due to adverse drug reactions: a report from the Boston Collaborative Drug Surveillance Program. *Arch Intern Med.* 1974;134:219–223.

21. Bates DW, Cullen DJ, Laird N, et al. Incidence of adverse drug events and potential adverse drug events—implications for prevention. *JAMA.* 1995;274:29–34.

22. Jick H. Adverse drug reactions: the magnitude of the problem. *J Allergy Clin Immunol.* 1994;164:659–662.

23. Budnitz DS, Pollock DA, Weidenbach KN, et al. National surveillance of emergency department visits for outpatient adverse drug events. *JAMA.* 2006;296:1858–1866.

24. McDonnell PJ, Jacobs MR. Hospital admissions resulting from preventable adverse drug reactions. *Ann Pharmacother.* 2002;3:1331–1336.

25. Burnun JF. Preventability of adverse drug reactions (letter). *Ann Intern Med.* 1976;85:80–81.

26. Bosh TK, Schulz L, Swerlein A. Identification of preventable adverse drug reactions using medical record E-codes (abstract). Presented at: 49th ASHP Annual Meeting, Washington, DC. June 2–8, 1992.

27. Porter J, Hershel J. Drug-related deaths among medical inpatients. *JAMA.* 1977;237:879–881.

28. Melmon KL. Preventable drug reactions—causes and cures. *N Engl J Med.* 1971;284:1361–1368.

29. Andrews EA, et al., International Society for Pharmacoepidemiology. Guidelines for good epidemiology practices for drug, device, and vaccine research in the United States. *Pharmacoepidemiol Drug Saf.* 1996;5(5):333–338.

30. Cobert B. *Manual of Drug Safety and Pharmacovigilance.* Sudbury, Mass: Jones and Bartlett; 2007:11–13.

31. Friedman MA, Woodcock J, Lumpkin MM, et al. The safety of newly approved medications: do recent market removals mean there is a problem? *JAMA.* 1999;281:1728–1734.

32. Guideline for Industry. The extent of population exposure to assess clinical safety: for drugs intended for long-term treatment of non-life-threatening conditions. http://www.hc-sc.gc.ca/dhp-mps/prod-pharma/applic-demande/guide-ld/ich/efficac/e1-eng.php. Food and Drug Administration. Wyeth-Ayerst Laboratories announces the withdrawal of Duract from the market. *FDA Talk Papers.* June 22, 1998. Available at: http://www.fda.gov/bbs/topics/ANSWERS/ANS00879.html. Accessed December 12, 2008.

33. Furber CD, Levin AA, Gross PA, et al. The FDA and drug safety: a proposal for sweeping changes. *Arch Intern Med.* 2006;166:1938–1942.

Legal and Intellectual Property

Michel F. Snyder

The pharmaceutical industry, in the aggregate, spends upward of $30 billion on research and development.[1] As you can imagine, such an enormous output of resources would not be justified unless there were incentives in place to reward such research and development. Various intellectual property systems throughout the world provide an incentive to the pharmaceutical industry for vigorous research and development programs by providing a means through which a pharmaceutical company can protect its developments. This chapter provides an overview of the interface between the pharmaceutical industry and intellectual property protection, with the focus on the United States intellectual property system.

■ The Patent System

The United States Constitution, Article I, Section 8, states that "Congress shall have the power . . . to promote the progress of science and useful arts, by securing for limited times to . . . inventors the exclusive right to their . . . discoveries." This constitutional article provides the basis for the United States patent system. Accordingly, a patent is a limited monopoly to a particular invention, and as a legal monopoly, it is therefore a very valuable form of property. Patents are available for "any new and useful process, machine, manufacture, or composition of matter, or any new and useful improvement thereof."[2] Clearly, there are many developments in the pharmaceutical industry that fall into the various categories for which patents can be sought.

A patent does not give the patent owner the right to do and/or make anything. Rather, the patent right is a "right to exclude." A patent owner has the exclusive right, for a limited time, to exclude others from making, using, selling, or offering for sale the patented invention.[3] Even the owner of a patent may not be able to practice its own invention if doing so would infringe on the superior rights of another patent owner.

Accordingly, patent licensing and cross-licensing are common practices for exploiting inventions.

Conditions for Patentability

To obtain a patent on a new invention, there are four main conditions for patentability. The first is that the invention must be directed to "patentable subject matter," that is, within the scope of the types of inventions for which the patent system will allow protection. The scope of patentable subject matter has been broadly construed to "include anything under the sun that is made by man."[4] Patentable subject matter would include, for example, genetically modified microorganisms. However, abstract ideas, laws of nature, and natural phenomena are not patentable subject matter because these exist without any inventive act.[5]*

The second condition for patentability is that the invention must be useful, that is, it must have utility.[2] This is a very low threshold and is met by nearly any invention having even the slightest utility.[6]

The third condition for patentability is that the invention must be novel.[7] The novelty requirement essentially means that no single article or item in the "prior art" (eg, anything existing prior to the date of invention) discloses every element of the invention. When a single article or item in the prior art discloses every element of the invention, the invention is said to be "anticipated" and, therefore, unpatentable.

The fourth condition for patentability is that the invention must not be "obvious" to a person of ordinary skill in the art.[8] An invention is obvious if the differences between the invention and the prior art are such that the subject matter of the patent would have been obvious at the time the invention was made to a person having ordinary skill in the art to which said subject matter of the invention pertains.[8] Rather than looking at just one specific piece of the prior art as in the novelty inquiry, an invention may be found to be obvious by combining several different prior art references or items. For example, if it would have been obvious to one of ordinary skill in the art to combine different elements found in different prior art references to arrive at the invention, the invention is obvious and therefore not patentable.

All of the preceding conditions for patentability must be met to obtain a valid patent. Most countries' patent systems contain similar requirements.[†] Of the conditions for patentability discussed, obtaining a patent is often a struggle between the patent applicant (the person or company seeking the patent) and the United States

---

* "A principle, in the abstract, is a fundamental truth; an original cause; a motive; these cannot be patented, as no one can claim in either of them an exclusive right" (*Le Roy v. Tatham*, 55 US 156, 175 (1852)).
† Some countries have an "absolute novelty" system, where a patent may not be obtained if the invention is publicly disclosed any time prior to filing a patent application. In such countries, patent filing must come before any disclosure.

Patent and Trademark Office (USPTO) over the novelty and nonobviousness of the proposed invention.

Types of Patents

There are two primary types of patents relevant to the pharmaceutical industry. These are utility patents, which include process or method patents, and design patents.

Utility patents are often thought of as covering mechanical inventions such as machines. However, utility patents also cover chemical formulations and biotechnology. A utility patent protects the functional aspects of an invention. An example of a utility patent in the pharmaceutical field is US Patent No. 4,194,009 ("Aryloxyphenyl-propylamines for obtaining a psychotropic effect") and US Patent No. 4,314,081 ("Arloxyphenylpropylamines") (the original patents covering Prozac [fluoxetine]). The owner of the rights to these patents has a limited monopoly for the compounds claimed in the patents.

A process or method patent involves a series of steps directed to producing a useful result. A method of utilizing Prozac for treating anxiety is found in US Patent No. 4,590,213 ("Anti-anxiety method"). The invention of US Patent No. 4,590,213 is "a method for treating anxiety in a human subject in need of such treatment which comprises the administration to said human of an effective amount of fluoxetine or nor-fluoxetine or pharmaceutically acceptable salts thereof."

Design patents may be granted for any new, original, and ornamental design for an article of manufacture.[9] A design patent essentially protects the visual appearance of the design shown in the drawings of the patent. For example, a pharmaceutical manufacturer may wish to protect the appearance of its drug tablet so that the ornamental appearance cannot be copied. The pharmaceutical manufacturer may obtain a design patent covering the tablet's appearance. For example, Merck & Co., Inc., obtained a design patent on the appearance of one version of the Fosamax (alendronate sodium) tablet, as shown in FIGURE 10-1 from US Design Patent No. D380,825 ("Pharmaceutical tablet").

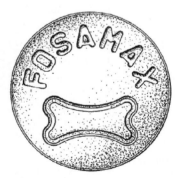

FIGURE 10-1 Fosamax.

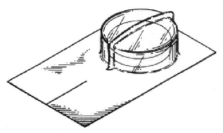

FIGURE 10-2 Blister package.

Design patents are often obtained for product packaging. Warner-Lambert obtained US Design Patent No. D253,515 for "Pharmaceutical blister package." Figure 1 of that patent is reproduced in FIGURE 10-2.

As can be appreciated, overlapping patents (eg, a utility patent and a design patent on the same product) provide for strong protection, potentially allowing a pharmaceutical company to dominate a particular market. A utility patent protecting a chemical compound coupled with a method patent directed to a method of treating a certain disease using that chemical compound will establish a potent monopoly and can box out competitors. In addition, design patents may cover both the appearance of the commercial version of the pharmaceutical tablet including the compound, as well as the packaging for the compound.

The Patent Process

The patent process generally begins with a development that is the result of extensive research. In the pharmaceutical industry, researchers are constantly working on new developments, whether they are new chemical entities, variations of existing chemical entities, or new medical devices. When a new development reaches a certain stage of progress, a pharmaceutical researcher or company can file a patent application for the development. The patent application must contain a complete disclosure of the invention in such detail as would enable a person of ordinary skill in the art to practice the invention.[10]

A patent application is generally prepared by a patent attorney or patent agent. Patent attorneys and patent agents are members of the Patent Bar, which means that they have passed the Examination for Registration to Practice in Patent Cases Before the US Patent and Trademark Office (USPTO) ("Patent Exam"). Only an attorney or agent who has passed the Patent Exam may practice before (correspond with and sign documents submitted to) the USPTO when prosecuting a patent on behalf of another person.*

---

*A party may appear before the USPTO "*pro se*," that is, without representation or representing themselves. However, this is not recommended because the rules for prosecuting a patent are highly technical in nature.

Once a patent application is submitted to the USPTO, it receives a filing date. That filing date is critical because both the date for considering whether something is "prior art" to the invention as well as the life or term of the patent (if one eventually issues) are measured from that date. The filing date will be used in certain circumstances to measure whether or not previous inventions disclosed in patents or printed publications are prior art.

With regard to the patent term, the longer the patent term, the longer the period of time that a pharmaceutical company will have a monopoly over a particular invention. Currently, the patent term is 20 years from the earliest priority date[11]* of the patent.[12] That term begins to run from the date that a patent application is filed and does not take into account the time a patent application is prosecuted through the USPTO. Accordingly, most patents issue "losing" approximately 2 years from their term, with such time taken up prosecuting the patent. The average effective patent life expectancy for pharmaceuticals is 11.5 years.[13]

Because of the tremendous increase in patent application filings each year, the USPTO faces a backlog in its review process. Patent pendency—the amount of time a patent application is waiting for examination before a patent is issued—averages more than 2 years.[14] In more complex technology areas, average pendency stands at more than 3 years.[14] Accordingly, filing a patent application is only the beginning of the process.

Several months after filing a patent application, a patent examiner in the USPTO will review the patent application filing. The patent examiner will conduct a search of the relevant prior art and consider whether the invention in the patent application is useful, novel, and nonobvious in view of the prior art. The patent examiner will then issue an *office action* with an explanation of the patent examiner's view of the invention.

A patent applicant has several options upon receiving an office action from the patent examiner. If the examiner has rejected the invention based upon prior art, the applicant can amend its patent to overcome the examiner's rejections. If there is allowable subject matter, the applicant can accept the allowable subject matter, and a patent will eventually issue. In US patent practice, the applicant can then continue its patent process by filing what are known as *continuation* or *continuation-in-part* patent applications.[11] Such applications claim priority from the earlier or "parent" application. Continuation practice provides a means for a patent applicant to continue to pursue a broad reading of its invention.

As can be appreciated from the foregoing, the patent process is not a simple one. It is often time-consuming and can be quite expensive. However, these are small trade-offs for a potential limited monopoly that could control a billion-dollar-a-year drug.

---

*Patents can claim priority from or relate back to earlier patent applications, such as continuation or continuation-in-part patent applications.

Patent Term Extension and the Pharmaceutical Industry

The Drug Price Competition and Patent Term Restoration Act of 1984 (also known as the Hatch–Waxman Act) amended 35 USC §156 of the Patent Act to provide for the extension of the normal 20-year patent term, if the product that is the subject of the patent is required by federal law to be approved before it is commercially marketed. The Hatch–Waxman Act recognizes the realities of the federal approval process in connection with the pharmaceutical industry. Both the Food and Drug Administration (FDA) and the US Department of Agriculture (USDA) require extensive trials, testing, and reviews of new human and animal drugs to determine both the safety and efficacy of the drugs.[15,16*] The drug approval process includes the submission of years of testing data prior to the federal government approving a drug for use in the United States.

Patent term extension means what it says—the term of a patent may be extended, taking into consideration the regulatory process that prevents a company, at least for a period of time, from receiving an immediate reward for a pharmaceutical invention.[17] Upon a proper application and the requisite showing that a pharmaceutical invention has been held up during the governmental regulatory process, it is possible for a pharmaceutical patent applicant to get back some of the time lost to the regulatory process as an extension on the life of the patent.[18] The Patent Office will make a determination of whether the patent term can be extended based on the information provided in the application for extension.[19] The Patent Office may contact the regulatory agency for information regarding the invention. After reviewing the information provided by the regulatory agency, if the Patent Office determines the patent to be eligible for an extension of the term, a calculation is made as to the length of extension for which the patent is eligible under the appropriate statutory provisions and criteria.[19,20] Extending the life of a patent can have a huge financial impact. Barring competition for even 1 year could translate into profits in the millions or even billions of dollars.

■ Trademarks

A trademark, or brand name,[†] is any distinctive word, phrase, logo, symbol, design, picture, styling, or a combination of one or more of these elements. A trademark is used by a business to identify itself and its products or services to consumers and to set itself and its products or services apart from other businesses. In that way, a trademark designates not only a product, but the source of the product. Thus, it is said that a trademark is a "badge of origin."

---

*See also Kefauver–Harris Amendments of 1962, Pub. L. No. 87-781, 76 Stat. 780 (1962), codified as 21 USC §321.

† The *brand* or *proprietary* name of a drug is the trademark name used by a particular company. The *chemical* name is based on the drug's chemical structure. The *generic* name is the name selected by the United States Adopted Names Council.

Trademarks are critically important to the pharmaceutical industry for many reasons. Consumers rely on branding to select goods or services based on their experiences. Over the course of use, a valuable good will is established between the source of the goods and the consumer. Accordingly, when a consumer has a good experience with a particular brand, the consumer will return to that brand or recommend that brand to others. The trademark, then, signifies a source that instills confidence in a consumer.

Trademarks are also important in distinguishing one company's goods or services from another to protect consumers from confusion. Because trademarks signify a particular source, if the trademarks of two products are too close, confusion or blurring may occur between the marks, the goods, or the services. This could result in not only brand confusion, but catastrophic effects when pharmaceutical agents are confused.

Drug naming, in particular, is an area where the pharmaceutical industry must take great care. Above and beyond source or brand confusion, if two drugs having similar names are confused, devastating medication errors could potentially occur. Medication errors based on name confusion can occur between brand names, between generic names, and even between brand and generic names. Accordingly, although all pharmaceutical products require brand names, prescription drug naming has its own unique set of legal issues.

Selecting a Drug Name

The generic name of a drug, which is a nonproprietary name that by definition cannot function as a trademark, is usually created for drug substances when a new drug is being tested. The generic name is selected by the United States Adopted Names (USAN) Council[21] according to principles developed to ensure "safety, consistency, and logic."[22] The USAN has developed a nomenclature scheme that includes, in part, an established *stem* that represents a specific drug class. For example, the arthritis medications celecoxib, valdecoxib, and rofecoxib are generic names containing the *–coxib* stem.[22] Practitioners will recognize many other examples of stems common across drug classes.

When a pharmaceutical company engages in testing of a new chemical compound, the company submits up to three proposed generic or nonproprietary names to the USAN for approval.[23] Once the USAN selects a generic drug name, the USAN collaborates with the World Health Organization to ensure that the generic name will be acceptable in foreign countries through the INN naming process.

In addition to the generic name, and more important from a marketing standpoint, pharmaceutical companies create a brand or trademark name, which is proprietary and may be used only by a particular company. That name will be the one associated with the pharmaceutical company that created the chemical entity (ie, the source of the goods) and will be thought of as the brand name. Pharmaceutical companies go to great efforts in selecting memorable and effective brand names. In addition, pharmaceutical companies must take care to avoid selecting a brand name that is confusingly similar to an existing drug name, whether another brand or a generic name.

Of course, trademarks must be selected for all of a pharmaceutical company's goods and services, not just for its prescription drugs, but over-the-counter preparations and any ancillary products. Each of these trademarks must be distinct from competitors' trademarks. In practice, it may be necessary for a pharmaceutical company to select literally hundreds of trademarks each year, many of which will be rejected for various marketing or legal reasons. At the end of the day, a trademark is chosen that will be the "badge of origin" for a particular product or group of products and that may be the foundation of a multi-million-dollar advertising campaign.

Types of Trademarks

A *trademark* includes any word, name, symbol, or device, or any combination used, or intended to be used, in commerce to identify and distinguish the goods of one manufacturer or seller from goods manufactured or sold by others, and to indicate the source of the goods. In short, a trademark is a brand name.[24] A *service mark* is any word, name, symbol, device, or any combination used, or intended to be used, in commerce to identify and distinguish the services of one provider from services provided by others and to indicate the source of the services.[24] A *certification mark* is any word, name, symbol, device, or any combination used, or intended to be used, in commerce with the owner's permission by someone other than its owner used, or intended to be used, in commerce to identify and distinguish the services of one provider from services provided by others and to indicate the source of the services.[24] A used, or intended to be used, in commerce to identify and distinguish the services of one provider from services provided by others and to indicate the source of the services.[24] A to certify regional or other geographic origin, material, mode of manufacture, quality, accuracy, or other characteristics of someone's goods or services or that the work or labor on the goods or services was performed by members of a union or other organization.[24] A *collective mark* is a trademark or service mark used, or intended to be used, in commerce by the members of a cooperative, an association, or other collective group or organization, including a mark that indicates membership in a union, an association, or other organization.[24]

Trade dress, which is protected under Lanham Act §43(a), 15 USC §1125(a), has been defined as the "total image or overall appearance of a product."[25] Trade dress refers to a product's label, packaging, color, or even the ornamental appearance of a product itself. For example, most drugs come in packaging and with labeling having a distinct appearance that is associated with a particular pharmaceutical company. In addition, a drug may have a unique shape or color or combination of shape and color that is associated solely with one pharmaceutical company. These forms of trade dress further distinguish one company's goods from those of its competitors, by appearance alone.

For example, Merck & Co., Inc., obtained US Trademark Registration Nos. 1,901,353 and 1,901,352 each for a "medicinal preparation for use in hypercholesterolemic therapy"; see FIGURE 10-3. These trademark registrations protect "octago-

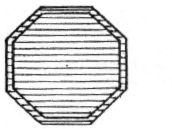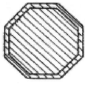

FIGURE 10-3 Octagonal tablets.

nal shaped tablets" for hypercholesterolemic medication, namely, the drug sold under the brand name Mevacor, in two different strengths. Johnson & Johnson obtained US Trademark Registration No. 2,442,526 for the packaging for the drug Pepcid AC, and US Trademark Registration No. 2,141,785 for the appearance of the tube for Clean & Clear facial cleanser and soap. From a consumer perception standpoint, a product's appearance and/or packaging is just as important as its name.

The Trademark Process

Trademark rights in the United States flow from use in commerce,* not from registration; this means that a party obtains "common law" rights as soon as a trademark is used in commerce.[26] Parties may also seek to register their trademarks with the United States Patent and Trademark Office (USPTO) to obtain a federal trademark registration.

There are several advantages to obtaining a federal trademark registration. A federal registration does the following: allows the trademark owner to sue in federal court for trademark infringement[27]; allows the trademark owner to seek to recover profits, damages, and costs from an infringer[28]; establishes constructive notice of ownership of the registered mark[29]; creates a presumption of validity of the registration, its ownership, and the exclusive right to use the registered mark in commerce in connection with those items specified in the registration[30]; constitutes prima facie evidence of the validity of the mark[30]; and allows the owner to use the federal registration symbol ®.

In the United States, a party may file a trademark application before it actually begins using the trademark in commerce. Such an application is called an *intent-to-use application* because an applicant must verify that it has a bona fide intent to use the trademark in commerce at a later date.[31] The intent-to-use application provides a constructive date of first use as of the date of filing, which may be significant if there is a contest over priority with another trademark owner.

---

* "The term *use in commerce* means the bona fide use of a mark in the ordinary course of trade, and not made merely to reserve a right in a mark" (15 USC §1127).

The process for obtaining a federal trademark registration begins with filing a trademark application with the USPTO listing the trademark and the goods or services with which the trademark is being used or will be used.[31] Today, most trademark filings are done electronically using the USPTO's Trademark Electronic Application System (TEAS).[32] The USPTO provides an electronic form that is filled out by the applicant or the applicant's attorney.

Once the application is electronically filed, it is assigned to a trademark examining attorney, who will review the trademark. There are several statutory rules for determining whether a trademark is registerable.[33] The primary areas of review are whether the trademark is descriptive of the goods or service and whether the trademark would create a likelihood of confusion* with another trademark that has been previously registered or applied for.[33] Also, the trademark examining attorneys must ensure that the identification of goods or the recitation of services are acceptable under the USPTO rules.[34]

The trademark examining attorney issues an office action listing any refusals or requirements. The first such office action is generally issued within approximately 6 to 8 months from the filing date of the application. A trademark applicant has a 6-month nonextendable deadline to respond to any issues raised by the examining attorney in the office action.[35]

If accepted, a trademark is "published" in the federal *Official Trademark Gazette* for opposition.[36] This means that any third party or member of the public who believes they may be damaged by the registration of the subject trademark may file an opposition to the registration of the trademark. An opposition proceeding is essentially a trial held before the administrative Trademark Trial and Appeal Board (TTAB), where an applicant's right to register its trademark is decided.

Once a federal trademark registration certificate is issued, it remains in force for 10 years.[37] However, if the party seeks to maintain its federal registration, the party must file a declaration stating that the trademark is still in use in commerce between the fifth and sixth years after the date of registration of the trademark.[37] This keeps the federal trademark register free of stale trademarks that are no longer in use. A trademark renewal is due at the end of 20 years from the date of registration.[38]

Trademarks are important to any pharmaceutical company in protecting its product lines, including the names and the appearance of its goods. Trademarks rights are particularly significant in that, in theory, trademark rights can last for an unlimited du-

---

*Whether a likelihood of confusion exists between two conflicting marks is determined by reviewing a multifactor test that takes into consideration *inter alia* the similarity or dissimilarity of the marks in their entireties as to appearance, sound, connotation, and commercial impression; the relatedness of the goods or services as described in an application or registration or in connection with which a prior mark is in use; and the similarity or dissimilarity of established, likely-to-continue trade channels. *In re E. I. du Pont de Nemours & Co.*, 476 F.2d 1357, 177 USP.Q. 563 (C.C.P.A. 1973).

ration, so long as the trademark is continuously used in commerce and does not lose its effectiveness as a designator of source.

■ References

1. Congress of the United States, Congressional Budget Office. *Research and Development in the Pharmaceutical Industry*. CBO Study. October 2006. Available at: http://www.cbo.gov/ftpdocs/ 76xx/doc7615/10-02-DrugR-D.pdf. Accessed December 12, 2008.
2. 35 USC §101.
3. 35 USC §271.
4. *Diamond v. Chakrabarty*, 447 US 303 (1980).
5. *Le Roy v. Tatham*, 55 US 156, 175 (1852).
6. United States Patent Office Manual of Patent Examining Procedure (MPEP), §2107.
7. 35 USC §102.
8. 35 USC §103.
9. 35 USC §171.
10. 35 USC §112.
11. 35 USC §119.
12. 35 USC §154.
13. Lichtenberg FR. *Benefits and Costs of Newer Drugs: An Update*. Cambridge, Mass: National Bureau of Economic Research; June 2002. NBER Working Paper No. 8996.
14. United States Patent and Trademark Office. *Performance and Accountability Report: Fiscal Year 2005*, at 4. Alexandria, Va: USPTO.
15. Federal Food, Drug, and Cosmetic Act of 1938.
16. 21 USC §301 (1938).
17. MPEP §2700, *et seq*.
18. 37 CFR §1.740.
19. 37 CFR §1.750.
20. 35 USC §156(c).
21. American Medical Association. *United States adopted names*. Available at: http://www.ama-assn .org/ama/pub/category/2956.html. Accessed January 6, 2009.
22. Rados C. Drug name confusion: preventing medication errors. *FDA Consumer*. 2005, July–August. Available at: http://www.fda.gov/fdac/features/2005/405_confusion.html. Accessed January 6, 2009.
23. American Medical Association. *How to apply for a name*. Available at: http://www.ama-assn .org/ama/pub/category/2960.html. Accessed January 6, 2009.
24. United States Patent and Trademark Office. Trademark FAQ. Available at: http://www.uspto.gov/web/ offices/tac/tmfaq.htm. Accessed January 6, 2009.
25. *Two Pesos, Inc. v. Taco Cabana, Inc.*, 505 US 763, 765 n.1 (1992).
26. 15 USC §1127.
27. 15 USC §1114.
28. 15 USC §1117.
29. 15 USC §1072.

30. 15 USC §1057.

31. 35 USC §1051.

32. United States Patent and Trademark Office. Trademark electronic Application System. Available at: http://www.uspto.gov/teas/index.html. Accessed January 6, 2009.

33. 15 USC §1052.

34. Trademark Manual of Examining Procedure (TMEP) §1400.

35. United States Patent and Trademark Office. Office actions and how to respond to them. Available at: http://www.uspto.gov/web/trademarks/workflow/oa.htm. Accessed January 6, 2009.

36. 37 CFR §2.80.

37. 15 USC §1058.

38. 15 USC §1059.

Sales and Marketing

Richard Randall

It is highly likely that, as pharmacists, all who read this book will eventually encounter a sales representative from a pharmaceutical company. Someone you may or may not meet is a marketer from this company. But marketers are certainly there in the background supporting the sales representative, and you will deduce that they are certainly the creators of the advertising and other materials that you will see in relation to the pharmaceutical products.

Thus, this chapter addresses marketing and sales in the pharmaceutical industry. Although several departments in a pharmaceutical company may interact with specific customers, the sales organization is all about direct relationships with the client. The marketing organization is the internal company conduit that organizes and distributes the diversity of resources in the pharmaceutical company out to customers. Marketing does this through a variety of channels, including the sales team. Strictly speaking, both marketing and sales do refer to such functional organizations within companies in the industry, but they can refer as well to sets of processes. This chapter probably concentrates more on the latter and takes you behind the scenes as to what happens in a pharmaceutical company by opening up the marketing and the sales processes.

■ The Marketing Processes

Marketing has four basic processes. These are analysis, planning, implementation, and control. The general flow of these processes is in this same sequence. A marketer starts with analysis of variables such as the disease, the market, the product, the competition, and the customers. He or she then synthesizes this information into a plan for the marketplace, which includes marketing strategy and promotional strategy. The plan also includes what further clinical development needs might be required from the research departments to sustain the strategies in the future. Implementing the plan begins with a marketing promotion program that includes direct-selling resources for the sales team and indirect resources, such as advertising materials and education programs. The final process is a means of control, or monitoring, of the implementation. This usually involves gathering data to measure the degree of success of the execution of the plan against predetermined metrics, and this would include data on usage patterns, customer feedback to questionnaires, and, of course, sales results.

In practice, these four processes are not entirely separate and sequential, and many elements run in parallel. In addition, these marketing processes work together as a continuous loop. The results of the control, or monitoring, process force the marketer back to further analysis, reexamination of the plan, and, if necessary, restructuring of the implementation, which then is monitored once more.

So, let's examine each one in more detail and describe some of the linkages to other chapters in this book.

■ Marketing Analysis

Marketing analysis starts with gathering data from the external marketplace and data internal to the company, which includes the key facets of the pharmaceutical product. I start with the former where marketers in the pharmaceutical industry rely on two types of external data to generate analyses: secondary data and primary data.

Secondary Data

This area can be very robust and uses data that are gathered by sources other than the marketer or the market research team in the company supporting the marketer. Thus, the term *secondary data* is used because someone else has generated or gathered the information for their purposes. The disadvantage is that the data may or may not have been collected and reported for the exact same use as the marketer anticipates. Nonetheless, the advantage of these data is that they are usually plentiful, and, although some private sources can be expensive, many public ones can be had for no to little cost.

Clearly, most of the information on the disease to be treated by the pharmaceutical product will initially come from the published literature, textbooks, and other sources such as ongoing teaching and educational programs in university centers. So, this is the starting point for the marketer in understanding the disease and its consequences, and how it is currently managed both with pharmacologic treatment and nonpharmacologic interventions. Many of the diseases managed today in the developed world have published treatment guidelines that are issued by specialist societies in that domain. For example, the diagnosis and management of certain cardiac conditions have practice guidelines published and updated from time to time by the American College of Cardiology and the American Heart Association in conjunction with overseas colleagues, such as the European Society of Cardiology. These guidelines usually provide an opinion on uses of the current pharmaceutical products for treating the condition.

Although the management of the disease in the real marketplace does not always follow the textbooks and guidelines, these documents do provide a good blueprint for what the teaching experts in the field are recommending. What the marketer is honing in on is where the disease is reasonably well treated, and where there is dissatisfaction or any unmet need. Against this latter point, the marketer will later compare and contrast the clinical results of his or her pharmaceutical product.

The other sources of secondary data are more quantitative and include surveys of the market size in patient terms, prescriptions and dollar sales of pharmaceutical products, and the market share of specific products, including products that will directly compete with the marketer's product. Many of these data come from private vendors who are in the business of collecting the data and then marketing their services. In the main, pharmaceutical companies who subscribe to these databases or syndicated surveys then all have access to much the same basic market information; that is, assuming they all have the same purchasing budget. How they analyze the data and how they interpret their own summaries are where the variance occurs between companies.

Whether from vendors or from published research literature, the marketer is also able to capture estimates of what the cost burden of the disease is in the marketplace, including that to specific customers. Other private sources can provide business intelligence information on competitors and their products, including estimates of promotional spending and types of promotion occurring in the marketplace. What the marketer is attempting to glean from these quantitative sources is size of any opportunities, as well as patterns of use and correlations between such things as competitive activity and changes in the key parameters in the marketplace. Thus, the marketer can look at a static situation at a chosen point in time or review dynamic changes if the data are gathered repetitively over several periods of time.

Primary Data

This is the area where the marketer commissions for himself or herself the collection of data. Thus, the term *primary data* is used because the information is intended to be gathered in a manner that directly addresses the issue at hand. This is a great advantage in interpreting the analyses. The disadvantages are time and budget constraints, both of which may considerably restrict the sample size. Such restriction could be particularly problematic for quantitative conclusions. The methods of collecting such primary data might be the same as secondary data and can include observation of activities and conducting surveys. Experiments could also be used.

The types of qualitative primary data of interest to the marketer are those that help him or her understand the why behind the what. As discussed earlier, a great deal of information on what is happening in the market can come from secondary data. However, the best means to understand the reasons for marketplace trends, usage of current products, or how a new product may fare is to actually observe users in action or, better yet, ask them specific questions. Although surveys can be and are done through remote means, such as mail and Internet, face-to-face questioning sessions are often done as individual interviews or group focus discussions. The former has the advantage of avoiding an influence bias from others present but suffers from the length of time required to generate answers from a large enough sample. The group focus session has advantages in quickly stimulating thought processes across the group but suffers from the potential that some participants may be reluctant to raise contradictions publicly between colleagues.

The good marketer employs several methods to understand such factors as awareness of the subject at hand, unaided and aided recall of specifics on diseases or products for treating these diseases, the why behind beliefs and preferences of various methods of management, actual past experiences with products, and, importantly, future intentions. These face-to-face methods also lend themselves well to proposing concepts and gauging reactions, both positive and negative, to new aspects of the marketer's product. Thus, much of the individual or group sessions are done using open-ended questions that seek in-depth answers.

With large enough sample sizes, some of the methods described for generating qualitative primary data can be used to attempt to quantify patterns and future intentions. Structuring questions for a response along a scale of agreement or disagreement also provides a level of quantification. There are also private vendors who will set up panels and do repetitive observations and surveying over time to determine dynamic changes. With comprehensive enough information, correlations between cause and effect can be drawn. A change in market share of products has occurred and the most likely explanation is that a competitor introduced new information through a promotion campaign. Experimentation also attempts to draw out cause and effect, and this is particularly used by the market researcher to understand the effectiveness of various means of promotion and whether the cost for such promotion is justified.

So now, from both the secondary data and the primary research, the marketer has a picture of the disease and patients, the customers who will treat them and use pharmaceuticals, the marketplace of the current products, and a pretty comprehensive understanding of attitudes and beliefs. He or she also has a clear image of the profile of his or her product and has already gauged reaction by customers to its key aspects. Now it is time to pull it all together and make recommendations for how this product will actually be marketed and sold. It is time to enter the planning process.

■ Marketing Planning

In this part of the process, the marketer and his or her team recommend the marketing strategy, the marketing objectives, the promotional strategy, and the promotional objectives. Later I cover in more detail the differences between these two strategies and two sets of objectives. But, in short, the marketing strategy defines where the product will eventually participate in the market, and the promotional strategy defines what will be said about the product at each stage along the way.

Marketing Strategy and Marketing Objectives

The marketing strategy defines the market in which the product will be used and the manner in which the product will be used versus other competitors or other management methods. For example, a new pharmaceutical product X will be the first choice of antibiotic therapy for the prevention of infection following surgery of Y disease. To fully realize the marketing strategy over the longer term and then sustain this strategy by addressing anticipated future changes in the marketplace, the marketers work with the scientific and clinical teams in the pharmaceutical company to plan further clinical development studies on the product. In that sense, the marketing strategy is not stated for the current time, but is stated as a direction for achieving a desired future state during the lifetime of the product. It is not constrained entirely to the current clinical research, the current knowledge and thoughts about the disease, and neither is it constrained entirely to the current product label. It is a statement that drives the long-term application of internal company research and development resources toward a future product label and a future stature in the marketplace. Therefore, as a consumer of such development resources, it needs to be considered by the company in the context of the long-term corporate strategy.

Marketing objectives set the course for the desired success in the marketplace as a whole and provide observable benchmarks for this penetration into the target market. Thus, examples of marketing objectives would be numbers of prescriptions both new and refill, number of patients both new patients and returning patients. The market shares of these prescriptions and patients would also be marketing objectives. Certainly, for the marketer the sales objectives for the product are a central marketing objective. Therefore, much of the quantitative secondary data described earlier finds a home in both setting marketing objectives and providing ongoing measurable results versus these goals.

Promotional Strategy and Promotional Objectives

The promotional strategy is the communication platform. It is what will be said about the product and to whom. To continue the example of product X earlier, it will be promoted to surgeons as highly effective against the spread of organism Z, a chief cause of postsurgical infections in patients with disease Y, and it will have significantly less side effects than the current competitors. Thus, from the promotional strategy flow the key messages that will be conveyed to customers. These include more specific statements surrounding its efficacy both in vivo and in vitro, what is meant by less side effects, and key information on how to administer. The messages also need to include information for the healthcare provider that outline critical boundaries for the product's clinical use, such as warnings, precautions, contraindications, and side effects that do occur and under what known circumstances. The promotional strategy is based in the current world and must, most certainly, be consistent with the current product label. It also drives the application of resources—this time marketing and sales resources—in the near term.

Promotional objectives are the goals the marketer sets for acceptance of the product in the mind of the customer, or in the minds of customer groups. Therefore, at the outset, objectives for awareness of the new product and the ability to recall it and its attributes are of importance. As time progresses, the marketer is interested in setting goals for beliefs about the product; preferences over other products and why; intentions to try the product; and finally actual trial of the product. Thus, much of the qualitative primary research discussed earlier now comes to play in setting promotional objectives and in providing the vehicles going forward for measuring progress against these objectives. The marketing processes become ever more intertwined.

Labeling Needs and Clinical Development Needs

It has been mentioned earlier that the marketer in the pharmaceutical industry must work closely with the clinical and regulatory teams in the company. How these teams operate is discussed in other chapters of this book. However, feedback from the marketing team to these groups about developments in the marketplace and results of secondary or primary market research will keep the research and development teams abreast of marketplace changes and, of course, product acceptance.

Although it is not the place of the marketer to design clinical or other scientific studies, nor to influence the conclusions of these programs, it is the responsibility of the marketer in the company to direct the clinical and regulatory teams toward what the marketplace is demanding in real time. With a long product life cycle and lengthy lead times for conducting clinical trials, it is even more important that the marketer help the company predict marketplace trends and events several years in advance. Because promotion of the product must mesh with the product labeling, the labeling needs of the future are as critical as the labeling of the current period.

Reimbursement and Pricing

Reimbursement and pricing are covered elsewhere in this book. The matter of pricing of pharmaceuticals today is one that has become highly controversial and constantly in the public arena and, therefore, part of the political forum. It is also one that is governed by laws in many countries. This is especially true of selling pharmaceuticals to government agencies themselves. The marketer must balance all of these factors versus the data that he or she sees in the marketplace with the feedback and competitive demands of customers. Where the marketer must weigh in is for the setting of a price for a product and for the conditions under which that price will be reimbursed, both based on value offered—not value offered in a vacuum, but value versus other available options, both pharmaceutical and nonpharmaceutical, in the marketplace. Chapter 13 on pharmacoeconomics and outcomes research is devoted to helping determine cost to benefit value. But I emphasize once again the need for the marketer to develop a tight rapport with the research and development teams to demonstrate medical value from studies. In that same rationale, he or she must do the same with the pharmacoeconomics team for economic value. Finally, the marketer must develop a good working rapport with the financial, legal, regulatory, government affairs, sales, and managed care customer teams in the company to coordinate planning for this area.

■ Implementation of the Marketing Plan

The execution of the marketing plan is probably the most exciting part of marketing. Although again it must be emphasized that the four processes of marketing do not all take place in a strict sequential set, the first two processes of analysis and planning are all about doing the homework. Then comes the challenging time of setting the plans in motion by putting theories and hypotheses into practice. The success in this phase depends on multiple factors. These include the inherent strength of the analysis and planning phases and the skills of the marketing team to provide implementation leadership to a large number of people in the company. It also includes the ability of the diverse areas of the company to implement the plans in a coordinated fashion, as the realities of the market and the competitive responses come to bear.

The Promotion Plan

The promotional strategy discussed earlier defines what will be communicated. The promotional plan defines how. Although strategies tend to stay relatively constant over time, plans change in real time with the realities of the marketplace.

Some of the more common elements of the promotion plan or promotion program are journal advertising, mailings, and consumer advertising, also known as DTC, or direct to consumer advertising. Much of the latter is seen regularly on television but also is evident in consumer magazines and on the Internet. DTC is generally expensive because one does need to advertise to an audience that is broader than the patient base that actually might use the product. However, there are means to help focus the approach. For example, certain health conditions may occur mainly in elderly men and there are research vehicles and surveys available to help determine the reading and television patterns of this profiled population. DTC does come with some controversy in the health community, with the argument being that patients place undue demands on healthcare providers to prescribe the latest product they just saw in an advertisement. There is now pressure mounting to prohibit DTC in the early years of marketing until greater experience with side effects has been gleaned. Nonetheless, the general public today does wish to know more about the prescription product they are taking or may take, and they wish to engage physicians and pharmacists in such a dialogue. They see DTC or other lay healthcare articles as a means to prepare for such conversations.

From a purely business perspective, there are ways to measure the effectiveness of pharmaceutical DTC advertising and correlate this expenditure to success or not in the promotional mix. The same is true of journal advertising to the healthcare professionals, which has been a staple for some time, and which is much more focused than that to consumers. The journals for placing ads for a cardiovascular pharmaceutical or communicating to pharmacists are quite obvious, as are many of the websites that healthcare providers visit regularly. In that latter vein, the pharmaceutical companies of today all have their own websites, where product and other therapeutic information may be found. Some companies also sponsor non-product–oriented Internet sites as services to the healthcare community, where links to a variety of disease and disease management information may be found. All of these advertising elements come as expense lines in the marketer's budget, which is not unlimited and will need to be justified within the corporate expenditure. Therefore, trade-off decisions are constantly made as to which elements will be supported.

Other major expenses in the promotion plan are those around educational programs. Traditionally, these have included symposia, colloquia, and lectures. The difference in these mainly is the larger audience size and a lengthier set of speakers at the symposia end, down to a single speaker and a much smaller audience with a lecture. All of these are formally presented from a podium to a seated live audience. However, various evening, lunch-time, or breakfast-oriented sessions may simply involve a roundtable format where information from the presenter is meant more to generate a group discussion. The cost to the marketer for such educational events involves not only the event itself, but the cost of producing and distributing slide sets, the cost of training the speakers, and the honoraria for the speakers' time.

Over the last number of years, the double factor of increasing time demands on physicians coupled with the ever increasing number of these programs conducted by the pharmaceutical industry has driven down the per event attendance numbers at these live face-to-face forums. The reality now of being able to generate a reasonably sized live audience to hear a live speaker at that exact time and place has not made many of these sessions cost effective for today's marketer. The age of computer and electronic media, however, has to some extent rescued the situation. Remote programs, where the speaker can be virtually anywhere, and so can the audience, have been conducted for years through telephone conferencing. This, however, required that each member of the audience had a set of slides on site. Today, the speaker and the audience need simply to connect online at the same time and through networking software can see slides and ask questions in real time. Web cameras can complete the picture, literally.

Many of the preceding elements of the promotion program are usually referred to as nonmanpower promotion elements or indirect-selling elements because a number of these are able to be conducted through vehicles other than the sales organization. A qualifier is that in many cases the live educational events are indeed organized through the sales force. Other nonmanpower promotional expenses include telemarketing, press announcements, and professional relations for key specialty societies.

Clearly a large piece of the promotion plan for the marketer is how to engage the sales organization assigned to promote the product in a face-to-face manner to healthcare professionals. Development of literature for the sales force, such as the selling aids or detail aids, occupy a large amount of the marketer's time and budget. All of these direct-selling materials need to comply with the product labeling, and therefore pharmaceutical companies have some internal means to control the development and distribution of these materials. This might involve a system within the company that has representation from marketing, the clinical or medical teams, the regulatory teams, and legal counsel to approve the text, layout, and graphics of these materials. This same system would probably oversee nonmanpower materials as well. The sales force would also be supplied with materials directed to pharmacists and physicians for assisting their patient clientele, such as patient education materials, lay leaflets on how to administer the product, and lay package circulars.

By no means exhaustive of the list, but completing the picture of sales force materials might be disease guidelines, clinical reprints, formulary kits for hospitals or managed care institutions, and, importantly, starter product material, known as samples. On this latter subject, to whom samples may be distributed and the conditions under which samples may be distributed are regulated by law in many countries. Deviation from these prescribed rules or diversion of samples can result in serious consequences. Thus, accurate records of samples distributed to sales representatives and subsequently distributed to healthcare providers, as well as the description of the sample request, are required. Finally, the marketer must account for training materials and training costs for the sales force for the promotion of his or her product.

So, now that the marketer has set the stage and prepared the materials and direction for the sales organization, it is time for face-to-face communication by the sales force to its customers. Let's turn our attention to the various selling teams that a pharmaceutical company may employ.

Sales Forces

All pharmaceutical companies do not organize their sales forces in the same manner, and neither does any one company have the same organizational structure continuously. Nevertheless, a number of common principles apply in the market.

Most sales representatives are responsible for more than one product. Many years ago that could have been a fairly large number of products "in the bag." This term came from the literature and samples that representatives carried in their detailing briefcase or detail bag. Sales representatives today are probably responsible for detailing or promoting up to only three or possibly four products. In some cases, they may have only one product of responsibility. Most commonly a representative is assigned to geography, or a territory, and is responsible for discussing the product to customers in that territory. However, in some cases, particularly managed care representatives or hospital representatives, representatives are assigned by customer accounts. Sales representatives report to a manager, who in turn reports to a director or other more senior management position in the company. For pharmacists, it is not uncommon to see representatives and to have their manager and even the more senior company people accompanying them.

For large pharmaceutical companies, there is probably more than one representative from that company in that same territory. One obvious reason is the large portfolio of products from that company. But it is not at all uncommon for more than one representative in the same territory to have responsibility for the same product. Larger volume products with large numbers of prescribers dictate more representatives in that same area to promote the product. This, in many cases, can cause issues with physician offices and pharmacies and the perception and even the reality of too many representatives from the same company calling on them. It also places responsibility on the shoulders of the representatives of that company to coordinate efforts and to have meaningful reasons to be in that same office not long after a colleague had just been there. Much of this may be self-correcting over the next few years as the rapid expansions of major pharmaceutical company sales forces is starting to reverse. Notable companies have already announced reductions. The driving force behind these reductions, beyond customer saturation by an excess of representatives, is the pressure to reduce costs in the face of the industry-wide slowdown in the rate of approval of new chemical entities.

The two broad types of sales forces are primary care and specialty. The former type is usually the larger within a large pharmaceutical company and calls on and provides services to primary care physicians in their offices, clinics, or in the hospitals. They probably have the responsibility to call on the local pharmacies in their territory as well. Because the customer audiences are more generalists, multiple products of responsibility are the norm for the larger companies. The primary care sales organization details the product to physicians and pharmacists and provides them with literature. They also help organize smaller venue educational programs in the local area or help customers join into the remote educational programs electronically. They help customers connect with others in the company to help answer questions or assist with other matters. The sales representatives also are charged with reporting back to the company incidents of adverse reactions in a timely manner and with assisting customers with product complaints. Many times representatives are asked by customers to help underwrite the local professional society functions and, depending on the request, help channel it to the correct party in the company. They are the primary representative of the company in the area for handling requests by physicians for product samples.

The specialty sales forces comprise a variety of sales teams responsible for select groups of customers. These certainly include sales forces that call on physicians trained in that specialty disease area, such as cardiologists, infectious disease specialists, rheumatologists, and so on. Having only one product of responsibility is not uncommon for such a specialty representative. The roles and functions of these specialty sales representatives mirror to a large extent those of the primary care representatives. However, the discussion and services are much more detailed around the disease and depth of information on the product. Use of published reprints is a staple in discussions. The specialty sales representatives used, or intended to be used, in commerce to identify and distinguish the services of one provider from services provided by others and to indicate the source of the services.[24] They probably also are charged with speaker training for educational programs.

The specialty sales forces also include hospital sales representatives, where again they are assigned to key hospital accounts in a geography. There are a large number of hospitals in the country and, in the main, most pharmaceutical companies dedicate a hospital sales organization to only a select number, usually the larger ones. Thus, the urban hospitals, particularly those teaching hospitals associated with medical schools, are their accounts, as are government hospitals on military bases and those for veterans. The role of the hospital sales force is similar to that of the specialty teams in provision of product information and services. However, they also have to interact with administrative and other officials in the institutions to discuss matters such as hospital formulary status. Thus, they work closely with members of the hospital formulary committee, which almost always includes key members of the hospital pharmacy staff. For smaller community hospitals, and those in rural settings, these hospital responsibilities might be assigned to either a specialty sales representative, a primary care sales representative, or one of their managers.

Finally, there may be specialty representative teams who call on major managed care customers, on long-term care providers, on wholesalers and chain pharmacy headquarters, or are responsible for government accounts such as the Department of Defense, Department of Veterans Affairs, the Bureau of Indian Affairs, or federal and state agencies for Medicare and Medicaid. Beyond provision of services and product information, a primary role of these representatives is dealing with formulary listing, purchasing decisions, and the negotiation of rebates and discounts as appropriate and permitted with these customers. In this regard, a whole different nature of support from the marketing team and other company departments is necessary. Greater discussion of these specialty markets including government, managed care, hospitals, and contracting is in other chapters of this text.

So, now the implementation stage of marketing and sales has been set in motion. Is it succeeding? It is time to monitor the results and to better control the outcome.

■ Control of the Marketing Plan

The realities of the marketplace have by now shown themselves in abundance. All customers may not have reacted entirely as predicted from market research. New managed care or government decisions may have taken place. Different sets of treatment guidelines may have been issued. The new product is now being used across the spectrum of patients in the day-to-day practice of physicians, which does not always mirror the restricted situation of controlled clinical trials. And, unfortunately for the marketer, the competition has almost certainly responded.

Monitoring is all about revisiting the marketing objectives and promotional objectives, and redoing the secondary and primary research to evaluate the actual results versus the planned objectives. The control phase is about adapting the marketing plan accordingly and adjusting the implementation. Thus, the final phase of the marketing process is really circling back to the first phase and beginning the cycle once more. It is a process not a destination.

■ Other Aspects

Much of what has been discussed in this chapter is oriented to the US market and to marketing processes in a major research-oriented and branded pharmaceutical company. Before this chapter ends, I make a few short comments on the marketing of generics, the commercial marketing and sales emergence of smaller biotech companies, and the marketing of pharmaceuticals in other countries. More detailed discussion on some of these aspects takes place in other chapters in this book.

In the early 1980s, less than one-fifth of all prescriptions in the US market were for generic drugs. Managed care was limited or even unknown in many parts of the country and was only just starting to develop some controls on prescribing. A branded originator product might even retain reasonable market share years after patent loss. In 1984, Congress passed the Drug Price Competition and Patent Term Restoration Act. This act eliminated much of the duplicative testing necessary to obtain approval in the United States for a generic copy of an innovator drug and it allowed any testing still required to be conducted before the patent for the innovator drug expired. Thus, it set the stage for more companies to have the ability to develop generics, all of which could potentially gain approval right at patent expiration.

This act, and the growth of managed care and its much more effective systems to control prescribing, have changed the face of the US market. Two decades later, roughly one-half of all prescriptions in the United States are for generics. Another approximately 10% are for what are known as branded generics, which are mainly novel dosage forms of off-patent products plus some generic products sold with a trade name. The market share today of an originator product is virtually eliminated within a few months of patent loss. Although the total annual sales value of the US generics in the early 2000s was around $20 billion, the growth rate is expected to take it to around $50 billion by the end of the decade.

The marketing of generics first revolves around assurance of sustained quality, batch after batch, and assurance of reliable supply to the customer. Once those determinants for entry to the generic market have been satisfied, then the ability to compete on price becomes the deciding competitive factor. This price competition influences which generic brand or brands a pharmacy, a hospital, or a managed care organization will carry from among what are usually a large number of options on large-volume products. However, this plethora of low-cost choices provides a competitive backflush onto the marketer of brand-name, innovative products. In many disease conditions, healthcare providers have a current therapeutic option of using a generic. Thus, the challenge for the marketer of any new or in-line innovative product is to constantly have to demonstrate value commensurate with what is almost certainly a significantly higher price than the generic. Therefore, we need to revisit the earlier discussions on reimbursement, pricing, clinical data, and pharmacoeconomic data, also discussed elsewhere in this text.

For the past several years, many smaller biotech companies have been making their impact in the areas of research and development of new chemical entities. Some estimates place the number of biotech organizations involved in research and development in the United States at well over a 1000 companies. The two largest dollar growth subsegments of the overall US pharmaceutical market of recent years are the generic drugs just discussed and the sales of drugs from the biotech research engines. The latter is estimated at anywhere up to $50 billion annually.

Some large biotechnology companies rank among the largest of pharmaceutical firms. However, many biotech products, researched by the smaller companies, have simply been licensed to larger pharmaceutical companies for them to sell commercially. Thus, in many cases for the practicing pharmacist, the sales representative that visits for the new biotech product has been one in the same as that for products out of the large companies' research pipelines. That has been changing and will continue to do so. Many smaller biotech companies are now making the business decision to go it alone commercially in the market, or at the very least to partner in the market with other larger companies. The implication for the healthcare provider is that more and more new pharmaceutical products will be marketed and sold to them by sales representatives from companies unknown to them previously.

Marketing and selling of pharmaceuticals in foreign markets could probably be broken simplistically into two sets of countries. The first comprises those countries around the world where the processes of marketing and sales of pharmaceutical products are essentially similar to those in the United States. These include, for example, the other two major North American markets of Canada and Mexico. It also includes many of the European Union countries and some other western European countries that are outside of the EU, such as Norway and Switzerland. You must include Japan, which is the world's second largest pharmaceutical market in dollar terms next to that of the United

States. You could probably also include places like Australia and some of the larger South American countries, like Brazil. Others could arguably be on the list, but the ones mentioned allow you to see the profile of this basket of countries that are the developed world major economic players.

These countries are where global pharmaceutical companies concentrate their marketing and sales efforts because these countries, along with the United States, generate roughly 80% of the dollar sales in the world pharmaceutical market, with about one-half of this coming just from the United States. This percentage dominance results from the higher prices in these countries and certainly does not take into account the number of units sold throughout the world. To say that the marketing and selling are similar is not to say that the regulatory approval requirements and the pricing and reimbursement requirements to come to market are exactly the same in these countries, because they are not. Neither are the postapproval regulations the same by which various oversight agencies in these countries monitor promotion, overall usage, and postmarketing pricing. But once the pharmaceutical company has met these requirements, the general processes of marketing and selling to healthcare professionals have more similarities to the United States than dissimilarities. For example, in some countries the treatment of some patients may take place more often in hospitals than it would in the United States. In other countries, injectables are more widely used by physicians in the setting of their offices than they would be in the United States.

Marketing to the second set of countries means marketing to about five-sixths of the world population. Russia is a large country, and both China and India have well over a billion people each. These countries, and those in Africa and other parts of eastern Europe, Asia, and the Americas, do indeed use pharmaceuticals. However, the marketing of pharmaceuticals in some of these countries tends to be dominated by indigenous pharmaceutical companies. Furthermore, the homegrown Indian pharmaceutical companies are in fact becoming the world powerhouses for marketing of generic drugs, including generics sold in the United States. Many over-the-counter (OTC) products around the world, such as vitamins, have origins from Chinese companies. In these and other smaller countries, the global research-oriented pharmaceutical companies may sell through local distributors.

This is not to say that the innovative research companies are not laying down their own footprint in this second set of countries. However, there are challenges to them in many of these places. Patent protections are very loose, if not nonexistent. As with other technology, laws and effective systems are not always in place to prevent piracy. There is low pricing to the point of the extreme in some of these countries. When large segments of the populations exist on less than $1 or $2 a day, the market demands this. In other countries, this low pricing is government mandated. Clearly, this can and has created moral and social issues for the supply of certain medicines to those world populations who truly need it but cannot pay for it. Witness the challenges of supplying AIDS medicines to Africa.

But in the main, the research, development, marketing, sales, and payroll cost structures of the global pharmaceutical companies make it an enormous challenge for their marketers to compete effectively outside the developed world. Companies from India and China are major suppliers to the third world developing countries because their cost structures allow them to compete more effectively in low-price markets.

■ The Interview

You have now read this chapter, you have graduated, and you have decided to apply for a product manager position in the marketing department at a major pharmaceutical company. Your background has allowed you to reach the interview stage. At some point, the interviewer poses the following scenario and asks you a question:

"Our company is about to launch its next major product. We believe that it will be a breakthrough and plan to promote it as follows . . . [*fill in any set of statements*]. Do you think this is what you would do?"

What is your answer?

Go back to the beginning of this chapter on marketing processes. You could explain to the interviewer that you would probably start by reviewing the analyses that have been done on the product, and then, you would look at the detailed plans that will address the product. Put all of this into your own words. But understand that the interviewer is not looking for concurrence or debate on the statement. How could you be expected to evaluate the marketing process, when you have no knowledge of the context? If you attempt to directly do so, you are unlikely to make the next cut! The interviewer is looking for your skills on how you would approach the problem or handle the issue, that is, your marketing and sales processes!

■ Additional Resources

Bennett A. US biotech industry poised for growth. IDG News Service. November 13, 2003. Available at: http://www.itworld.com/Tech/4535/031113usbiotech/. Accessed December 12, 2008.

Conducting market research with primary data: http://iws.ohiolink.edu/moti/ res_prim.html

Congress of the United States, Congressional Budget Office. *How Increased Competition From Generic Drugs Has Affected Prices and Returns in the Pharmaceutical Industry*. CBO Study. July 1998. Available at: http://www.cbo.gov/ showdoc.cfm?index=655&sequence=0. Accessed December 12, 2008.

Division of Drug Marketing, Advertising, and Communications: http://www .fda.gov/cder/ddmac/

Generics still nagging Pfizer: http://www.thestreet.com/newsanalysis/pharmaceuticals/_msnh/10350811.html?cm_ven=MSNH&cm_cat=FREE&cm_ite=NA

Health Market Science: http://www.healthmarketscience.com/abouthms/

Impact Rx: http://www.impactrx.com/index.asp?section=products

IMS Health: http://www.imshealth.com/ims/portal/pages/homeFlash/us/0,2764,6599,00.html

Innovations in Healthcare Analytics: http://www.sdihealth.com/

Law reins prescription drug spending: http://news.moneycentral.msn.com/ticker/article.aspx?Symbol= US:MRK&Feed=AP&Date=20070205&ID=6438764

Marketing Teacher. Promotion. Available at: http://marketingteacher.com/Lessons/lesson_promotion.htm. Accessed December 12, 2008.

Office of Generic Drugs: http://www.fda.gov/cder/ogd/

Pollack A. Pfizer to lay off 10,000 workers. January 22, 2007. Available at: http://www.nytimes.com/2007/01/22/ business/22cnd-pfizer.html?ex=1327122000&en=b8ce628b49ce0fd4&ei=5088&partner=rssnyt&emc=rss. Accessed December 12, 2008.

Prescription Drug Marketing Act of 1987: http://thomas.loc.gov/cgi-bin/bdquery/z?d100:HR01207: @@@D&summ2=m&%7CTOM:/bss/d100query.html%7C

Primary data sources: http://ollie.dcccd.edu/mrkt2370/Chapters/ch3/3prim.html

The principles of marketing: marketing principles: http://www.marketingprinciples .com/articles.asp?cat=419

Richards E. *Regulation of Labeling and Promotion.* Available at: http://biotech.law.lsu.edu/cphl/slides/ Regulation%20of%20Labeling%20and%20Promotion.ppt#256,1,Regulation%20of%20Labeling %20and%20Promotion. Accessed December 12, 2008.

Rosen M. The deconstruction of "Big Pharma." WTN News. February 12, 2007. Available at: http:// wistechnology.com/article.php?id=3694. Accessed December 12, 2008.

Rosen M. The world's leading biotech companies. WTN News. March 6, 2006. Available at: http:// wistechnology.com/article.php?id=2748. Accessed December 12, 2008.

SK&A Healthcare Information Solutions. Analytical physician office profiling. Available at: http://www .skainfo.com/physician_analytical_survey/physician_research.php. Accessed December 12, 2008.

Sources and uses of secondary data: http://oassis.gcal.ac.uk/rms/irm/sd.html

Steinbrook R. For sale: physicians' prescribing data. *N Engl J Med.* 2006; 354(26):2745–2747. Available at: http://content.nejm.org/cgi/content/full/ 354/26/2745. Accessed December 12, 2008.

Top line industry data: http://www.imshealth.com/ims/portal/front/indexC/ 0,2773,6599_5264_0,00.html

Three key principles of sales and marketing in service industries: http://www.mover.net/cam/CanadianMover/ F02W03/Myles.html

Finance

Brian Kearns

■ Finance and Accounting

The corporate finance component has two somewhat separate, but related functions. It is responsible for maintaining control over and information about the real-time financial status of the firm, mainly with an accounting effort, and secondly, it works with senior management in examining investment opportunities, securing financing when needed, searching for economies and leading the planning activities.

Every dollar spent or received must be recorded and the aggregates of these numbers become the reports that management uses to inform business decisions. Recording and processing these cash flows is the accounting task.

Analyzing these numbers to identify trends, patterns, problems, or opportunities is the work of the corporate finance side. For example, if an opportunity is seen, corporate finance is expected to determine what amount of resources would be required and the cost of each option.

Corporate Finance

Departments of corporate finance are departments responsible for providing the funds required for a corporation's ongoing activities. This finance function is not only responsible for providing these funds, but it is also responsible for managing the funds held by the firm and for planning for expenditures of the funds in the future on assets and other needs. Within the US pharmaceutical industry, a corporate finance department is responsible for generating or raising the cash to be used to pay for clinical studies, research and development, and marketing, among other items as well.

Pharmaceutical company finance departments function in the same role as finance departments in almost any other organization or business enterprise. Corporate finance usually involves the application of a toolbox of techniques to balance the risk and reward of certain business activities. This function is ordinarily focused on the business's future and is often highly involved in strategic planning and financial planning.

In a majority of instances, finance and accounting are managed in the same department. Although the functions of accounting and finance are closely related, some distinctions may also be made. In general, financial accounting is more concerned with the reporting of historic financial information whereas corporate finance is more focused on the future needs of an enterprise. A more detailed definition of accounting may be helpful.

Accounting

Accounting is responsible for the measurement, disclosure, and provision of assurance about financial information primarily used by managers, investors, tax authorities, and other decision makers to make decisions about resource allocation within companies, organizations, and public agencies. The term derives from the use of financial accounts. Accounting is also widely referred to as the "language of business." This area is becoming ever more complex as new governmental and standards agencies add new tasks to protect investors.

Financial accounting is undertaken by all firms and is one branch of accounting. Historically, it has involved the mechanisms by which financial information about a business is recorded, classified, summarized, analyzed, interpreted, and communicated. The resulting information is generally publicly accessible. Conversely, *management accounting* information is used within an organization and is usually confidential and accessible only to a small group of mostly higher echelon decision makers. Tax accounting is the accounting activity required to comply with jurisdictional tax regulations. *Tax accounting* involves working with federal, state, and local tax authorities to ensure that the proper amount of taxes is paid when due (and no more).

There exist numerous professional standards bodies for accountants throughout the world. Many of these allow their members to use titles indicating their membership or qualification level. The most recognized example in the United States is the Certified Public Accountant (CPA). It is quite similar to the Chartered Accountant in the United Kingdom.

Auditing is a separate but related discipline, with two subspecialties. There is internal auditing and external auditing. External auditing is the activity where an independent auditor examines an organization's financial statements as well as additional accounting records so as to be able to express an opinion on the truth and fairness of the statements and the internal accountant's adherence to Generally Accepted Accounting Principles (GAAP). The Big Four auditors are the largest multinational external auditing firms and are PriceWaterhouseCoopers, KPMG, Deloitte, and Ernst & Young. Previously, there were more of these firms, but their numbers have shrunk as a result of mergers. Internal auditing works to provide information for management usage and is typically carried out by auditors employed by a company, and sometimes by external service providers, who act as if they were internal auditors.

Accountants strive to prepare accurate financial reports that are useful to managers, regulators, and to other stakeholders such as shareholders, creditors, potential creditors, investors, or owners. Financial managers in such a corporate finance department analyze data prepared by accountants and make recommendations to senior management on how best to improve business performance and financial metrics. Accurate and timely financial advice assists top management in making sound business decisions that will increase the health and financial well-being of a pharmaceutical company.

Finance and accounting are responsible for the following:

- Ensuring compliance with regulatory authority regulations and policies
- Establishing and maintaining internal controls over financial reporting
- Maximizing long-term stakeholder value
- Safeguarding corporate assets
- Providing guidance for strategic planning

Financial Planning

In common parlance, a *financial plan* is usually seen as a budget, a plan for spending and saving future income. Such a budget allocates future income to various types of expenses, such as rent, utilities, or R&D, and also reserves some income for short-term and long-term investment or savings. A financial plan may also be an investment plan, which allocates savings to various assets or projects expected to produce subsequent income, such as a new product line, shares in an existing or new business, or real estate.

In business, a financial plan can refer to the three primary financial statements (balance sheet, income statement, and cash flow statement) created within a business plan. A financial forecast or financial plan may also refer to an annual projection of income and expenses for a firm or for only a division, department, or subsidiary. A financial plan can also be an estimation of cash needs and the basis for a decision on how to generate that cash, such as via borrowing or issuing additional shares in a firm. Additional information is provided in the next section regarding strategic planning and forecasting.

Equity Financing

An example of corporate finance is the sale of stock by a company to institutional investors such as an investment bank, which, in turn, sells the shares to the public. The stock gives its owner a part ownership in that company. If one purchases one share of ABC Inc., and it has 100 shares outstanding (held by investors), that investor is a 1/100 owner of that company and therefore owns 1/100 of the net difference between assets and liabilities on the balance sheet. In return for the stock, the company receives cash, which it uses to expand its business in a procedure referred to as *equity financing*. Equity financing combined with the sale of bonds (or any other debt financing) is called the company's capital structure.

■ Introduction to Strategic Planning

Wise strategic planning is one of the most valuable functions undertaken by an organization. Without strategic planning, operating the organization is like taking a ride without a map or goal in mind, and as too many persons could say, there is the distinct possibility of going around in circles. Such a path does not help shareholders, managers, or the trading partners of a firm.

Business managers, entrepreneurs, and executives are frequently so occupied with current issues and threats that they sometimes lose sight of their ultimate objectives. That is the rationale for a business review or a strategic plan. Strategic planning is an absolute necessity. This may not be a recipe for success, but without it, a business is much more likely to fail. A sound plan should accomplish the following:

- Provide a basis for more detailed planning
- Serve as a framework for decisions or for securing support/approval
- Explain the business to others to inform, motivate, and involve
- Assist benchmarking and performance monitoring
- Stimulate change and become a building block for the next plan[1]

The process is strategic because it involves preparing the best way to respond to the circumstances of the organization's environment, whether or not its circumstances are known in advance; nonprofits often must respond to dynamic and even hostile environments. Being strategic, then, means being clear about the organization's objectives, being aware of the organization's resources, and incorporating both into being consciously responsible in a dynamic environment.[2]

The process is about planning because it involves intentionally setting goals (ie, choosing a desired future) and developing an approach to achieving those goals.[2]

The process is disciplined in that it calls for a certain order and pattern to keep it focused and productive. The process raises a sequence of questions that helps planners examine experience, test assumptions, gather and incorporate information about the present, and anticipate the environment in which the organization will be working in the future.[2]

Finally, the process is about fundamental decisions and actions because choices must be made to answer the sequence of questions mentioned previously. The plan is ultimately no more, and no less, than a set of decisions about what to do and why to do it. Because it is impossible to do everything that needs to be done in this world, strategic planning implies that some organizational decisions and actions are more important than others are—and that much of the strategy lies in making the tough decisions about what is most important to achieving organizational success.[2]

Approach to Strategic Planning

A critical review of past performance by the owners and management of a business and the preparation of a plan beyond normal budgetary horizons require a certain combination of mindset and disposition. Yet, there is a need for a few words of caution: Being tied too tightly to a specific strategic plan can be severely detrimental to a firm or organization. As events, environmental variables, and internal activities change, it frequently becomes necessary to modify the strategic plan based upon the latest inputs of data. There is nothing bad or negative about changing plans. Failure to do so can potentially cause greater harm than good for a firm.

So, expecting greater horseshoe sales in the future while the automobile makes ever greater inroads into the transportation market makes no sense whatsoever. Even if a firm makes only one product—horseshoes—it should recognize trends and modify and expand its product lines accordingly.

Analyzing Strengths, Weaknesses, Opportunities, and Threats: SWOT Analysis

A group should list as many features in each of the following four categories. Some examples might be as follows:

Strengths

- The company is well regarded.
- The firm has sufficient cash reserves.
- The manufacturing facilities are state-of-the-art.
- The firm is seen as a market leader.

Weaknesses

- We are entering a recession.
- Offshore producers can beat our prices.
- Our sales force is young and inexperienced.
- Some technology is rapidly making our products obsolete.

Opportunities

- We have long-time superb relations with our suppliers.
- Our customers speak highly about us.
- The leading competitor has serious IRS problems.
- Another competitor has unstable labor relations.

Threats

- An Asian company recently began selling here.
- Our best salesman just retired.
- New technology could make our product obsolete.
- Competitor was just purchased by a Chinese firm.

The Mission

The purpose and function of a business are often expressed in terms of its mission, which indicates the purposes of the business, for example, "to design, develop, manufacture, and market specific product lines for sale on the basis of certain features or price to meet the specified needs of certain customer groups through predetermined distribution channels in particular geographic areas." A statement along these lines indicates what the business is about and is infinitely clearer than saying: "We're in printing," or "we're here to make a profit."

The Vision

A preliminary step is the development of a realistic vision for the firm. It must be presented as a picture of the business for the future, in 3 or more years time in terms of its likely physical appearance, size, activities, and so forth. Consider future products, markets, customers, processes, location, staffing, and so on.

Key Results Areas

Most companies have 10 to 15 key results areas (KRAs), areas in which the organization must achieve success to grow and prosper. The company's objectives and tactics can be grouped into these key areas, making it easier to process and prioritize objectives, allocate resources, and coordinate with other areas.

These are developed from the SWOT analysis. Following are some examples of KRAs[3]:

- Increase revenues
- Keep pace with the competition
- Improve efficiency and productivity
- Achieve and maintain superior customer service
- Capitalize on emerging trends

Developing Business Strategies

After the SWOT review is completed, a series of tactics usually suggests itself, for example:

- Build on strengths
- Resolve weaknesses
- Exploit opportunities
- Avoid threats

Why Strategic Plans Fail

No treatment of this subject would be complete without mention of the fact that some strategic plans fail. The major reasons are as follows:

- Strategy was defined incorrectly.
- The plans lacked detailed implementation steps with tasks, schedules, and responsibilities.
- Goals were not stated in clear and quantifiable terms.
- Planning did not involve input of key managers.

■ Pricing

The prices charged for pharmaceutical products have been the subject of public policy scrutiny for many years. Politicians wishing to demonstrate their concern for the welfare of citizens have periodically determined that the prices charged for medications provide a relatively risk-free platform to show concern and gain public visibility. In response, the pharmaceutical industry goes into a defensive posture and defends the need for research as its only reason for such prices. The net result, inevitably, is that the industry loses ground, either through a damaged public image or through the loss of some pricing freedom.[4]

The unique nature of pharmaceuticals, being the product of profit-seeking corporations but considered by many to be a "public good," has resulted in major differences between pharmaceutical markets and the so-called free markets.[4]

The topic of pharmaceutical pricing is further complicated by the variety of pricing levels that may be referred to. The highest price is usually referred to as Average Wholesale Price (AWP). Purchasers of pharmaceuticals often receive credits or discounts against this AWP price for such items at cash discounts, chargebacks, and rebates. This section attempts to explain some of these pharmaceutical pricing issues.[4]

Chargebacks

In simple terms, a chargeback is the difference between the manufacturer's price to the wholesaler and the contract price to the customer. Wholesalers submit chargeback requests to the manufacturer on a regular basis (daily or weekly). Each chargeback request may contain thousands of line items for review. A typical drug manufacturer processes millions of chargeback requests per year and transfers hundreds of millions of dollars per year in chargeback payments. There are frequent discrepancies in the requested chargeback amount, creating a very onerous and tedious validation process. This section lays the groundwork for understanding the chargeback process in the pharmaceutical industry.[5]

According to SAP, one of the world's leading providers of business software, the pharmaceutical contracting and related chargeback process is complicated, but can be better handled through a collaborative approach among all participants.

The Business Scenario Map, shown in FIGURE 12-1, is designed by SAP for the pharmaceutical industry. "It shows you how different companies—a manufacturer, a wholesaler,

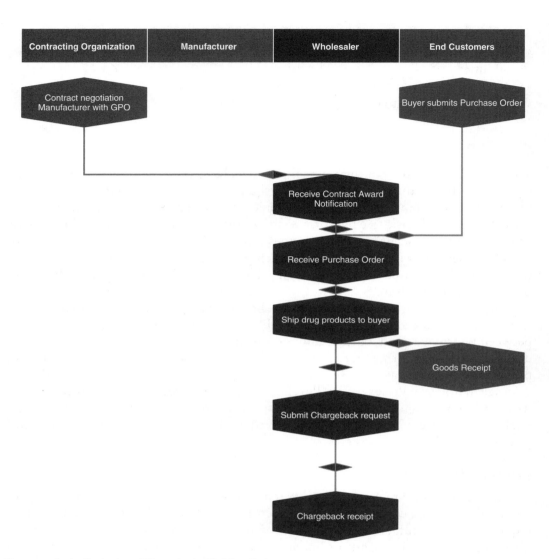

Pharmaceuticals: Contracts and Chargebacks (Collaborative)

FIGURE 12-1 Business scenario map.

a group purchasing organization buyer—use the business Internet to negotiate the best contract prices and settle the resulting chargebacks. The map illustrates the benefits of collaboration. The result is increased processing accuracy which saves times and money" for all.[6]

The buyers of pharmaceuticals, such as a hospital or a drugstore,

may join a group purchasing organization (GPO) to negotiate a better price for purchasing large volumes of drug products. The GPO negotiates with manufacturers to obtain the best contract prices for its members. A typical drug manufacturer may have to negotiate thousands of contracts per year with hundreds of different GPOs. These GPOs may contain over 100,000 individual members.

To simplify the distribution of their drug products, manufacturers also negotiate selling drug products in large quantities to wholesalers at specified catalog prices. The wholesalers then stock their multiple distribution centers with the drug products. Buyers purchase the drug products from wholesalers at the agreed GPO contract prices. The chargebacks occur when the wholesaler sells the drug product at a contract price lower than what he or she paid. The chargeback is the difference between the manufacturer's price to the wholesaler and the contract price to the customer. The wholesaler will submit a chargeback request to the manufacturer.

There are frequent discrepancies in the requested chargeback amount. One of the main reasons for the discrepancies is buying group membership. In the pharmaceutical industry, a customer may belong to one or more buying groups that have different contracts with the manufacturer. The buying group to be in effect for purchasing from the manufacturer is chosen annually by each customer, and then notification is sent by Electronic Data Interchange (EDI) or via the Web as a bid award to wholesalers. When a customer orders from a wholesaler, it is charged the contracted price and the wholesaler submits a chargeback for any price difference to the manufacturer. The manufacturer replies by EDI or through the Web with the amount of credit and any reason for discrepancy.[6]

Rebates

There are currently three federal programs that provide assistance with the cost of medications, the Medicaid Drug Rebate Program, the Federal Supply Schedule (FSS) program, and Medicare.

Medicaid Drug Rebate Program

Medicaid is a state and federally funded program that covers the medically indigent. Medicaid offers prescription drug coverage, which includes guidelines that set the amount of reimbursement to the pharmacies and manufacturers.

Because Medicaid prescription drug coverage is state run, drug plans differ from state to state. Patients covered by Medicaid generally receive their medications from private independent pharmacies. Medicaid-covered consumers may be required to make a nominal copayment at the time of purchase. The Medicaid program then reimburses the pharmacy a set amount for the prescription drug. This amount is usually a fixed percentage less than the estimated acquisition cost. In this manner, the state pays the actual acquisition cost, plus a slight retail markup. Medicaid programs also employ formularies, restricting the drugs for which they will reimburse.

The Omnibus Budget Reconciliation Act of 1990 (OBRA 90) includes a provision to create the Medicaid Drug Rebate Program. This program is also administered by the Centers for Medicare and Medicaid Services (CMS), whose objective is to obtain discounts on pharmaceutical products dispensed to Medicaid patients. Pharmaceutical companies are required to have an agreement with the Department of Health and Human Services for this program, which includes obtaining a minimum discount of 15.1% on branded and 11% on generic pharmaceuticals dispensed to Medicaid recipients. Any price discounted greater than these rates is called the Best Price. Currently, more than 500 pharmaceutical companies participate in this program.

As of January 1, 1996, the rebate for covered outpatient drugs included innovator and noninnovator drugs. The rebate for innovator drugs is calculated by using the larger of 15.1% of the Average Manufacturer Price (AMP) per unit or the difference between the AMP and the Best Price per unit and adjusted by the Consumer Price Index for Urban Consumers (CPI-U) based on launch date and current quarter AMP. The calculation for noninnovator drugs is based on 11% of the AMP per unit. AMP is defined as the average price paid to manufacturers by wholesalers for drugs distributed to the retail class of trade. Pharmaceutical manufacturers calculate AMP at the end of each calendar quarter to help them determine the amount of rebates owed to state Medicaid programs for the manufacturer's drug products dispensed in that quarter.

Manufacturers need to consider all of the rebates, discounts, and price concessions that they provide to retail pharmacy customers, such as prompt-pay discounts, volume discounts, and cash discounts, when performing the AMP calculation. Pharmaceutical manufacturers also need to include the value of any free goods that they provide to retail pharmacies.

An example of how to calculate AMP is as follows: A manufacturer earns $100 in revenue by selling 1,000 units to a retail pharmacy and paid $40 in discounts to these customers; thus, AMP is calculated as $100 – $40 / 1,000 units = 6 cents/unit.[7]

In addition to the programs just mentioned, there are other programs run by the federal, or state or local governments. They are smaller, usually, and we will not go into detail about them here. Some of these include the Indian Health Service, for Native Americans residing on reservations, and public health clinics run by cities or counties, among others.

Public Health Services Program Overview

Under this program the manufacturer agrees to charge a price to those who are eligible that will not exceed the amount determined under a legislative procedure. Section 340B of the Public Health Service Act functions as the nation's safety net to manage the cost of serving vulnerable and low-income patients. This program limits the cost of covered outpatient drugs to certain federal grantees, federally qualified health center look-alikes, and qualified disproportionate share hospitals. Those who participate in this federal program can see a significant savings on pharmaceuticals.

Federal Supply Schedule Program Overview

The Federal Supply Schedule (FSS) is a federal government program that purchases pharmaceuticals and other various healthcare products for its own use. The Veterans Administration administers this program and purchases more than $2 billion in pharmaceuticals annually for itself and other governmental entities such as the Department of Defense, the Coast Guard, and the Indian Health Service.

Medicare Part B Overview

The Medicare Prescription Drug Improvement and Modernization Act of 2003 was enacted to provide individuals with disabilities and seniors with prescription drug benefits. To ensure appropriate pricing, the Centers for Medicare and Medical Services (CMS) requires that manufacturers submit their average sale price on a quarterly basis. A manufacturer's chief executive officer (CEO), chief financial officer (CFO), or another corporate delegate must certify the accuracy of these calculations. These prices are used by CMS to reimburse physicians for Medicare Part B drugs, which are not paid on a cost or prospective payment basis. This ensures that CMS is getting a reasonable, current rate for the drugs it purchases.

Private Sector Pricing*

Three different distribution methods link prescription drug manufacturers with consumers:

- *Cash customers.* This type of arrangement involves cash-paying customers, who either have an indemnity insurance (which reimburses out-of-pocket costs) or who do not carry any insurance benefit. Cash customers typically pay the highest prices for pharmaceuticals because they do not have the bargaining power to negotiate better pricing with manufacturers or retail outlets. Usually, they pay at least the

---

* This section is taken from and modified with permission from von Oehsen WH III, Ashe M, Duke K. Pharmaceutical discounts under federal law: state program opportunities. *Am J Health Syst Pharm.* 2003, March 15;60(6):551–553.

average wholesale price (AWP), which is the manufacturer's list price. Cash customers need to shop around to find the lowest prices for drugs.

- *Pharmacy benefit managers (PBMs)*. PBMs are third-party administrators who manage drug benefits for large groups of people, such as insurance plans or self-insured companies. Their huge negotiating power ensures that they get optimal discounts for their subscribers. These discounts, which are honored by both participating pharmacies and preferred manufacturers, can save subscribers 20–40% off of the Average Manufacturer Price.
- *Institutional purchasers*. Institutional purchasers are organizations such as hospitals and health maintenance organizations (HMOs) that generally own and operate their own pharmacies. Institutional purchasers generally receive favorable pricing because they purchase directly from manufacturers instead of procuring through retail markets. Depending on the volume of pharmaceuticals, institutional purchases can generally negotiate discounts of 20–40% below AWP.

Federal Drug Discount Programs*

In contrast to pharmaceutical sales in the private sector, federal purchasers benefit from a complex array of regulations that produce deeper discounts. There are five different federal drug discount programs:

- *Medicaid Drug Rebate Program*. As previously discussed, federal Medicaid law mandates that pharmaceutical companies pay state Medicaid agencies a 15.1% rebate for the AWP for brand name drugs and an 11% rebate for generics. In addition, the Medicaid net price is further reduced by either an inflationary or Best Price adjustment. This means that Medicaid prices will almost always be better than any prices negotiated by the private sector. Medicaid net prices are generally about 40% below AWP.
- *340B Program*. Section 340B of the Public Health Service Act ensures that federally funded clinics, health departments, and hospitals are eligible for below-market discounts. Although the program provides for the same discount structure as the Medicaid Rebate Program, it often is able to negotiate subceiling prices, thereby creating greater discounts. Additional savings are generated because this program does not have to compensate for any retail drug markups and dispensing fees. Generally, the 340B Program prices are about 50% of AWP.
- *Federal Supply Schedule (FSS)*. The FSS is a schedule of contracted prices for frequently used supplies and services available to federal agencies, as well as other gov-

---

* This section is taken from and modified with permission from von Oehsen WH III, Ashe M, Duke K. Pharmaceutical discounts under federal law: state program opportunities. *Am J Health Syst Pharm*. 2003, March 15;60(6):551–553.

ernment entities including US territories and tribal governments. Although there are no laws creating price ceilings for these entities, the government often leverages deals by using a "favored customer" price as a negotiating point. Although it often obtains below-market pricing, the FSS prices are generally slightly higher than the 340B pricing components.

- *Federal Ceiling Price (FCP).* The FCP refers to the maximum price pharmaceutical manufacturers can charge for FSS-listed brand name drugs to the Veterans Administration, Department of Defense, Public Health Service, and the Coast Guard (often referred to as the Big 4). FCP pricing is required to be at minimally 24% below the nonfederal average manufacturer price. FCP are generally slightly below 340B prices.
- *VA contract.* Big 4 purchasers are permitted to negotiate prices below the FCP points. The VA has been especially successful at generating better pricing through the use of a national formulary to rally greater purchasing power. The VA has contracted prices that are up to 65% below AWP.

Discount Pricing Opportunities for States*

State-level entities looking for better pricing for their own drug assistance programs should model their legislation based on current federal discounting laws. States need to take the following three steps to secure best pricing guidelines:

1. *Stay within the Best Price Exemption.* The Medicaid Drug Rebate Program discourages brand name pharmaceutical manufacturers to give deep discounts to many customers. A discount below the minimum increases the rebate obligations that manufacturers will owe to state Medicaid agencies. Federal law mandates that states are allowed to purchase pharmaceuticals at prices below the best prices available to the private sector. Any agreements with the private sector, including bulk purchasing or outsourcing, could endanger these discounting opportunities.
2. *Set price limits.* Many state drug assistance programs already get discounted prices that are comparable to the Medicaid net prices because they require pharmaceutical companies to give equivalent rebates. Many states are considering legislation that could give them access to FSS, 340B, or FCP pricing schedules, thereby further increasing product discounts.
3. *Negotiate subceiling prices.* If a state chooses to mandate price limits through legislation rather than through contract negotiation, it may have the ability to

---

* This section is taken from and modified with permission from von Oehsen WH III, Ashe M, Duke K. Pharmaceutical discounts under federal law: state program opportunities. *Am J Health Syst Pharm.* 2003, March 15;60(6):551–553.

achieve even lower prices through use of a formulary. Using a formulary could leverage additional rebates from manufacturers whose drugs are included on it. States could also provide incentives for patients who have Medicare to seek care and subsequent pharmacy services at a 340B clinic or hospital, thereby using federally brokered pricing discounts.[8]

Now let us review the other major functions of a typical finance department, with the understanding that each firm may be somewhat slightly different.

Multiple pressures imply multiple roles for the finance function, including the following:

- *Scorekeeper*. Processing transactions and maintaining accounting records at low cost and delivering efficient month-end reporting processes.
- *Communicator*. Explaining the business story to internal and external stakeholders.
- *Diligent caretaker*. Ensuring effective operation of governance and control in matters of financial management and operations.
- *Business partner*. Providing the business with insight and advice on competitive issues, developing strategy and plans, operating as business advisor, and challenging the complexity of the business model.[9]

One additional area of recent developments regarding regulatory compliance relates to a relatively new law known as Sarbanes–Oxley.

Sarbanes–Oxley Act of 2002

The Sarbanes–Oxley Act of 2002 (also known as the Public Company Accounting Reform and Investor Protection Act of 2002 and commonly called SOX) is a federal law passed in response to recent corporate accounting scandals, including those at Enron, WorldCom, and Tyco International. These scandals mounted increasing distrust of corporate accounting and reporting practices. This wide-ranging group of new laws establishes new or enhanced standards for all US public company management and boards of trustees, as well as public accounting firms.

The first part of the SOX established a new quasi-public agency called the Public Company Accounting Oversight Board (PCAOB). This board is charged with regulating accounting firms in their roles as auditors of public companies and disciplining as necessary. The act increases financial disclosure rules, internal control assessment, and corporate governance. Major provisions of this act include the following:

- Financial report certification by both CEOs and CFOs
- Requirements that any stock exchange–listed company has a fully independent audit committee, which supervises the relationship between the corporation and its auditor

- The degree of independence an auditor must maintain, including bans on certain types of work for the audited corporation and a precertification by the company's audit committee on any other work that is not audit related
- Ban on most types of personal loans to any corporate executive or director
- Faster reporting on any insider trading
- Significantly larger fines and longer maximum jail sentences for executives who knowingly misstate financial documents

The Sarbanes–Oxley Act is intended to give investors confidence that accounting and auditing principles are stringent enough that the corporate scandals of the early 21st century cannot occur in the future.

■ References

1. PlanWare. *Developing a strategic plan.* BRS, Inc. Available at: http://www.planware.org/strategicplan.htm. Accessed January 6, 2009.
2. Bryson JM. *Strategic Planning for Public and Non-Profit Organizations: A Guide to Strengthening and Sustaining Organizational Achievement.* 3rd ed. San Francisco: Jossey-Bass; 2004.
3. Plicastro ML. *Introduction to Strategic Planning.* Washington, DC: US Small Business Administration; 2002.
4. Kolassa EM. *Elements of Pharmaceutical Pricing.* Binghamton, NY: Haworth Press; 1997.
5. Center for Business Intelligence: http://www.cbinet.com/show_conference.cfm?confCode=PC07036&field=workshop
6. Pharmaceuticals: Contracts & Chargebacks (Collaborative): http://www8.sap.com/businessmaps/iv_182A9570F4EB11D3875B0000E820132C.htm
7. International Pharmaceutical Compliance Summit. *Overview of Government Price Reporting Requirements.* Pharmaceutical Pricing, Payment and Reimbursement Symposia. March 30, 2005.
8. von Oehsen WH III, summarized by Ashe M, Duke K. Pharmaceutical Discounts Under Federal Law: State Program Opportunities.
9. PriceWaterhouseCoopers. *Finance.* Available at: http://www.pwc.com/extweb/service.nsf/docid/75EB298244B82EA3852570140054ACB8. Accessed January 6, 2009.

■ Additional Resources

Bradford RW, Duncan JP, Tracy B. *Simplified Strategic Planning: A No-Nonsense Guide for Busy People Who Want Results Fast.* Worcester, Mass: Chandler House; 2000.

Fogg CD. *Team-Based Strategic Planning: A Complete Guide to Structuring, Facilitating and Implementing the Process.* New York, NY: American Management Association; 1994.

Goodstein L, Nolan T, Pfeiffer JW. *Applied Strategic Planning: How to Develop a Plan That Really Works.* New York: McGraw-Hill; 1993.

Olsen E. *Strategic Planning for Dummies.* New York, NY: John Wiley; 2006.

Pharmacoeconomics and Outcomes Research

Albert I. Wertheimer

Until 25 years ago, there were just enough drugs manufactured to meet worldwide demand, and essentially everything produced was sold. But today, there is more industry capacity and more generic and branded competitors and manufacturers needing to find a specific niche where their product is the most cost-beneficial one on the market. Many of the major pharmaceutical companies believe that outcomes research will profoundly affect their corporate image and their future corporate identity.[1]

In the "good old days," physicians selected a drug for a patient and the patient took the prescription to the pharmacy, paid for it, and received a bottle of pills or capsules. No one looked over the shoulder of the physician and no one dictated which drug should be used. That scenario described what used to be the norm in fee for service medicine practice. In that environment, the physician performed some service for the patient, and the patient paid for it from his or her own pocket.

That individual patient (or consumer, to the economist) had no bargaining power or market leverage. The patient paid the price that was demanded and purchased what was selected for him. If he were to make a fuss about the price or the nature of the service, he would likely be told to find another physician because the loss of one "customer" would not have a material impact on the physician's income.

The advent of indemnity health insurance did not change the scenario very much because the insurer did not know what had been done or prescribed, often for weeks or months after the date of the service provision when the patient submitted the paid receipts for reimbursement.

All of that changed in the 1970s when health maintenance organizations (HMOs) were founded to provide prepaid, closed panel health care. Now the HMO could create a formulary or practice algorithms for its participating physicians. They would use drug A from among the five competing products. The HMO would receive a discount, which it could use to lower costs and therefore lower premiums to remain competitive. This was an example of a cost-minimization process.

That crude drug selection process to earn a volume or quantity discount from the manufacturer in the 1970s has evolved into the current, sophisticated process of using pharmacoeconomic methods to select the most cost-beneficial product among all options as the preferred formulary drug for managed care organizations (MCOs).

The cost calculations today consider global costs of physician visits, the need for imaging, laboratory tests, hospital admissions, treatment of adverse events, and so forth. The most cost-beneficial drug has a lower copayment to provide a financial incentive for the patient to accept that drug product.

■ Definition

Outcomes research is a term originally used to describe a particular line of health services research that focused on identifying variations in medical procedures and associated health outcomes.[2] It consists of three components: clinical, economic, and humanistic outcomes. According to Kozma and colleagues,[3] *clinical outcomes* are defined as medical events that occur as a result of disease or treatment. *Economic outcomes* are defined as direct, indirect, and intangible costs compared with the consequences of medical treatment alternatives. *Humanistic outcomes* are defined as the consequences of disease or treatment on patient functional status or quality of life.

Pharmacoeconomics is defined as a social science concerned with the description and analysis of the costs of pharmaceutical products and services and their impact on individuals, healthcare systems, and society.[4] Because pharmacoeconomics is a social science substantially concerned with events in clinical practice, it overlaps with a branch of medicine called outcomes research. Pharmacoeconomics is that subset of economics that deals with pharmaceuticals and includes economic outcomes.

Because of the changes in the marketplace, pharmaceutical manufacturers have established outcomes research/pharmacoeconomics/pricing departments. Naturally, the scope, depth, and focus of these vary by company. The larger, research-intensive multinational firms maintain full capacities in these areas internally, whereas the smaller firms outsource this work to outside consulting firms that specialize in this area.

The larger firms have departments that can exceed 50 persons. The staff is usually a mix of physicians, pharmacists, and finance, economics, and business graduates. Of course there are also statisticians and database use/computer experts.

Such a department calculates a cost–benefit equation and has data that may be used by the sales force in detail visits or in making presentations to managed care formulary committees or purchasing staff within the United States. Abroad, the data are used when negotiating with the government health authorities in setting a price for the product in that country.

■ History of Outcomes Research

Early proponents of outcomes measurement focused on its value as an indicator of quality. In 1914, Ernst A. Codman, a surgeon, noted that hospitals were reporting the number of patients treated but not how many of the patients benefited from treatment. He argued that all hospitals should produce a report "showing as nearly as possible what are the results of the treatment obtained at different institutions. This report must be made out and published by each hospital in a uniform manner so that comparison will be possible."[5]

In 1966, Donabedian readdressed Codman's concept of quality,[6] creating the term *outcome* as part of his *structure, process, and outcome* paradigm for quality assessment. Donabedian had a broad definition of *outcome*: "Although some outcomes are generally unmistakable and easy to measure (death, for example), other outcomes, not so clearly defined, can be difficult to measure. These include patient attitudes and satisfactions, social restoration and physical disability, and rehabilitation." He believed that "outcomes, by and large, remain the ultimate validators of the effectiveness and quality of medical care."

From the 1970s to mid-1980s, concerns about lack of oversight grew as advanced technology was applied to a greater number of patients, resulting in exploding healthcare costs. Many writers noted that the increase in costs did not necessarily bring improved patient outcomes. Archie L. Cochrane was one of them. He warned in his book that "cure is rare while the need for care is widespread, and that the pursuit of cure at all costs may restrict the supply of care."[7] He noted the "very widespread belief that for every symptom, or group of symptoms, there was a bottle of medicine, a pill, an operation, or some other therapy which would at least help."[5] If all of these therapies were applied without evidence of benefit, the system would become bankrupt. He also advocated the randomized clinical trial as the best way of determining effectiveness.[5]

By 1988, government, other third-party payers, patients, and physicians were all seeking improvements in the delivery of health care and objective evidence of value for money. Paul M. Ellwood wrote about a plan to link treatment and outcome data in a massive database to facilitate "outcomes management."[8] He believed that studying the outcomes of large numbers of patients—including standardized survival, disease status, quality of life, and cost information—could improve patient care and inform national policies.

■ Other Types of Outcomes Besides Clinical Outcomes

There are three types of outcomes: clinical, economic, and humanistic. The vast majority of interest, research, and publications involve clinical and economic outcomes. Clinical outcomes are reported in the clinical studies, clinical trials, and in the clinical literature. This is where we learn the percentage of conditions resolved, the extent of adverse events, and other findings of relevance to clinicians.

Humanistic outcomes encompass quality of life and patient satisfaction. Insurers and other payers have very little interest in this matter and there is minimal research support for studies in this realm.

The interest of insurers, managed care organizations, and other payers involves economic (sometimes referred to as financial) outcomes for decision making regarding formulary placement or copayment tier status.

Economic Outcomes

Cost Analysis

Pharmacoeconomics focuses on the cost and economic aspects of drug use decision making. The clinical outcomes are combined with cost/price data to calculate relative efficiency. The basic calculations involve cost analysis. This is further explained as follows:

- Cost of care
- Burden of illness

A cost of care analysis is an enumeration of the healthcare resources consumed—in this case, drugs, pharmacy services, and so forth—and the dollar costs of providing care to a given patient population over a given time period. The outcomes resulting from the care are not considered.[4]

A cost of illness analysis normally falls under the umbrella of other outcomes research rather than of pharmacoeconomics. In a classical cost of illness analysis, the total cost that a particular disease imposes on society is expressed as a single dollar amount. Burden of illness, in essence, is the same thing as cost of illness except that the emphasis is placed on the more tangible component costs rather than on an aggregate dollar figure. Thus, the total direct medical costs of treating an illness, the number of deaths, hospitalizations, lost work days, and so forth, are the variables of interest in a burden of illness analysis.

Cost Outcomes Analysis

The basic tools of pharmacoeconomic analysis involve four equations used as appropriate. Each has a specific purpose, in comparing similar or identical alternative therapeutic choices, in investigating the cost per clinical unit of benefit, etc.

- Cost-effectiveness
- Cost utility
- Cost minimization
- Cost–benefit

Humanistic Outcomes

Humanistic outcomes are mainly of real interest to patients only. HMOs have little interest whether one drug causes stomach cramps more than another, or one drug leaves a metallic taste in the mouth. Nevertheless, humanistic outcomes play a role where the cost and effectiveness of two drug products are essentially identical. In such instances, the option favored by patients will be selected.

- Quality of life
- Patient preference
- Patient satisfaction
- Willingness-to-pay

■ Types of Pharmacoeconomic Evaluation

Cost-Effectiveness

Cost-effectiveness analysis compares two (or more) alternative treatments for a given condition in terms of their monetary costs per unit of effectiveness.[4] The unit of effectiveness can be any "natural" unit—such as percent lowering of LDL-C, major coronary events, number of lives saved, or years of life saved. The unit of cost (currency and year) and effectiveness must be the same for the treatments compared. Cost-effectiveness analysis is used to decide among two or more treatment options.

Cost Utility

A cost utility analysis is performed in the same way as a cost-effectiveness analysis except that the unit of effectiveness is quality-adjusted life-years (QALYs) or another measure of utility.[4] Consider that the outcome of a treatment may be a prolonged life but with a degree of disability, or a reduced probability of disability without prolongation of life. The value or *utility* that individuals or society place on different life outcomes can be qualified using a number of techniques.

Because the endpoint is in practice always expressed as cost per QALY saved, cost utility analysis can be used to compare not just alternative therapies for the same disease but therapies for different diseases, and rankings of the cost utilities can be drawn up.[4] Such rankings can be useful in selecting investments when, for example, a government wants to choose among installing highway guard rails, hiring additional food inspectors, or vaccinating seniors for flu.

Cost Minimization

A cost minimization analysis is a cost-effectiveness analysis in the special case in which the effectiveness of the treatment is the same.[4] Once the effectiveness (expressed in whatever natural units are appropriate) has been determined to be equivalent for the alternative treatments, is it not considered further and the analysis focuses entirely on

TABLE 13-1	Types of Pharmacoeconomic Evaluation	
Methodology	Cost Unit	Outcome Unit
Cost-effectiveness	Dollars	Natural units or unit of effect
Cost utility	Dollars	Quality-adjusted life-years (QALYs) or other utility
Cost minimization	Dollars	Natural units assumed to be equivalent in comparative group
Cost–benefit	Dollars	Dollars

the costs, with the aim of determining which treatment minimizes costs. A cost minimization analysis is, in effect, a cost of care analysis in which alternative treatments are compared. Unlike a true cost of care analysis, however, the outcomes are taken into account and must be shown to be equivalent.

Cost–Benefit

Like cost-effectiveness analysis, cost–benefit analysis compares the costs and outcomes of alternative therapies; unlike cost-effectiveness analysis, however, the outcomes in a cost–benefit analysis are expressed in monetary terms. For example, the outcome of the treatment in question is first expressed in terms of life-years saved or quality-adjusted life-years saved, and this is then translated into an equivalent monetary amount— under the human capital approach, this amount is the present value of a person's lifetime productivity. Because both the costs and the effects of the treatment are expressed in the same units, they can be directly compared. Any cost–benefit ratio of less than 1.0 is cost beneficial. (See TABLE 13-1.)

■ Different Types of Outcomes Research Study Designs

Pharmacoeconomic studies usually require data both on costs and effectiveness. The effectiveness data are taken from epidemiologic or medical research studies. The design of every medical research study can be classified according to a few fundamental mutually exclusive dichotomies (see TABLE 13-2).

Retrospective Study Design

A retrospective study means when data are being collected, the events being studied have already occurred. This case happens only when the study is an observational one. Retrospective economic analyses have been performed on clinical trials that did not originally include an economic component. These studies are limited by the lack of some patient-specific information (eg, out-of pocket costs) and the potential for incomplete

TABLE 13-2	Outcomes Research Study Designs		
Investigator Involvement	Study Design		
	Observational		Experimental
Time Perspective	Prospective	Retrospective	Prospective
Time Sampling	Longitudinal or cross-sectional	Longitudinal or cross-sectional	Longitudinal

data recorded in medical records. Quality-of-life information for patients who receive new therapeutic strategies may not be retrievable retrospectively. Even with comprehensive data for specific sites, such as medical records for a study center, economic data are frequently missing or incomplete. However, beside the limitation mentioned, it is indeed less expensive and time consuming.

Prospective Study Design

A prospective study means when data are being collected, the events being studied have not occurred yet and will be studied as they happen. Prospective economic evaluation can be included in all phases of the clinical development process—phases 1 through 4. Because prospective economic studies of clinical trials are based on random assignment of patient populations to treatment groups, it protects against biases in patient assignment and ensures appropriate comparison groups for the assessment of new therapeutic strategies. Often, in prospective economic studies, the resources required to care for patients are recorded in the clinical case report forms, whereas the costs of the resources are collected outside the clinical trial. Although prospective study is more accurate and favored by researchers, it is very costly and time consuming.

■ Why Are Outcomes Research and Pharmacoeconomics Done by the Pharmaceutical Industry?

Advanced knowledge and technology have resulted in improved medicines and increased healthcare costs. However, they do not necessarily result in improved patient outcomes. Government, other third-party payers, patients, and physicians are all seeking improvements in the delivery of health care and objective evidence of value for money. As a result, outcomes research and pharmacoeconomic analysis become a requirement when drug companies seek approval to market a drug in the country or get onto the formulary of a third-party payer.

In Europe, especially in western Europe, the authority in charge of drug approval in many countries requires outcomes research and pharmacoeconomic analysis reports as a part of the document to demonstrate the value of the drug. Especially in the markets of countries in which drug products are subject to price regulations and reimbursement controls, there is a need for companies to justify price premiums for innovative products on the basis of cost-effectiveness and other pharmacoeconomic analyses.[9,10]

In the United States, although the Food and Drug Administration (FDA) does not require outcomes research and pharmacoeconomic analysis reports for its review for the approval of a drug, drug companies still need to have these reports to demonstrate the value of their drugs to get onto a third-party payer's formulary. If the report shows a great value of the drug, the drug can not only get onto the formulary, but also be a first-tier or second-tier drug.

Most MCOs maintain a formulary committee, sometimes called a P&T (Pharmacy and Therapeutics) committee, that evaluates new drugs shortly after they are approved for marketing and routinely reviews the clinical literature to determine whether preferred drug choices should be modified. This is likely to occur when a patented, branded drug loses patent protection and less costly generic versions appear in the marketplace.

A typical P&T committee may place a new drug into one of three categories:

1. Drug is inferior or no more than equal to existing therapies.
2. Drug has some advantages over existing therapies.
3. Drug is a significant improvement and should be adopted for use immediately.

A category 1 drug will only find its way to a formulary listing if its advantage is a reasonable price decrease. Category 2 drugs may or may not be included depending on pricing and deals, and category 3 drugs will almost always be included in the formulary.

During the 1990s, each MCO, HMO, and insurer had its own forms to be completed by the manufacturer for formulary consideration, but a standard form was produced by the Academy of Managed Care Pharmacy that today is nearly universally employed.

■ Not All Drugs Work for 100% of Patients

Assume that there is a patient with hypertension. When she goes to a doctor, the doctor has three angiotensin converting enzyme inhibitors (ACEIs) to use. Drug A has low effectiveness, but its price is low, too. Drug B has superior effectiveness, but it costs a lot more. Drug C has medium effectiveness and cost. All of them cause patients to cough as a side effect; however, the chance of each of them varies (see TABLE 13-3).

According to the data, the cost of the treatment with drug C will be $5,550/month, while that with drug B and drug A will be $4,800 and $5,575, respectively, for 100 patients. Once the decision has been made to use drug B (as shown in the calculation in the FIGURE 13-1), drug B will be inserted into the hypertension algorithm, where a drug is called for. An example of this treatment protocol is shown in FIGURE 13-2, where the physicians see an evidence-based protocol optimal for the treatment of hypertension.

Drug Names	Cost for ACEIs (per day)	% Effectiveness	% Cough	Cost for Cough Medicine (per month)	Cost for 2nd Medication (per day)
A	$0.80	70%	15%	$20.00	$1.50
B	$1.25	90%	5%	$20.00	$1.50
C	$1.00	75%	10%	$20.00	$1.50

TABLE 13-3   Information on Drugs A, B, and C

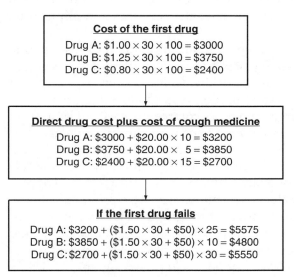

Cost of the first drug
Drug A: $1.00 × 30 × 100 = $3000
Drug B: $1.25 × 30 × 100 = $3750
Drug C: $0.80 × 30 × 100 = $2400

Direct drug cost plus cost of cough medicine
Drug A: $3000 + $20.00 × 10 = $3200
Drug B: $3750 + $20.00 × 5 = $3850
Drug C: $2400 + $20.00 × 15 = $2700

If the first drug fails
Drug A: $3200 + ($1.50 × 30 + $50) × 25 = $5575
Drug B: $3850 + ($1.50 × 30 + $50) × 10 = $4800
Drug C: $2700 + ($1.50 × 30 + $50) × 30 = $5550

FIGURE 13-1 Cost of using drugs for 100 patients.

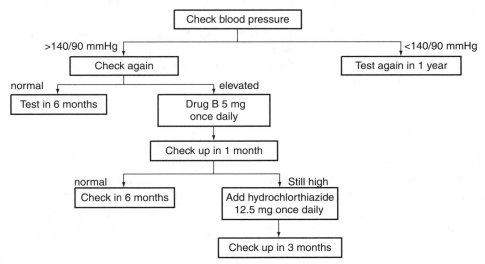

FIGURE 13-2 Protocol for treating hypertension.

■ Piggyback Pharmacoeconomics on Clinical Trials

Pharmacoeconomic analysis early in the drug development process can provide valuable input into: (1) the design of clinical and nonclinical development programs (what information is collected and when); (2) project selection and termination decisions (portfolio management); and (3) the optimal pricing strategy.[11] Drug development involves many resources and many choices. Pharmacoeconomics can be used to aid resource allocation decisions, which means it can help manufacturers develop more efficient products in a more efficient manner. For a pharmaceutical company, pharmacoeconomic analysis in phase 3 development can support both external and internal decision makers, which means maximizing sales revenues and minimizing costs.

Today, pharmaceutical companies consume a significant amount of resources in the development of new drugs. From a survey of R&D costs of 68 randomly selected new drugs from 10 pharmaceutical companies worldwide, it has been estimated that the average cost per new drug is now US$802 million (year 2000 value).[12] The key factor pushing up R&D costs include larger and more complex clinical trials, shifts in the therapeutic product mix toward targeting more expensive chronic and degenerative illnesses, and increased expenditure on technological and labor inputs. Early pharmacoeconomic activities can reduce the amount of money spent on the entire R&D portfolio through the early elimination of unattractive projects and a focus on opportunity costs where resources saved are relocated to more attractive projects.[11]

Costs increase tremendously as a drug moves through the development phases. Earlier decisions to terminate development of drugs that will eventually fail would significantly reduce costs. It has been shown that shifting 5% of all clinical failures from phase 3 to phase 1 could reduce clinical development costs by up to 7.1%.[13] This is an important reason to begin pharmacoeconomic studies early so that the economic prospects of a new drug candidate can be evaluated before undertaking costly phase 3 trials.[14]

Ideally, economic models of therapy are developed in phase 1, pilot testing data collection instruments are completed in phase 2, pivotal assessment of therapies is completed in phase 3, and assessments of different comparative agents or "real-world" effectiveness studies of therapies are completed in phase 4.[15]

■ Other Issues

At the moment, the FDA has no regulations regarding the use of pharmacoeconomic data, but it is likely to enact some shortly. Most observers agree that would be a good move to demand rigor in the studies.

Because it is perfectly legal and a wise policy for a pharma company to maximize its profits, it can conduct substudies of various categories of patients until it finds a group where its drug excels compared to others. If it is found to be superior for postmenopausal women aged 70 and older, the drug will be promoted as especially formulated for that patient population.

European Social Security authorities have fought back by introducing "reference pricing" for drugs. If the previous standard therapy cost 1 Euro per day, the new drug will have to demonstrate some significant advantage in clinical outcomes or patient satisfaction to be granted a higher price. If the drug can prove no clinical superiority, its rationale for formulary inclusion will have to be a price discount compared to the older product.[16]

The issue of perspective cannot be ignored in pharmacoeconomic calculations. Any study has to be done from a single perspective. Usually, the four possible perspectives used are payer, provider, patient, and society. As you can see immediately, the loss of wages is a significant cost to the patient, but an irrelevancy for the managed care organization. Most calculations are done from the payer (insurance company, MCO) perspective.

Pharmacoeconomics and outcomes research remain dynamic and exciting areas within pharmaceutical companies. You can expect to see continuing refinements in methodologies and greater precision in calculations enabling health care to make rational, evidence-based decisions in drug selection.

■ References

1. Wyse R. Outsourcing—a growing force in health economics. *Scrip Mag.* 1996:40–44.
2. *Medical Outcomes and Guidelines Sourcebook.* New York, NY: Faulkner & Gray; 1996.
3. Kozma CM, Reeder CE, Shulz RM. Economic, clinical, and humanistic outcomes: a planning model for pharmacoeconomic research. *Clin Ther.* 1993;15:1121–1132.
4. Morrison A, Wertheimer AI. *Pharmacoeconomics: A Primer for the Pharmaceutical Industry.* Philadelphia, PA: Temple University; 2002.
5. Codman EA. The product of a hospital. *Surg, Gynecol Obstet.* 1914;18:491–496.
6. Donabedian A. Evaluating the quality of medical care. *Milbank Q.* 1966;44(suppl):166–206.
7. Cochrane AL. *Effectiveness and Efficiency: Random Reflections on the Health Services.* London: Nuffield Provincial Hospitals Trust; 1972.
8. Ellwood PM. Shattuck Lecture: Outcomes management: a technology of patient experiences. *N Engl J Med.* 1988;318:1549–1556.
9. Davies L, Coyle D, Drummond M, et al. Current status of economic appraisal of health technology in the European Community: report of the network. *Soc Sci Med.* 1994;38(12):1601–1607.
10. Drummond M, Rutten F, Brenna A, et al. Economic evaluation of pharmaceuticals: a European perspective. *Pharmacoeconomics.* 1993;4(3):173–186.
11. Miller P. Role of pharmacoeconomic analysis in R&D decision making: when, where, how? *Pharmacoeconomics.* 2005;23(1):1–12.
12. DiMasi JA, Hansen RW, Grabowski HG. The price of innovation: new estimates of drug development costs. *J Health Econ.* March 2003;22(2):151–185.

13. DiMasi JA. The value of improving the productivity of the drug development process: faster times and better decisions. *Pharmacoeconomics*. 2002;20(suppl 3):11–29.

14. Grabowski HG. The effect of pharmacoeconomics on company research and development decisions. *Pharmacoeconomics*. May 1997;11(5):389–397.

15. Schulman KA, Linas BP. Pharmacoeconomics: state of the art in 1997. *Ann Rev Public Health*. 1997;18:529–548.

16. Wertheimer AI, Navarro RP. *Managed Care Pharmacy: Principles and Practice*. Binghamton, NY: Haworth Press; 1999.

Public Affairs

James Russo

■ Introduction

Public affairs departments typically comprise several component divisions such as state and federal governmental affairs, public relations, trade and professional relations, investor relations, policy analysis, and community relations. The terminology employed varies quite widely. The objective of a public affairs department is to establish and maintain contact with academic institutions, relevant professional and business/industry groups, patient organizations, and the media. Such a department promotes the image, views, and good works of the industry to opinion leaders, the media, and others and protects and represents the interests of the industry. Public affairs departments function both individually and through liaisons to organized trade associations that represent the entire industry.

The primary organizations representing the various segments of the pharmaceutical industry in the United States are the Pharmaceutical Research and Manufacturers of America (PhRMA), which represents about 35 of the major pharmaceutical and biotechnology companies; the National Pharmaceutical Council (NPC), which represents a smaller number of research-intensive pharmaceutical manufacturers; the Generic Pharmaceutical Association (GPhA), representing the generic manufacturers; and the Consumer Healthcare Products Association (CHPA), representing the sellers of over-the-counter medications. In addition, other organizations represent various aspects of the industry, such as clinical research organizations and animal health product makers, but they are not featured in this chapter.

Above all, pharmaceutical manufacturers have an immense task to tackle: the very negative public opinion of the industry as being uncaring firms only interested in large profits. There is a high priority to inform thought leaders and the public in general about the companies' social investments, their products' ability to replace more costly or less effective interventions, and the potential negative effects of excessive regulatory effects on the industry's ability to innovate.

■ Inside the Department

The activities in a public affairs department can be broadly divided into two categories. The first category is routine responsibilities that are conducted regularly and that may be seen at all such companies. The second category can be broadly described as the need to respond to unpredictable events. When there is a product recall or when there is publicity about problems with one company's products or when an officer or other representative of the company gets into some trouble or difficulties, it falls to the public affairs department to deal with the media and with the efforts of the company to put things right—or, minimally, to put a positive "spin" to diminish the negative consequences of the event. Good media relations are essential to a successful public affairs department, and therefore such departments maintain regular contact with the various media that cover the industry. And they provide periodic media training for key executives and department heads who may be called upon to speak for the company from time to time.

Within the area of governmental affairs, there are a number of functions that a public affairs department is responsible for. For example, it is necessary to establish and maintain good relations with the various governmental and regulatory agencies, including the legislative bodies. The company's government affairs staff, therefore, uses a variety of services to reach state and federal regulatory agency personnel as well as legislators and their staffs. These may be in the form of periodic seminars in which these persons are invited to learn some of the latest developments about the pharmaceutical sector and may also take the form of newsletters and other mailings. Good relations with legislators also may include support of candidates' reelection campaigns through donations by the company as well as encouraging donations from the employees through the company political action committee (PAC). Another way of helping legislators is to provide information or background for a speech or presentation. And, of course, the company may ask legislators who represent districts in which the firm has plants and employees to introduce legislation favorable to the firm's needs or to oppose bills the company cannot support. Legislators normally welcome the opportunity to show their constituents that they are active on behalf of their employers, particularly regarding jobs.

Oftentimes, legislators and public affairs personnel work together on mutually beneficial matters. For example, there may be some policy that the company would like to make illegal and the legislator may oblige the company and assist with that issue if he or she also sees that there is some merit in this activity for the voters. Similarly, a pharmaceutical manufacturer will want to have good relations with the career personnel at the various regulatory agencies because the patent office, Food and Drug Administration, the Federal Trade Commission, Environmental Protection Agency, and other regulatory agencies have considerable say about the future of all companies.

When new legislation or regulatory changes are proposed—at either the state or the federal level—it is the public affairs department's responsibility to advise management about the impact of the proposal on the company's interests. If the analysis indicates that it will have no impact or a salutary one, the firm may elect to take a passive attitude toward it or to actively support its adoption. However, if the analysis projects negative consequences, then it will become the obligation of the department to resist the enactment of that legislation with the legal and acceptable tools available to it. This may include preparation of testimony to be presented at public hearings; discussions with staffers and company experts to seek changes in the bill or regulation the company can support; coordination with other interested companies through trade associations; and collaboration with allied organizations, for example, medical, pharmacy, and patient groups.

Another major function or focus of a public affairs department is in the area of donations or charitable contributions. (This function is separate from political contributions, which are usually managed from the firm's government affairs offices.)

In recent years, there has been substantial growth in pharmaceutical companies' support of international relief agencies and other developmental assistance organizations, on a worldwide basis. The contributions may be in the form of cash grants or in-kind services or donation of pharmaceutical products. In-kind services might include the loan of company specialists (eg, experts in supply chain management, transportation, quality control) to local governments or humanitarian agencies after a disaster to help the community get back on its feet as soon as may be practically possible. In-kind services also include the loan of equipment or a service. For example, a pharma company may print some educational materials for an organization or for the survivors in a disaster area.

The last—but often most important—kind of contributions are the actual products that a pharmaceutical manufacturer makes and sells. Traditionally, such donations were made out of surplus inventory—products that the firm expected to sell but that the market has not absorbed. However, as new and more precise techniques have enabled manufacturers to very closely approximate demand, smaller and smaller quantities of excess or surplus products are available. More and more firms are now manufacturing specifically for the client humanitarian organization without interfering with the quantity available for sale in their regular courses of business. One indicator of the growth of the research-based pharmaceutical industry's activities in this area is provided by the Partnership for Quality Medical Donations, an alliance of leading medical product makers and humanitarian agencies advancing the health and welfare of persons in the least developed countries and victims of disasters through coordinated donations of money and pharmaceutical products.

■ Public Relations

The corporate contributions office may also manage the firm's scientific awards programs, but more often they are directed by the research and development division.

Drug firms fund some of the most prestigious awards in clinical medicine as well as fellowships and research experience opportunities. The Washington-based drug industry trade organizations provide even more investments in this realm.

When you read an editorial or op-ed article in the lay press asserting that the life of a US patent on a new medication is not long enough to yield sufficient return on its investment, or that greater surveillance is needed to keep foreign products from being imported into the United States, or how some child was miraculously saved by a new experimental drug, it is often likely that one of these companies or its trade association was involved in giving the story to reporters or in some other way "seeding" the story.

In the area of public relations, the pharmaceutical industry does the same things every other private sector organization (and, increasingly, agencies of the federal government) does to advance, improve, or defend its "image." Thus, the company and/or its trade associations provide news stories to journalists and media representatives, fill requests for interviews from journalists, and accept opportunities to address community and professional groups regarding issues and events affecting the pharmaceutical industry. Thus, when counterfeit products are discovered or a widely prescribed medication must be withdrawn in the wake of unexpected adverse effects, the industry attempts to balance the negative news, to the extent that the firm can demonstrate its responsiveness to the problem. Unquestionably, however, such news can all but erase any successes the firm may have had in creating a favorable image of the therapeutic benefits the firm's research programs have achieved for patients.

Only recently can you see several areas where the drug firms' government relations, public relations, and media intervention activities have come in to play. For example, in early 2007 the Congress of the United States, having been taken over by Democrats for the first time in a dozen years, attempted to introduce direct federal government negotiation of pharmaceutical prices, using its enormous purchasing power on behalf of Medicare Part D beneficiaries. The industry prefers to avoid this based on its experience in Europe, where such negotiations are *de rigueur* and significantly lower prices are routinely realized. Through a very active effort (including, for example, outreach to newspaper editorial writers nationwide) the industry made the case for the existing system, under which individual insurance firms administer the Medicare drug program and realize substantial price reductions. As this chapter was being completed, the industry had secured favorable editorials from key newspapers, including the *Washington Post* and the *Wall Street Journal*, and in the initial Senate vote on the bill, government price negotiations were rejected.

Another issue is the frequent news in the lay press touting less costly—and often identical—Rx drugs available in Canada and Mexico. Typically, these human interest stories portray seniors on fixed incomes chartering buses to take them across the borders to buy large supplies of life-sustaining prescription medicines at big savings. Predictably, there have been calls in Congress for legislation and regulations to legalize "reimportation" of such drugs safely and create pathways for generic biological products as well.

These moves also are resisted by the large pharmaceutical and biotechnology manufacturers. In each of these cases, there is a need to tell the industry's side of the story and attempt to create support from voters and legislators so that whatever public policies are developed on this subject will not be adverse to the industry's future vitality.

■ Investor Relations

Investor relations is also a critical area for the pharmaceutical industry as it is for any industry. The investing public must feel that the industry has a bright future and is worthy of investment and that there are promising future prospects. When shareholders read a report about their company's "dry" new product pipeline or that managed care organizations are pressing hard on drug prices, the company's investor relations staff generates information for shareholders and the media to put the stories in context. This effort is among the most sensitive of all the company's communications work. Almost every word and figure used in the context of investment matters can affect investment decisions and will be given close scrutiny by investors and regulators.

Sometimes, for example, when the company's research portfolio is at issue, the company may convene press conferences where industry-based scientists can talk about their work or the possible implications of a new scientific breakthrough in the fight against a particular disease and perhaps some information about the impact on the overall financial or clinical burden of illness in the country. Investor relations departments are also expected to provide visits to pharmaceutical facilities for securities analysts and business writers covering the company.

Key to all of these functions is the public affairs department's ability to provide early intelligence on and to analyze and track a wide array of information and data. The basic objective is to build and maintain the department's capacity to protect management from surprises; provide the time, competence, resources, and—most important—sound judgment needed to allow the firm to avoid policies and activities that lead to adverse outcomes; and when adversity occurs, manage it in a way that preserves the firm's reputation and its ability to work the problem through.

■ Government Relations

How do these departments function? In the information arena, data and conversations must go in both directions. Public affairs personnel are vigilant regarding pending and proposed legislation and upcoming reports in the media and scientific discoveries and breakthroughs in other companies and related industries. This information is passed up the chain of command where decisions are made as to whether or not any company activities are called for or whether, as is the case sometimes, it is best to let sleeping dogs lie.

In the last couple of decades, firms have learned that they must monitor legislative developments at the state level, as well as the federal, because states have increasingly been taking actions to address issues such as runaway Medicaid costs. Many firms now have representatives at the state capitals, or at least some of the major states. The purpose is the same as at the federal level, that is, to acquire early warning on developing issues, prevent or minimize negative outcomes, and facilitate and bolster understanding of the company's importance to the state as an employer, taxpayer, or provider of essential products and services—in short, to advance the image, status, and reputation of the company and the industry. These representatives are the eyes and ears of the company, providing advance notice for any initiatives where the company would want to take a stance. Similarly, the allied professions (medicine, pharmacy, nursing, etc.) have representatives to cover their interests, and the various statewide professional societies hold conferences and meetings where new developments or other market intelligence of possible value to the company is discussed.

■ Media Relations

Typically, public affairs departments offer several varieties of communications skills: media experts, usually with backgrounds in journalism, who build relationships with key journalists to ensure that they know someone in the company who will respond and try to be helpful; speech writers, who prepare senior executives' presentations on public policy matters; policy specialists, who develop analyses and policy statements on key issues, such as national health insurance and corporate responsibility matters; and writers, who draft press releases and brochures and handle routine consumer issues.

One of the company's most important public affairs jobs is the selection of spokespersons, who must be media-trained and available on short notice when news breaks. In most companies, individual executives are strongly encouraged to decline opportunities to comment to the press ad hoc until a well-thought-out position is agreed to. The unfortunate effect of this desire to control what is said often conflicts with the media's deadline needs—and results in a story saying the company had "no immediate comment," with its implication, to many readers, of guilt or evasiveness.

An additional, often quite discrete part of the corporate affairs department serves the investment community—arranging business press and analyst interviews, answering questions from individual shareholders and institutional holders of the stock, and preparing the speeches that are presented to shareholders at the annual meeting of shareholders. The investor relations department's responsibilities also include preparation of the company's most important documents, the quarterly and annual reports to shareholders, with all the crucial financial data and image-building content they must provide.

Finally, investor relations produces the corporate equivalent of a Broadway musical every year, the annual shareholders meeting. These events are not really about financial reporting (virtually all of the business information is public before the meeting occurs). Rather, they are designed to give shareholders and all who attend a favorable perception of the stature, momentum, and outlook of the firm and its senior management.

■ Intelligence Gathering

Because it is not possible to have a staff that reads every newspaper and magazine and listens to the proceedings of every state legislature, many firms use the services of outside organizations that provide everything from newspaper and magazine clipping services to early warnings about investigatory hearings on drug prices being planned in far-off state capitols. These firms provide reports to a client on any topic or term that the client specifies. The client may receive newspaper clippings, recordings from radio or television shows, and reports or proceedings from conferences or other sessions. Some such firms provide political counsel as well as information services, offering guidance on legislative procedures, potential allies within the state who have shared interests, and so forth.

■ Purchasing Influence

How do public affairs departments spend their money? Perhaps the largest single category of cost is outside expertise, for example, consultants in Washington and in state capitals who help the company articulate its positions effectively to the true decision makers. Similarly, the firm may provide unrestricted grants to influential university professors and researchers and other opinion leaders in academia; these may take the form of appointments to speakers' bureaus, consultant panels, or advisory boards. Public affairs also manages the company's political donations to political parties and individual candidates.

The phenomenal rise and importance of public policy institutions over the past couple of decades—the think tank industry—is a major factor in pubic affairs departments as well. They frequently support demonstration projects and studies whose results might be expected to further their causes. Donations and other support are also provided to patient groups and professional societies to help defray the cost of their journals, newsletters, annual conferences, and educational seminars. Sometimes, a company provides its scientists or clinicians as speakers at these meetings, or in other cases money is donated to assist an organization in its work.

■ Measuring Success

To evaluate the effectiveness of a public affairs organization, you need only look at what its mission or mandate is to determine whether it is successful. Did the candidates that the company support win? Was the company able to defeat or postpone potentially negative legislation? Was legislation the firm desired signed into law? Were goals regarding public opinion met? These matters can be evaluated in determining whether a public affairs department was successful and whether funding should be continued or increased.

■ Threats to the Pharmaceutical Industry

All industries face both predictable and some unpredictable threats. For example, the pharmaceutical industry has for many decades been attacked by animal rights groups that oppose all experimentation on laboratory animals. Others are dedicated to reducing patient outlays for prescription drugs, whether through importation of drugs, mandatory use of generic drugs, weakening or elimination of patents, price controls, or profit regulation.

■ Who Works in a Public Affairs Department?

There is wide variation among companies, but many public affairs executives are attorneys, political science graduates, journalists, and ex-congressional staffers. Others have backgrounds in business, social sciences, history, and liberal arts. Others have climbed the corporate ladders through sales or marketing, transferring product-related skills to marketing the corporation as a whole.

■ The Value of a Public Affairs Department

It is difficult to be precise in the matter of quantifying the value of a public affairs department. You can safely say that if the pharma firms did not view these departments as of real value, they would not exist, or at least would not exist in their present form.

So far, the discussion has been limited to the United States. However, every industrialized nation has a pharmaceutical industry and, within each firm, a public affairs department. Similarly, each has a national trade association that looks after the common good. Indeed, some threats are universal, such as drug counterfeiting and compulsory licensing. To address the various global issues, a global association is required. For the drug makers, it's the International Federation of Pharmaceutical Manufacturers Associations (IFPMA) located in Geneva. There, pharmaceutical manufacturers collaborate on the shared challenges of the day.

This brief exploration of pharmaceutical industry corporate affairs departments suggests that their operations are well organized and skillfully staffed and financed to advance this industry's public affairs objectives. It seems fair to ask, therefore, why this industry shows up so badly in every poll of public opinion over the last several decades.

How can an industry whose research has borne so much fruit, whose products do so much to prevent disease, improve survival, raise the quality of life, and hold so much promise, be ranked with tobacco companies and the gun lobby? Clearly, if there were any simple answers, the question would not be asked. But a few questions may be worth exploring:

- How much would public opinion improve with universal drug insurance—and would improved perception of the industry help reduce pressure on prices and patents?
- How much does the industry communicate with opinion makers about its record on corporate responsibility? Would *sustained* outreach to opinion leaders on the industry's support of humanitarian causes change attitudes?
- Is the industry willing to put as much creative effort into changing public perceptions as it is in promoting its products?

Drug companies' public affairs operations are as competent as any in the business world. And, as the preceding questions suggest, their success will be made more likely—and the industry's place in the public square will be enhanced—with more open communication on behalf of the industry.

Generic Drugs

Kathleen Jaeger

America's generic pharmaceutical industry is perhaps the single most significant contributor to affordable health care in the United States. Founded on the simple concept that competition can fuel both innovation and savings, this highly complex balancing act has provided more than two decades of increased access to prescription medicines for employers, healthcare providers, and consumers, particularly the poor, elderly, and underinsured.

Generic pharmaceutical manufacturing in the United States predates the inception of the modern generic industry, which began formally in 1984 with the enactment of the Drug Price Competition and Patent Term Restoration Act of 1984 (commonly known as the Hatch–Waxman Act, in recognition of its primary sponsors, Senator Orrin Hatch of Utah and Congressman Henry Waxman of California). These legislators, and others, recognized the need for creating a regulatory approval process that permitted market entrance of lower-priced, US Food and Drug Administration–approved generic pharmaceutical products following the expiration of the patents on brand-name pharmaceuticals.

The Hatch–Waxman Act, although challenged throughout its history by numerous efforts by brand pharmaceutical companies to capitalize on unintentional loopholes that limit competition, has stood the test of time. Today, the savings provided by generic pharmaceutical competition for brand-name pharmaceuticals exceeds tens of billions of dollars each year.

■ The History

Prior to the approval of the Hatch–Waxman Act, a number of entrepreneurs recognized the potential for manufacturing and marketing generic versions of brand pharmaceutical products. Many of the founding companies of the industry were created to provide consumers with access to simple antibiotic products. Some manufacturers even served as contract manufacturers for brand pharmaceutical companies. This recognition of the value of creating an industry based on providing more affordable versions of brand-name drugs, and its potential to create significant savings for consumers, served as the foundation for the complex legislative compromise of Hatch–Waxman.

The Hatch–Waxman Act opened the floodgates for generic competition for pharmaceutical products, creating the modern generic pharmaceutical industry. However, in the early days of the industry, the potential for companies to earn millions of dollars with generic products resulted in a crisis that virtually destroyed the generic industry 4 years after Hatch–Waxman. In the late 1980s, some unscrupulous manufacturers falsified applications, going so far as to alter branded pharmaceuticals and submit these products as their own. Then, in 1988, a government subcommittee uncovered attempts by unscrupulous manufacturers to bribe FDA employees to gain preferential treatment in the processing of generic drug applications. The industry was rocked by the scandal and the resulting congressional hearings and adverse publicity virtually destroyed public confidence in the fledgling industry, and the very agency charged with regulating it.

In May of 1992, the Generic Act was enacted. The Generic Act, a result of the legislative hearings and investigations into generic drug approval process irregularities, gave the FDA new authority to impose debarment and other penalties on individuals and companies that commit certain illegal acts relating to the generic drug approval process. In some situations, the Generic Act required the FDA to debar (ie, not accept or review Abbreviated New Drug Applications [ANDAs] for a period of time) a company or an individual who has committed certain violations. It also provided for temporary denial of approval of applications during the investigation of certain violations that could lead to debarment and also, in more limited circumstances, provided for the suspension of the marketing of approved drugs by the affected company. Last, the Generic Act allows for civil penalties and withdrawal of previously approved applications.

Today, the generic industry is stronger for having survived the scandal of the late 1980s. The subsequent strengthening of the regulations that govern the generic pharmaceutical industry's ability to manufacture and market products restored public confidence in the quality of generic medicines. In fact, consumer confidence in generic pharmaceuticals as a valued, cost-effective component of health care in the United States has continued to grow significantly over the intervening years. Today, generic pharmaceutical products are a trusted source of affordable health care by physicians, pharmacists, and consumers.

■ Generic Pharmaceutical Industry Growth

More than one billion prescriptions are filled with generic medicines every year. Generic pharmaceuticals represent an increasing proportion of medicines dispensed in the United States. In 1984, the US generic pharmaceutical industry had total US sales of approximately $220 million. In calendar year 2006, the US generic pharmaceutical industry had total US sales of approximately $54 billion.

As sales revenues have grown, so too has the usage of generic pharmaceutical products by American consumers. In 2006, unbranded and branded generics (generic drugs that for marketing reasons are sold under a trade or brand name rather than the name of the active ingredient) represented 63% of the total prescriptions dispensed in the United States, but only 20% of all dollars spent on prescription drugs. In 2006, the average prescription filled with a brand-name product cost $111.02; the average cost for a prescription filled with a generic drug was $32.23.

Growth in the generic pharmaceutical industry has been driven by state and federal government, employers, third-party payers, and consumers working to reduce healthcare costs; increased acceptance of generic medicines by physicians, pharmacists, and consumers; and the availability of an increasingly broad number of generics as the result of the ongoing annual expiration of patents on brand drugs.

The generic pharmaceutical industry is highly competitive. As patents for brand-name products and any related market exclusivity expire, a generic will seek FDA approval to enter the marketplace. Often, generics will enter the market on the same day the brand drug loses exclusivity.

Generic pharmaceuticals represent a much larger percentage of total drug prescriptions dispensed than their corresponding sales percentage. The lower percentage of total dollar sales, compared to the percentage of prescriptions dispensed, reflects the substantial discount at which generic pharmaceuticals are sold. This discount tends to increase as the number of generic competitors increases for a given product.

In the early years of the generic pharmaceutical industry, it often took months, if not years, for generic competition to gain a significant portion of market share. However, in recent years, the ability of generic competition to capture a leading share of the market for a pharmaceutical, and the subsequent rapid decline in price to consumers, has escalated dramatically. Today, generics can capture 80–90% of the market for a specific drug within weeks. And generic drugs that in years past entered the market at a 30% discount to the brand product, and gradually dropped to a 70–80% discount over time, can drop dramatically within weeks. It is a reality that some generic products, in highly competitive environments can enter the market already discounted to 80% or more of the brand price.

These lower prices not only provide an immediate benefit to the consumer, and the insurance payer, government, or employer, but lower prices also increase access. The ability to purchase a more affordable generic medicine has been shown to increase patient compliance with their drug regimen, an issue of particular concern with chronically used medicines, particularly with the infirmed and elderly.

■ Understanding Generic Pharmaceuticals

Generic pharmaceuticals are the chemical and therapeutic equivalents of brand-name drugs. When a medicine is first developed, the pharmaceutical company discovering the product and bringing it to the market for the first time is granted a period of patent protection on that medicine. On average, blockbuster products enjoy protection from about a dozen patents, with each patent running from 20 years from the date of the filing of that patent application with the Patent and Trademark Office (PTO). The brand companies also enjoy market exclusivity—a market monopoly protection that is mutually exclusive of patent protection and which is provided through the Hatch–Waxman Act. Novel medicines (commonly referred to as new chemical entities [NCEs]) are awarded 5 years of market exclusivity, with new pharmaceutical products securing 3 years.

When the patents and market exclusivity expire, typically other pharmaceutical companies can then seek approval from the FDA to market an equivalent product under its chemical, or "generic," name. Sometimes generic versions of patented products may enter the market before the expiration of a patent if that patent is shown to be invalid or if the generic version does not infringe on the patent.

Generic pharmaceuticals are occasionally referred to as "copycat" drugs, suggesting that generic pharmaceutical manufacturers simply copy the formula of the brand-name pharmaceutical process. Nothing could be further from the complex, science-based reality that is the modern generic pharmaceutical product. Years of research and millions of dollars are invested in identifying and sourcing the active ingredient for a generic pharmaceutical, in formulating a generic product that does not violate patents or brand company intellectual property, and in the clinical studies conducted to ensure that the generic version will have the same safety and efficacy as the brand-name product.

The FDA requires that the generic pharmaceutical manufacturer prove that its generic version of the product meets the following requirements:

- Contains the same active ingredient(s)
- Is identical in strength, dosage form, and route of administration
- Has the same indications, dosing, and labeling
- Is bioequivalent
- Meets the same batch-to-batch requirements for strength, purity, and quality
- Is manufactured under the same strict Good Manufacturing Practice regulations as the branded pharmaceutical

Sometimes the generic manufacturer may be prohibited from adopting the same color or shape because of patents protecting the brand drug. These cosmetic differences in no way affect the safety or effectiveness of the generic version.

The FDA requires all manufacturers and their facilities to adhere to specific guidelines, called Current Good Manufacturing Practices (CGMPs), no matter what the drug and no matter who the manufacturer. In addition, the FDA scientists, chemists, and microbiologists reviewing generic medicines have the same qualifications as those reviewing the brand drugs.

All pharmaceutical manufacturers, whether brand or generic, are subject to extensive regulation by the federal government, principally by the FDA, and, to a lesser extent, by the Drug Enforcement Agency (DEA) and state governments. The Federal Food, Drug, and Cosmetic Act, the Controlled Substances Act, and other federal statutes and regulations govern or influence the testing, manufacturing, safety, labeling, storage, record keeping, approval, pricing, advertising, and promotion of the products. Noncompliance with applicable requirements can result in fines, recalls, and seizure of products. Under certain circumstances, the FDA also has the authority to revoke drug approvals previously granted.

When a generic drug meets FDA requirements for pharmaceutical and therapeutic equivalence, it is approved and receives an "AB Rating." This rating allows the generic drug to be substituted for the branded product when a prescription is presented to the pharmacist for dispensing.

Abbreviated Drug Approval Process

FDA approval is required before any new drug can be marketed. The development of a new, brand pharmaceutical product involves scientific discovery. Using a number of R&D techniques, a brand pharmaceutical company will screen chemical compounds for potential use in treating a specific disease. Once a promising molecule or chemical compound is discovered, it enters the development phase.

There are essentially four phases in the development process of a new brand pharmaceutical product as defined by FDA regulations in the United States. The first phase—preclinical research—involves laboratory and animal testing of the compound that is primarily aimed at establishing safety and efficacy. If successful, the innovator can then file an Investigational New Drug (IND) application with the FDA, seeking approval to move the compound into a three-phase process of human testing.

At the successful completion of lengthy human clinical trials, the developer files a New Drug Application (NDA) submission with the FDA seeking to bring the new compound to market. The process required to establish safety and efficacy can take as long as 10 to 12 years and cost nearly one billion dollars. To recapture this investment, the brand company is typically granted a period of market exclusivity.

The generic pharmaceutical company, seeking to market an equivalent to a brand product (once the market exclusivity on the product has expired), uses a significantly less costly and faster process, the Abbreviated New Drug Application (ANDA) process. The generic manufacturer relies on the safety and efficacy data supplied by the innovator and has to prove to the FDA that its product is equivalent to the branded product.

Although the FDA waives the requirement of conducting complete clinical studies of the brand product prior to approval, it does require testing to prove that the generic drug provides the same dosage of the active ingredient at the same rate of absorption by the human body as the brand drug. These studies require the generic company to conduct bioavailability and/or bioequivalence studies.

Bioavailability indicates the rate and extent of absorption and levels of concentration of a drug product in the blood stream needed to produce a therapeutic effect. *Bioequivalence* compares the bioavailability of one drug product with another, and when established, indicates that the rate of absorption and levels of concentration of a generic drug in the body are substantially equivalent to the previously approved brand drug.

Bioequivalence studies are generally conducted in human volunteers. In a typical bioequivalence study, each subject receives both the brand drug and the generic test drug products in a randomized crossover design. Single doses of the test and reference drugs are administered and blood or plasma levels of the drug are measured over time.

Major Requirements for FDA Approval: Generic Drug

According to the FDA there are:

eight major parts of the generic drug approval process. The requirements that generic products must meet prior to approval include:

1. The basis for submitting an application for a generic drug is simply that there must be a previously approved drug which is the same as the proposed generic drug. The generic product must have the same active ingredients(s), route of administration, dosage form, and strength.
2. The generic firm must demonstrate that its product is bioequivalent to the brand-name drug. Bioequivalency is a critical factor in drawing a conclusion that the two products will produce similar activity or therapeutic results in a patient population.
3. In addition to having the same product characteristics, a generic drug firm's labeling must also contain information that is virtually the same as that of a previously approved product.
4. A generic drug application also must contain documentation of the complete chemistry, manufacturing, and controls of the drug product, for each step of the manufacturing process starting from the synthesis of the raw material used through the packaging and labeling of the finished product.
5. The generic application must assure that the raw materials used, as well as the finished dosage form, meet the specifications set forth in the United States Pharmacopeia (USP), the official drug compendium of this country.
6. The generic drug firm must also demonstrate, prior to approval that its product is stable under both extremes of temperature and humidity, then, after approval the firm must continue to monitor the product under room temperature conditions. Data also must be submitted to the FDA demonstrating that the proposed container closure system used to package the product is suitable and does not interact with the drug product. Additionally, firms manufacturing

injectable, ophthalmic, and other drug products purported to be sterile, must submit data supporting the stability and integrity of these products.

7. A firm submitting a generic drug application must provide a full description of all facilities used for the manufacture, processing, testing, packaging, labeling, and control of the drug product. All firms must certify that they are in compliance with regulations pertaining to CGMPs and undergo inspection by the FDA to assure compliance.

8. Before the Office of Generic Drugs (OGD) will approve a drug product, an FDA investigator generally conducts a product specific inspection to assure that the firm has actually followed the conditions set forth in their generic drug application and audits data used to support the application.

FDA's standards for bioequivalence (the same rate and extent of absorption into the body) have raised the most concern within the clinical community. A −20/+25% "rule" is used to compare the two products. The meaning of this rule is widely misunderstood. It actually represents acceptable bounds on the 90% confidence intervals around the ratio of the mean results for each of the two products.

In practice, because of human variability, this means that the actual results for rate and extent have to be very close. FDA did a study in the 1980s evaluating 224 bioequivalence studies that "passed" the −20/+25% rule. In these studies, the average observed difference in absorption between the brand name and the generic was about 3.5%. This study was repeated for the 127 bioequivalence studies done for generic drugs approved in 1997. The average observed difference in absorption in these studies was about 3.3%.

It is important to note that FDA applies an identical bioequivalence standard to brand name products when significant changes in manufacturing or formulation occur. Brand name drugs may undergo many such changes while on the market. FDA requires bioequivalence studies be performed to "bridge" the current product back to the product that was used in clinical trials. . . . The degree of regulatory control over rate and extent of absorption for any formulation is the same for a generic and branded drug.[1]

Among the requirements listed for drug approval by the FDA is that the generic company's manufacturing procedures and operations conform to CGMPs, as defined in the US Code of Federal Regulations. The CGMP regulations must be followed at all times during the manufacture of pharmaceutical products. In complying with the standards set forth in the CGMP regulations, a generic company must continue to expend time, money, and effort in the areas of production and quality control to ensure full technical compliance.

If the FDA believes a company is not in compliance with CGMPs, certain sanctions can be imposed upon that company including withholding from the company new drug approvals as well as approvals for supplemental changes to existing applications; preventing the company from receiving the necessary export licenses to export its products; and classifying the company as an "unacceptable supplier" and thereby disqualifying the company from selling products to federal agencies.

■ Generics Are the Same

For more than 20 years, generic medicines have proven their effectiveness in billions of prescriptions used by millions of patients. Since the Hatch–Waxman Act, the FDA has repeatedly assessed US generic medicines and found that patients can be assured that US generics are fully substitutable for the brand product.

In the late 1990s, the introduction of generic versions of blood thinners and drugs to treat epilepsy led a number of brand companies to seek support in more than two dozen states for legislation that would prevent automatic substitution of these products. The FDA responded to this initiative, at the request of various state legislators and members of the generic industry, with repeated positions that supported the automatic substitution of all FDA-approved generic drugs.

In 1997, Roger L. Williams, MD, Deputy Center Director, Center for Drug Evaluation and Research, US Food and Drug Administration, responded to a request from the National Association of Boards of Pharmacy to clarify FDA's position on generic substitution of Narrow Therapeutic Index Drugs, such as blood thinners and antiseizure medicines. Dr. Williams wrote:

> FDA is aware of the NTI initiatives that are occurring at the state level. These include, but are not limited to, the proposed legislation . . . the lobbying of state Boards of Pharmacy, the establishment of an organization to oppose NTI substitution, and the proposals by the State Drug Utilization Review Committee(s). . . . To date, we have not seen data to support such proposed changes.
>
> If one therapeutically equivalent drug is substituted for another, the physician, pharmacist, and patient have FDA's assurance that the physician should see the same clinical results and safety profile. Any differences that could exist should be no greater than one would expect if one lot of the innovator's product was substituted for another.[2]

As the controversy continued, in January 1998, FDA took the unprecedented step of writing to all healthcare providers to answer questions raised about substitution of generic products. Stuart L. Nightingale, MD, FDA's Associate Commissioner for Health Affairs, issued a "Dear Colleague" letter providing FDA's "comment on the issue of interchanging any brand-name drug with a therapeutically equivalent generic drug."

FDA felt compelled to issue the letter stating, "Certain individuals and groups have appeared recently before state legislatures, state boards of pharmacy, and drug utilization review committees to express concerns about the interchangeability of certain products they characterize as narrow therapeutic index (NTI) drug products."

Dr. Nightingale concluded, "Products evaluated as therapeutically equivalent can be expected to have equivalent clinical effect whether the product is a brand name or generic drug product."[3]

Finally, in December of 1999, FDA Commissioner Dr. Jane E. Henney wrote a column published in the *Journal of the American Medical Association (JAMA).*[4] Dr. Henney's column was written in response to questions that have been "raised recently about the ethics, safety, and effectiveness of generic substitutes for brand-name products." As a result of these questions, the FDA reviewed the data from 127 in vivo bioequivalence studies supporting the 273 generic drug applications approved in 1997. The results of the review confirmed the therapeutic equivalence of the generic products to the brand products. Dr. Henney concluded, "Practitioners and the public may be assured that if the FDA declares a generic drug to be therapeutically equivalent to an innovator drug, the two products will provide the same intended clinical effect."

Although anti-consumer and anti-competitive actions still result in attempts by some special interests to suggest that generics are not the same as brand products, this issue has lost traction with physicians, pharmacists, and consumers for the majority of generic medicines.

■ Future Opportunities with Biogenerics

Over the past several years, Congress and members of the biopharmaceutical, pharmaceutical, and generic pharmaceutical industries have been discussing opportunities to extend generic savings from traditional medicines into biopharmaceuticals. Although traditional pharmaceuticals are developed using a chemical process, biopharmaceuticals are derived from living cells. The debate has centered around developing a workable pathway for the FDA to review and approve affordable generic versions of biopharmaceutical products—biogenerics.

America's biopharmaceutical industry represents one of the most successful and fastest growing segments of US health care. Ten years ago, revenues for this industry were approximately $8 billion. In 2006, biologics had annual revenues that exceed $30 billion. By 2010, analysts estimate that biologic sales will exceed $60 billion.

More than 150 biopharmaceutical drugs are currently marketed, including human insulin, interferons, human growth hormones, and monoclonal antibodies. In 2005–2006, more than 30 new drugs were approved, compared to just 2 in 1982. There are more than 370 biopharmaceutical drug products and vaccines currently in clinical trials targeting more than 200 diseases including cancer, Alzheimer's disease, heart disease, multiple sclerosis, AIDS, and arthritis.

Biopharmaceuticals are a major driver of skyrocketing prescription drug costs. Six products—Procrit, Epogen, Neupogen, Intron A, Humulin, and Rituxan—each generated sales of more than $1 billion. And at least three new blockbusters are expected to join that list. The top three biopharmaceuticals—Neupogen, Epogen, and Intron A—cost patients $23,098, $10,348, and $5,850, respectively, each year.

Biogenerics hold great promise for millions of Americans. Legislative proposals under discussion would result in the creation of a workable approval pathway to bring safe and effective biogenerics, much as Hatch–Waxman did for traditional pharmaceutical products.

■ The Future of the US Generic Industry

All economic signs are pointing to continued growth for the US generic pharmaceutical industry, which in turn will create more opportunities for consumers and healthcare providers to save billions of dollars each year through the increased availability of affordable generic medicines. This growth will be driven by a variety of factors.

Today, there are enormous pressures to hold down healthcare costs in general, and prescription drug spending in particular. Generic pharmaceuticals will continue to offer payers the opportunity to hold down monthly insurance premiums, out-of-pocket costs, and drug spending related to Medicare and Medicaid programs.

In addition, a record number of pharmaceutical products will lose patent protection within the next 5 years. In fact, blockbuster products valued at $27 billion in 2007, and $29 billion in 2008, lost patent protection. One industry analyst has suggested that the total sales of drugs coming off patent will exceed $160 billion by 2015. This flood of patent expirations will create numerous opportunities for generic pharmaceutical manufacturers over the next decade. As a result of the large number of drugs expected to lose patent protection, analysts have predicted that the overall market for generic drugs could continue to grow at double-digit rates through the end of the decade.

The growth of the generic pharmaceutical industry is based upon the strength of innovation and intellectual property of the brand pharmaceutical industry. Without innovation, and the market exclusivity that is granted to brand companies as their incentive to invest in new drug discovery and development, the future of the generic industry would be very bleak. A Congressional Budget Office study in the late 1990s demonstrated that although generic competition was growing, investment by brand industry in new drug development also grew. The generic industry strongly supports appropriate market exclusivity, intellectual property, and the ability through market exclusivity of the brand pharmaceutical industry to recoup its investment in new product innovation, while continuing to invest in new product development.

It's been an extraordinary 20 years for the generic industry. The growing pains were tough, but the benefits to consumers have been enormous. With biopharmaceutical medicines now growing at an astonishing rate—almost twice the rate of traditional medicines, accounting for approximately $30 billion in US sales and about 12% of the total pharmaceutical market—all eyes will be on how the brand and generic industries deal with this emerging category of medicines. There is great promise ahead—promise for the pharmaceutical industry and consumers alike.

■ References

1. Galson SK. Personal letter to Bradley F., January 5, 2004.
2. Williams RL. Therapeutic Equivalence of Generic Drugs Response to National Association of Boards of Pharmacy. February 6, 1998. http://www.fda.gov/cder/news/ntiletter.htm.
3. Nightingale SL. Therapeutic Equivalence of Generic Drugs Letter to Health Practitioners. February 4, 1998. http://www.fda.gov/cder/news/nightgenlett.htm.
4. Henney JE. From the Food and Drug Administration. *JAMA*. December 1999;282(21):1995.

■ Suggested Reading

Berndt ER, Mortimer R, Bhattacharjya A, Parece A, Tuttle E. Authorized generic drugs, price competition, and consumers' welfare. *Health Aff* (Millwood). May–June 2007;26(3):790–799.

Cook A. *How Increased Competition from Generic Drugs Has Affected Prices and Returns in the Pharmaceutical Industry.* Darby, Pa: Diane Publishing Company; 1998.

Generic drugs go to market: effective, safe and less expensive. *Mayo Clin Health Lett.* September 2006;24(9):4–5.

Impurities in generic pharmaceutical development. *Adv Drug Deliv Rev.* January 2007;59(1):56–63.

Increasing the availability of generics. *FDA Consum.* September–October 2006;40(5):3.

Kanfer I, Shargel L, eds. *Generic Drug Product Development: Bioequivalence Issues.* New York, NY: Informa HealthCare; 2007.

Nitzki-George D. *Generic Alternatives to Prescription Drugs.* North Bergen, NJ: Basic Health Publications; 2003.

Scott AB, Culley EJ, O'Donnell J. Effects of a physician office generic drug sampling system on generic dispensing ratios and drug costs in a large managed care organization. *J Manag Care Pharm.* June 2007;13(5):412–419.

Shargel L. *Development of Generic Drug Products: Solid Oral Dosage Forms.* New York, NY: Informa HealthCare; 2004.

Sipkoff M. Employers want plans and PBMs to push hard for generics. *Manag Care.* January 2007;16(1):15–16.

Steinman MA, Chren MM, Landefeld CS. What's in a name? Use of brand versus generic drug names in United States outpatient practice. *J Gen Intern Med.* May 2007;22(5):645–648.

Swarbrick J, ed. *Encyclopedia of Pharmaceutical Technology: Film Coatings and Film-Forming Materials: Evaluation to Generic Drugs and Generic Equivalency.* 3rd ed. Vol. 6. New York, NY: Informa HealthCare; 2006.

Voet MA. *The Generic Challenge: Understanding Patents, FDA & Pharmaceutical Life-Cycle Management.* 2nd ed. Boca Raton, Fla: BrownWalker Press; 2008.

War on generic drugs. *Rev Med Brux.* September–October 2006;27(5):420–421.

Over-the-Counter Drugs

David Spangler

■ The Hypothetical

You've recently been transferred within QRS Health to a regulatory affairs role in the consumer healthcare division. You're already familiar with the science behind the company's product portfolio, but you need to look at things in a different light in your new role. Although you'll be working on existing nonprescription or over-the-counter (OTC) medicine brands, you will also be called in on meetings with colleagues on the Rx-to-OTC switch team and will interface with colleagues in marketing, sales and logistics, and general management. Your agenda for the next several days:

- Brush up on basic legal and regulatory framework for OTC medicines
- Take part in the preparations for a meeting of the Food and Drug Administration's (FDA) Nonprescription Drugs Advisory Committee, which will be meeting to review the company's Rx-to-OTC switch application for an overactive bladder disorder treatment
- Brainstorm with colleagues as the company considers a potential future Rx-to-OTC switch for a chronic condition
- Meet with one of the company lawyers for a primer on advertising law because you anticipate being called upon in the future to provide regulatory review for advertisements
- Get a briefing from a colleague in sales because you want to take a deeper dive into the retail environment to prepare for the next meeting with the potential future switch group

QSR Health uses an integrated manufacturing and quality division for both its Rx and OTC medicines. Safety monitoring is run through the same system for Rx and OTC medicines as well. You understand some of your competitors do things differently, with different systems for each, but your company's way seems to be more common. Basic corporate functions are shared as well—legal, finance, and administration, and so forth.

■ OTC Regulation

As we will learn as we go further into this chapter, OTC drugs are regulated by the Food and Drug Administration (FDA), the Federal Trade Commission (FTC), and state health departments, among others.

OTC Classification and the Importance of Labeling

Labeling is a crucial part of a drug's ability to be classified as nonprescription. Stepping back, this has been central to OTC status since the 1938 federal Food, Drug, and Cosmetic Act. Although the act did not explicitly require prescription status for any category of drugs, it included a requirement that the labeling of any drug bear "adequate directions for use," and it authorized the FDA to issue exemptions from that requirement. The FDA issued regulations for exempting drugs from the directions requirement if the label bore a statement, "Caution: To be used only by or on the prescription of a [physician, dentist, or veterinarian]."[1] In other words, at that time OTC status was the default status with prescription status as the exception.

In 1951, the Durham–Humphrey Amendments to the act made the prescription–OTC distinction explicit in law, with the basic definition for prescription medicines that remains in place today:

> A drug intended for use by man which
> (A) because of its toxicity or other potentiality for harmful effect, or the method of use, or the collateral measures necessary to its use, is not safe for use except under the supervision of a practitioner licensed by law to administer such drug; or
> (B) is limited by an approved application under section 505 [the section describing the approval process for new drugs] to use under professional supervision of a practitioner licensed by law to administer such drug; shall be dispensed only [upon a prescription].[2]

Note that in this approach, safety, efficacy, and basic Good Manufacturing Practices (GMP) remain the same as for prescription drugs. What differs are the emphases on higher confidence in safety, and methods or measures of use, which drives at labeling.

In very basic terms, FDA has described OTC labeling in the context of OTC Review monographs as needing to be clear, truthful, and not misleading. This information is to be in terms likely to be read and understood by the ordinary individual, including individuals of low comprehension, under customary conditions of purchase and use.[3] Although the regulation cited applies to OTC Review monographs, the principles described are universal for OTC medicines because they are in turn grounded in the Food, Drug, and Cosmetic Act.

Today, the package label the consumer sees at the point-of-sale is standardized, for both monographed and New Drug Application (NDA) medicines, under the Drug Facts rule.[4]* The purpose of the standardized format is to give consumers user-friendly cues to help them locate and read important health and safety information and allow quick and effective product comparisons, thereby helping consumers to select the most appropriate product.[5] The Drug Facts format follows a standard outline as follows (see FIGURE 16-1).

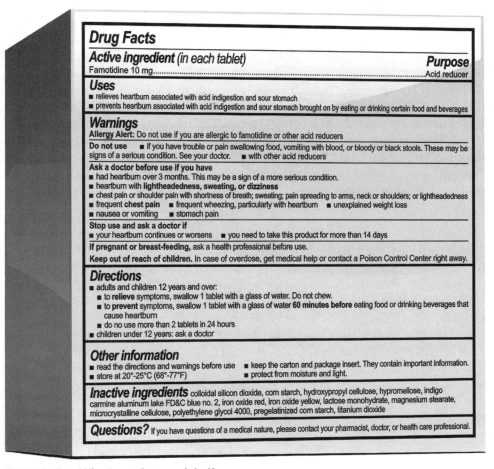

Drug Facts

Active ingredient (in each tablet)   **Purpose**
Famotidine 10 mg...Acid reducer

Uses
- relieves heartburn associated with acid indigestion and sour stomach
- prevents heartburn associated with acid indigestion and sour stomach brought on by eating or drinking certain food and beverages

Warnings
Allergy Alert: Do not use if you are allergic to famotidine or other acid reducers

Do not use   ■ if you have trouble or pain swallowing food, vomiting with blood, or bloody or black stools. These may be signs of a serious condition. See your doctor.   ■ with other acid reducers

Ask a doctor before use if you have
- had heartburn over 3 months. This may be a sign of a more serious condition.
- heartburn with **lightheadedness, sweating, or dizziness**
- chest pain or shoulder pain with shortness of breath; sweating; pain spreading to arms, neck or shoulders; or lightheadedness
- frequent **chest pain**   ■ frequent wheezing, particularly with heartburn   ■ unexplained weight loss
- nausea or vomiting   ■ stomach pain

Stop use and ask a doctor if
- your heartburn continues or worsens   ■ you need to take this product for more than 14 days

If pregnant or breast-feeding, ask a health professional before use.

Keep out of reach of children. In case of overdose, get medical help or contact a Poison Control Center right away.

Directions
- adults and children 12 years and over:
  - to **relieve** symptoms, swallow 1 tablet with a glass of water. Do not chew.
  - to **prevent** symptoms, swallow 1 tablet with a glass of water **60 minutes before** eating food or drinking beverages that cause heartburn
  - do no use more than 2 tablets in 24 hours
- children under 12 years: ask a doctor

Other information
- read the directions and warnings before use   ■ keep the carton and package insert. They contain important information.
- store at 20°-25°C (68°-77°F)   ■ protect from moisture and light.

Inactive ingredients colloidal silicon dioxide, corn starch, hydroxypropyl cellulose, hypromellose, indigo carmine aluminum lake FD&C blue no. 2, iron oxide red, iron oxide yellow, lactose monohydrate, magnesium stearate, microcrystalline cellulose, polyethylene glycol 4000, pregelatinized corn starch, titanium dioxide

Questions? If you have questions of a medical nature, please contact your pharmacist, doctor, or health care professional.

FIGURE 16-1   What's on the new label?

---

*FDA has granted temporary exemptions from the Drug Facts rule for one- or two-dose convenience size packages in certain circumstances and for sunscreens pending completion of issues in the sunscreen monograph. FDA has granted specific, circumscribed partial exemptions in two or three instances.

The Drug Facts rule includes very detailed requirements on type size, formatting, how to group warnings, and how to bullet list them, and so forth.[6] In the warning section in particular, companies and FDA have to pay particular attention to when and how to warn. Again, the goal is to write labels in terms that are likely to be read and understood, so warnings about hypothetical possibilities or that are in terms beyond a consumer's ability to understand and in turn act on are not helpful. Summing up a policy on when to warn, the agency has stated that warnings must be scientifically documented, clinically significant, and important to the safe and effective use of the product by the consumer.[7*]

One final difference surrounding labeling in the Rx and OTC markets is the time element. In the Rx world, figuratively speaking, a change in labeling approved by FDA on Monday could be posted electronically and available Tuesday. Contrast the OTC world: the figurative Monday change—either in an NDA or through an amendment to an OTC Review monograph (which would come through a rulemaking process)— would go to package engineering; to label or art design and review; to art and mechanical production; to printing and delivery of packaging components; to production; and finally to distribution, where the end consumer can ultimately look at the new label on the package on the shelf.[8] That's months. And what if your medicine is seasonal in nature: will you make it before the season starts? If not, the relabeled product may miss a year. In short, there's a good deal of complexity and planning with what otherwise might seem like a simple label change.

Routes to Market: Monographs or NDAs

The 1962 Kefauver–Harris Amendments to the FD&C Act, among other provisions, added a requirement that all new drugs, including those introduced from the 1938 act up to that time, be shown to be effective as well as safe. For prescription drugs (as well as some OTCs, although they were not the focus), the effectiveness for 1938–1962 drugs was evaluated under the Drug Efficacy Study Implementation (DESI) review. For OTC drugs, FDA started the OTC Review in 1972. Rather than limiting the OTC Review to 1938–1962 drugs, FDA included all OTCs introduced before 1974 and broadened the review to look at not only effectiveness but whether the ingredients reviewed are "generally recognized as safe and effective" (GRAS/GRAE)—the criteria for drugs not subject to an NDA—with the FDA's stamp of approval. Through the OTC Review, the FDA spells out not only its determinations on what ingredients are GRAS/GRAE, but under what conditions—that is, at what doses and with what labeling. The OTC Review looks at ingredients under category monographs (antacids, internal analgesics, nasal decongestants, etc.) rather than product by product. Therefore, individual products within the OTC Review do not need an individual license or authorization, so long as they meet the requirements of applicable monograph as well

---

*See also 47 Fed. Reg. 54750 (December 3, 1982).

as the laws and regulations of general applicability to all medicines—GMPs, inspections, packaging, listing products with the FDA, and so forth. The FDA took this approach because the agency was concerned that its resources were not suited to look at each and every of the approximately 100,000+ OTCs on the market (a figure that includes all package sizes, dosage form or strength variations, and national and store brands).[9]

The early years of the OTC Review involved outside expert panels that looked at studies and other information submitted after a call for data. The panels prepared panel reports, which were published by the FDA with the agency's thoughts in the form of a proposed monograph outlining conditions under which a category of OTC drugs is GRAS/GRAE, and outlining conditions excluded on the basis of the agency's conclusion that they would not be either GRAS or GRAE.[10]

After receiving comments and additional data on the panel reports, FDA published tentative final monographs, and ultimately final monographs. A number of final monographs are still pending, even where portions or aspects of them have been finalized. Through the OTC Review, industry submitted more than 20,000 volumes of data to the panels and the agency. Thanks to the OTC Review, the OTC industry was brought up to a modern scientific footing.

But the world of OTC medicines didn't stop with the onset of the OTC Review in 1972. OTC ingredients introduced since 1972 can still be included in OTC Review monographs on the basis of general recognition of safety and effectiveness (as triggered by their use for a "material time and material extent"[11]). As a practical matter, however, almost all OTC ingredients or dosages introduced since 1984 have come through the NDA route. The last ingredient or dosage to come through the OTC Review monograph route was in 1992. From a business perspective, the ability to gain data exclusivity based on clinicals essential to the approval of an OTC medicine has been a significant driver behind this shift. Considerations such as these are similar to those discussed for prescription drugs in the legal chapter. From the FDA's perspective, although a number of ingredients, indications, or dosages were switched to OTC status through the OTC Review monographs, the agency takes the position that the original OTC Review procedures were not developed to address post-1972 drugs and notes that the switches that came through the monographs were begun during the expert panel phase of the OTC Review.[12] The expert panel phase has long been completed.

■ Rx-to-OTC Switch

The Hypothetical

On the train ride to an off-site meeting, you run into your former boss, Ed, from a prescription division, and your friend Donna from marketing. Donna is on the team for the company's next hoped-for Rx-to-OTC switch.

Donna: "Won't your division lose out, Ed, when the switch goes through and it comes to consumer healthcare?"

Ed: "That's if the switch goes through. Besides, that's not how we think about it. It has had several years of prescription use to generate more safety data; it has a very good safety profile; and I understand the consumer healthcare folks have done a great job on the consumer behavior studies. Besides, with the patent expiring and data exclusivity up, we're on to the next new drug."

Donna: "True enough. I read something in the *Wall Street Journal* recently where the CEO of another company was talking about the chance consumer healthcare products have to live on forever thanks to the value of their brands. There are plenty of OTC medicines with brand names families have trusted for decades—even generations. That's without patents, without exclusivity."

Ed: "Yes, and you can thank us for starting to build that brand equity on the prescription side. Lose it and you won't get it back."

Donna: "What makes you so sure we're keeping your brand name? We might have found something more appropriate for the OTC medicine setting. . . . Just kidding, but we could."

Background

Advil, Imodium A-D, Gyne-Lotrimin, Tavist, Pepcid AC, Rogaine, Nicorette, Claritin, and Plan B are all examples of brands with active ingredients that began their lives in some form as prescription medicines. All told, nearly 100 ingredients, dosages, or indications have been introduced to the OTC marketplace through the Rx-to-OTC switch process. Although occasionally a pure switch occurs—that is, the new OTC is identical to the Rx parent in its method of use—most switches vary from the parent in some way. Either the indication is different (heartburn vs. ulcer treatment, for example), the strength varies, the dosage form is different, or they differ in some fashion.

Although there is nothing in the law to prevent an ingredient from being introduced directly as an OTC medicine, this is fairly rare because there would likely not be a sufficient safety profile for direct OTC introduction. In the vast majority of cases, a company would want, and the FDA would expect, sufficient use in the Rx market to fully characterize an ingredient's safety. For purposes of this discussion, I look at OTC introductions with an Rx parent history.

In looking at an Rx-to-OTC switch, a first area to consider is safety: is the margin of safety sufficient to allow the medicine to be sold without a doctor's supervision. The drug's safety profile will have been well characterized through clinical trials and Rx use so that even rare side effects should have become apparent. Beyond the basic safety profile, a switch sponsor and FDA during its review typically look at another layer of safety questions revolving around a product's use, such as the following:

- Does the Rx characterization of safety apply in a likely wider OTC population?
- Are there side effects of the drug that could be worsened or become more frequent in the absence of professional supervision?
- Would OTC availability be likely to delay a diagnosis/treatment of a more serious underlying condition than Rx availability?

On all of these questions, the real world of prescription experience is a more apt comparator than controlled clinical trials.

For efficacy, data from the Rx NDA will likely be a part of the switch NDA package. But where the switch is for a new indication, for example, new efficacy studies would be needed.

Different from prescription NDAs, the vast majority of today's switch NDAs also include label comprehension studies and actual use studies. Label comprehension studies usually involve an iterative testing process beginning with interview sessions and ending with quantitative studies with hundreds of respondents. The intent is to learn about clarity of key messages, identify areas of confusion, and compare wording alternatives.

Actual use studies seek to simulate a more naturalistic, consumer-centered use of a product. The focus here is typically on self-selection and deselection, that is, are people appropriately choosing the product and are people appropriately deciding to either not take product or to appropriately stop using it. Concordance with the product labeling or safety during actual consumer use can also be assessed through actual use studies.

The goal in these studies is to provide a venue that simulates, as best as can be done, the true OTC environment. Study design elements that help achieve this might include a mock store shelf, allowing study participants to purchase the study drug.

Whether through traditional efficacy or safety studies, information gathered during prescription experience, label comprehension studies, or actual use trials, the bottom line is to have a data-driven switch process. Whether an indication or a category of medicine should or shouldn't be switched isn't the question; whether there are data to address the product-specific questions that would otherwise prevent a switch is. It is that common thread that ties diverse medicines such as Advil, Imodium A-D, Gyne-Lotrimin, Pepcid AC, Rogaine, Nicorette, Claritin, Plan B, and many others together.

Advertising

The Hypothetical

After work, you're chatting with your friends Paul, a pharmacist and former classmate who works at a nearby hospital, and Donna, who recently moved from one of the major ad agencies to the QRS Health marketing department. Donna is opining favorably on one of your competitor's new ad campaigns.

> *Paul:* "No, Donna, you're just wrong. If they've got allergies, there's no way a simple pill will let them roll around in the flower pollen with a smile on their face. You guys all think you can sell something serious like medicine as though it were a box of cereal."

> *Donna:* "You're missing the point. Lots of things are serious beyond medicines. Insurance, taxes, buying a home—those are serious, significant issues that touch all of us, and you don't seem to have a problem with their advertising. You had to use pesticides in your college apartment—those have risks around them if misused."

> *Paul:* "Yes, but why aren't your ads more balanced?"

> *Donna:* "Think it through. When you turn on the television, you're not there for the ads. Not every program is the Super Bowl, where the ads have become part of the program and we read a column about the ads the next day. If there are 10 minutes, give or take, of advertising in an hour of television, that's probably 20-something ads, and that's if they're mostly :30s, not :15s. The best you can hope for is to cut through the clutter to get across one, maybe two, points. Think about how many ads you see that caught your attention, but you don't remember the product name. It's tougher than it looks."

> *Paul:* "But you see them again and again, and don't you guys spend upward of $3 billion on advertising?"

> *Donna:* "Yes we do, for Rx, OTC, and corporate ads. That's around three-quarters of what the financial services sector spends, and maybe two-thirds more than insurance. Those are serious too. The bottom line is we're trying to get people's attention to let them know we can help them."

What's your response?

Background

Unlike prescription medicines, authority over OTC medicine advertising rests with the Federal Trade Commission, rather than the FDA. Under the Federal Trade Commission Act, unfair or deceptive acts and false advertisements, including for medicines, are prohibited.[13]

Within companies, the marketing department will typically work with its ad agency on developing a core message or messages and creative concepts around it. At some point in the process, claims and other statements in a proposed advertisement need to be vetted for regulatory and legal clearance to ensure that they meet with relevant government and self-regulatory standards. In the case of government, the FTC's authority over advertising boils down to three basic standards: the prior substantiation doctrine, deception policy, and unfairness policy.

Prior Substantiation

Prior substantiation drives at whether an objective claim is true or not. Under this doctrine, the FTC requires that objective claims, whether express or implied, be supported by adequate substantiation before the ad is disseminated. *In re Pfizer*, which first articulated the standard, looked at the type of claim (eg, safety, efficacy, dietary, health), the product involved (eg, food, drug, other consumer product), consequences of a false claim (eg, personal injury, property damage, monetary damage), degree of reliance by consumers on the claims, and the type and accessibility of adequate evidence to support a claim.[14] In looking at substantiation for OTC medicines, the FTC generally looks to the FDA determinations or works with the FDA.[15]* In general, a claim needs to be supported by the level of substantiation it communicates to a consumer. For example, a claim that a product is "clinically proven" must be supported by clinical tests.

Deception Policy

The FTC's deception policy looks to real-life situations and how consumers would interpret an ad or, in more legal parlance, at practices that are likely to cause injury to consumers by affirmatively misleading their informed choice (this includes either misrepresentations or omissions).[16] For those used to a more health and FDA orientation, note that "injury" in the FTC sense is a much broader concept that includes economic or monetary harm as well as a safety, health, or adverse event–oriented harm.

The real life aspect of how the policy works is important because the FTC and the courts recognize there can be a harmless "puffing" aspect in some ads. As the Commission put it, "Perhaps a few misguided souls believe, for example, that all 'Danish pastry' is made in Denmark. Is it, therefore, an actionable deception to advertise 'Danish pastry' when it is made in this country? Of course not."[17]

Unfairness Policy

Distinct from deception, unfairness looks at circumstances under which a practice causes a consumer injury that is: (1) substantial; (2) not outweighed by countervailing consumer or competitive benefits that the practice produces; and (3) one that consumers could not reasonably have avoided.[16]† For the first factor and unlike deception,

---

*See also Bachrach EE. *Regulation of OTC Drug Advertising in the United States*. Unpublished manuscript, September 1995, on file at the Consumer Healthcare Products Association.

†Congress later acted to translate the International Harvester three-pronged definition into law. 15 USC §45(n): "The Commission shall have no authority under this section or section 57a of this title to declare unlawful an act or practice on the grounds that such act or practice is unfair unless the act or practice causes or is likely to cause substantial injury to consumers which is not reasonably avoidable by consumers themselves and not outweighed by countervailing benefits to consumers or to competition."

where the likelihood of an injury is the question, for unfairness, the extent of harm (again, monetary, safety, health, etc.) is the focus. A cost–benefit analysis is one way to think about the second factor, or, more simply, unmitigated = unfair. The third factor is centered on informed choice. As a practical matter, particularly given the strong role of the FDA in an OTC medicine's labeling, GMPs, and safety monitoring, the unfairness policy rarely comes into play for an OTC medicine.

Beyond the FTC, companies marketing OTC medicines have to be familiar with four other mechanisms used to ensure that OTC medicine ads are truthful and not misleading. First, companies have their own internal approval steps for advertisements, which typically include medical/scientific, legal, regulatory, and general management review.

Second, the major television networks have their own clearance, or program practices, departments, which must be satisfied with an ad before the network will accept it. Documentation to support claims can become important in this review.

Another mechanism is the National Advertising Division (NAD) of the Council of Better Business Bureaus. NAD investigates complaints based on staff identification, challenges by competitors, or complaints from other parties (including consumers or local Better Business Bureaus) based on the truth and accuracy of the advertisement. Once a complaint has been screened by NAD staff, both the advertiser and the complainant go through a judicial-style process, after which NAD prepares a final case decision that is published in the *NAD Case Reporter*. Decisions typically report on both NAD's views and the advertiser's plans to respond to the decision, such as supporting substantiation, modifying the ad, or discontinuing the ad. NAD refers cases to the FTC or other authorities as appropriate, including when an advertiser does not respond to a decision.

Fourth and finally, competitive forces play an important role in how companies approach their advertising. One CEO put it this way: "There is no doubt in my mind that the best cop on the beat is one's competitor. . . . They never sleep."[18] Looming behind statements such as that is the ability of firms to litigate under the Lanham Act, which creates a private right of action when an advertiser misrepresents its products or a competitor's product where the conduct causes a significant competitive injury.[19,20] For extended periods in the 1970s and 1980s, Lanham Act litigation between consumer healthcare companies was not uncommon.[21]

■ Retail Environment

While the OTC industry prepares drugs whose safety and effectiveness have been well established, and with labeling that meets FDA requirements for self-use by lay persons without the need for any professional (physician or pharmacist) supervision or assistance, the pharmacy profession is active in campaigning for pharmacist control of some OTC products.

The Hypothetical

You're continuing your conversation with Paul the hospital pharmacist and Donna from marketing.

Paul: "Another thing that bothers me about you guys is that it seems like you sell OTC medicines everywhere. If these are serious medicines, you should limit them to pharmacies where a pharmacist can be involved."

Donna: "If my boss were here, he'd give you a long lecture about the centuries-old history of a third class of drugs. Be thankful he's not. Seriously, it's not like the in-patient setting you work in where there's a team of professionals making decisions about patients. We're talking about millions of people making decisions in their everyday lives. Think about your friends from pharmacy school who ended up in the community pharmacy setting. Think about how many prescriptions they fill everyday, and the number of folks they get to counsel. They don't have the time to talk to each and every shopper in that store."

Paul: "But at least they're available if the consumer has questions. It's not like it's a gas station."

Donna: "Sure, but that's different than mandating it. Most OTC medicines are purchased from stores that have pharmacies, but that's by the consumer's choice. Besides, when is the last time you saw a fully stocked health and beauty aisle in the quicky-mart. They've got a handful of basic items for the sake of convenience. Medicines aren't an impulse buy."

Paul: "Do shopping data back that up?"

Donna: "Sure, we have data from check-out scanners and household diary panels, but that's proprietary between our company and the market research firm. Let's talk about something else."

Background

Another area where OTC medicines differ significantly from their prescription cousins is the retail environment. At its simplest: If you're in the airport with a headache, the opportunity to buy an OTC analgesic at Hudson News is a welcome option. There's no wait to see a doctor. There's no additional travel time to take a special trip to a pharmacy. Choice, cost, and convenience are all strengths of the open US retail environment for OTC medicines.

Occasionally suggestions arise that the United States should have a class of non-prescription medicines only available through pharmacists, which is often the case in other countries. In looking at this issue, the US Government Accountability Office examined

10 countries with a pharmacy or pharmacist-only class of medicines, plus the European Union,* and found no support for such a class, stating:

> *Thus, there is no evidence to show that the role that US pharmacists would have to play to support the appropriate use of an intermediate class of drugs (either fixed or transition) would be fulfilled reliably and effectively. The evidence indicates that at this time major improvements in nonprescription drug use are unlikely to result from restricting the sale of some OTCs to pharmacies or by pharmacists, nor are the safeguards for pharmacy- or pharmacist-class drugs that would have otherwise remained in the prescription class likely to be sufficient.[22]*

As a practical matter, even if the FDA were to assert authority to restrict the distribution of an OTC medicine to sale by pharmacists only, the impact and asserted value added of such a restriction would be run up against the fact that the FDA does not control the practice of pharmacy. As with the practice of medicine, the practice of pharmacy is a matter of state licensing and control.

In the company context, there are instances, however, where NDA sponsors have voluntarily committed to actions around distribution or product placement for OTC medicines. FDA's August 24, 2006, approval letter to Duramed concerning levonorgestrel (the emergency contraceptive Plan B) is a recent and prominent example of this. The approval letter and accompanying memos from FDA Commissioner von Eschenbach and CDER Director Galson note the voluntary nature of the restrictions agreed to by the sponsor, and they also reference the state and private-sector infrastructures to restrict certain products (not limited to medicines) to certain consumers.[23] The larger point is that, as discussed earlier in the Rx-to-OTC switch section, the specific issues that would otherwise prevent a switch are the questions that need to be addressed through data in a switch NDA. The place-of-sale is unlikely to answer these questions.

Selling to Retailers

Although OTC medicines can be sold in any retail outlet, the vast majority of OTC medicines are sold through three basic retail channels: mass merchandisers (many of which include in-store pharmacies that might have different hours from the store as a whole); grocery stores (again, many of which have in-store pharmacies); and community pharmacies. For the small handful of the largest retailers, larger consumer healthcare companies (or larger consumer package goods manufacturers in general) have sales account executives dedicated to that retailer. So, when launching a new

---

*The European Union differentiates between only two classes: prescription and nonprescription. EU member states may subdivide, and they do so in varying manners.

product, for example, the account team might bring in other colleagues from their company to talk about different aspects of the product.

For more midsized or independent retailers (or for more midsized or smaller manufacturers with larger retailers), a manufacturer could decide to use an outside firm specializing in sales execution or to sell through a health distribution company/wholesaler.

Returning to the opening hypothetical, a business impact of these approaches is that OTC medicines are more likely to be sold directly from the manufacturer to a retailer than prescription medicines would be. The further impact is that your colleagues in OTC sales will be focusing on retailers, while your colleagues in Rx sales will be focusing on health plans and physicians.

■ Conclusion: The Hypothetical Ends

As with the pharmaceutical industry as a whole, OTC medicines are grounded in science and are subject to many of the same regulations as prescription medicines. The differences from prescription medicines come most sharply into focus by first thinking about the consumer: the person who walks into the store and picks a medicine up off the shelf is the person driving things. That person is the one to whom your labeling is addressed. That person is the one making the decision that your product is appropriate for them and provides a good value at its price. That person is the one to whom your advertising must speak.

Your job is to establish and maintain consumers' trust with a safe, effective medicine, available at their convenience.

It's 2:25, and your switch brainstorming session starts in 5 minutes.

■ References

1. Temin P. The origin of compulsory drug prescriptions. *J Law Econ.* 1979;(22):91. Excerpted in PB Hutt, RA Merrill. *Food and Drug Law: Cases and Materials.* 2nd ed. Foundation Press, Westbury, NY; 1991.
2. Federal Food, Drug and Cosmetic Act §503(b)(1) (21 USC 353(b)(1)).
3. 21 CFR 330.10(a)(4)(v).
4. 64 Fed. Reg. 13254-302 (March 17, 1999) (Over-the-Counter Human Drugs; Labeling Requirements; Final rule). (Codified at 21 CFR 201.66.)
5. OTC Drug Facts rule, supra, at 13254.
6. 21 CFR 201.66.
7. 63 Fed. Reg. 56789 (October 23, 1998).
8. Consumer Healthcare Products Association, FDA. *Challenges to OTC Drug Product Marketing and Regulation.* Seminar Series. May 15, 2003. Available at: http://www.fda.gov/cder/Offices/OTC/FDA_CHPA_seminar_2003_may.pdf. Accessed December 15, 2008.
9. Over-the-Counter Drugs: Proposal Establishing Rule Making Procedures for Classification, 37 Fed. Reg. 85 (January 5, 1972).

10. 21 CFR 330.10 Procedures for classifying OTC drugs as generally recognized as safe and effective and not misbranded, and for establishing monographs.

11. Federal Food, Drug, and Cosmetic Act 201(p) (21 USC 321(p)).

12. 67 Fed. Reg. 3060 (January 23, 2002).

13. 15 USC §45 and §52.

14. Pfizer Inc., 81 F.T.C. 23 (1972).

15. Bachrach EE. Over-the-counter drug advertising: FTC and FDA concerns. *Food, Drug and Cosmetic Section Newsletter* (New York State Bar Association). 1990, September;7:7.

16. International Harvester Co., 104 F.T.C. 949 (1984).

17. Heinz W. Kirchner, 63 F.T.C. 1282 (1963).

18. LaMothe W. Over-Regulation v. self-regulation. *The Advertiser* (Association of National Advertisers). Fall 1991:24.

19. Lanham Act §43(a).

20. 15 USC §1125(a).

21. Mann C, et al. The big headache. *The Atlantic*. October 1988.

22. US Government Accounting Office. *Nonprescription Drugs: Value of a Pharmacist-Controlled Class Has Yet to Be Demonstrated*. GAO/PEMD-95-12. Washington, DC: US GAO; August 2005.

23. Center for Drug Evaluation and Research. Plan B (0.75mg levonorgestrel) tablets information. Available at: http://www.fda.gov/cder/drug/infopage/planB/default.htm. Accessed December 15, 2008.

Future Industry Trends

Thomas Jacobsen and Albert Wertheimer

The pharmaceutical industry is the total of its constituent companies. Both the companies and the overall industry change over time. This change results from changes in technology, development, taxation, wealth, and the characteristics of the marketplace. As new technologies enable the operation of a pharmaceutical production facility by computer, with very skilled technicians present, it then matters very little whether the plant is located in Basle or Botswana. If Botswana can provide uninterrupted electricity supply, stable business/economic climate, a minimum of corruption, and a relatively dependable transportation infrastructure, it could become the center of pharmaceutical production.

We can expect in the future to confront change at a rate greater than ever before in the history of the pharmaceutical industry. For the past 100 years, the research-based pharmaceutical industry was composed of ever larger firms located in only a handful of countries. However, during the beginning of the 21st century, a number of low-cost countries have became involved in quite a few tasks performed by pharmaceutical companies.

First came outsourcing of clinical trials, along with bioequivalency testing. This was followed by the importation of bulk active phamaceutical ingredients (APIs). More recently, finished dosage forms are coming to North America and western Europe from Asia and eastern Europe.

And most recently, basic research and drug discovery are being performed abroad. Well, if drug discovery, clinical development, and manufacturing are conducted offshore, it is a fair question to ask what the future of multinational pharmaceutical company might look like. If we extend these trends, it is likely that we will find pharma companies in the United States, the United Kingdom, France, Switzerland, and Germany as virtual companies with most tasks outsourced offshore to independent subcontractor companies or to their own foreign subsidiaries. The principal task maintained by the corporations will be promotion and marketing. Sales and marketing will probably remain local responsibilities because local staff understand the psyche, personality, and culture of the customers, usually physicians, better than people who are not local.

■ The Future Fear

Surely, most persons who think carefully about the future of the pharmaceutical industry do so with the realization of a possible massive catastrophe. That horror is the recognition that "modern medicine" really cures nearly no diseases other than infections. Diseases are controlled, or more accurately stated, the symptoms are controlled. Think about it: We do not cure diabetes or hypertension; we control blood glucose levels and we control blood pressure. This is accomplished through the use of daily medication regimens.

If patients fail to take their medications, the symptoms might return and progressive deterioration of health status might continue. So, the pharmaceutical industry today sells an enormous amount of maintenance medications to be used for symptom control of chronic diseases. But one of these days, some skillful biochemists will develop a novel molecule and delivery system to reinvent a well-functioning insulin production capacity for diabetic patients.

With patients' pancreases-producing insulin, much of the insulin industry, as well as the bulk of the syringe and needle industry and many manufacturers producing multi-billion-dollar oral agents, will find a major shortage of patients. The biotechnology industry has the potential to deliver a one-two punch to the chemical synthesis (called the small molecule) pharmaceutical industry. Granted, this event will not happen within the next 3 or 4 years, but it's not that far around the corner.

Perhaps, this partially explains why existing pharma companies are buying promising biotechnology startup companies. By this same token, we can expect pharma companies to revitalize their interest in the generic drug market. Novartis has shown the world that its generic division, Sandoz, can hold its own and contribute to overall corporate profitability.

It is likely that the industry will continue to synthesize chemistry-based drugs, participate in the generic drugs market, and join the biotechnology competition. In addition, there are at least two other spaces that should be profitable. One is as a specialist in end-of-life-cycle products, where a little extra marketing push can squeeze a few more years of sales and profitability from old, moribund products.

The other related area where industry people have knowledge and experience, and therefore see it as a possible expansion area, is in the selling of over-the-counter (OTC) drugs. Such OTC drugs are sold without the necessity of a doctor's order and may be purchased in nearly any type of retail outlet. OTC sales require different sales and marketing experience, but production and many other functions are identical to prescription drug manufacture and sales.

What follow are some examples of major trends that will surely affect the pharmaceutical industry.

■ Individualized Medicine

Ironically, current drug therapy is targeted toward the broadest population that is perceived to have the best response from it and yet 2500 years ago, Pythagoras observed the first instance of genetic polymorphism (hemolytic anemia) in individuals who were deficient in glucose-6-phosphate dehyrogenase.[1] Only over the last twenty 20 has there been a resurgence of research in identifying polymorphisms that either cause or affect the susceptibility to human disease.[2] The completion of the Human Genome Project and subsequent development of the HapMap enable us to understand the common patterns of human DNA sequence variation throughout the genome and provide valuable information for understanding disease.[3] The entire biopharmaceutical industry is based on less than 500 drug targets, although there are approximately 5000–10,000 genes that could be used as possible therapeutic targets. Although this potential seems massive, the percentage of these targets that will be therapeutically useful and pharmacologically manipulative is debated and remains to be determined.

Currently, physicians must play a guessing game as to which medication will produce the desired outcome with the least propensity for adverse events. Variability of drug response can take a variety of different forms, but new technologies allow predictive insight to produce the desired therapeutic effect. With the advent of pharmacogenetics (single genes) and pharmacogenomics (multiple genes) the genetic personalization of drug therapy is now possible. By collecting epidemiologic, genetic, clinical, and genealogical information, it is possible to uncover genes more effectively that predispose persons to disease, enrich the population that is likely to respond to the drug, and eliminate the nonresponder.[4]

The fundamental question is whether an initial random segregation of gene markers in the patient population prior to drug administration can be organized according to drug response in the same patients. Is the distribution of a given marker different between responders and nonresponders or between safe responders and adverse responders? If so, an association exists between drug response and segregated gene markers. This knowledge will in turn reduce trial and error physician prescribing; however, at present the impact on medicine is minimal at best, and the greatest challenges are to understand genotype-environmental factor interactions, the role of ethnicity, and the development of high-quality technologies.[5]

There are also several negative psychosocial issues that should be considered as well such as violation of privacy, the availability of testing, the complexity associated with the interpretation and explanation of results, and cost. The potential to reveal a predisposition to an illness may compromise insurability or may exclude workers from certain jobs. The balance of positives versus negatives should be weighed when considering the implications of pharmacogenetic testing because pharmacogenetics not only affects the individual but the population as a whole, which can result in strongly conflicting values and interests.[6] The application and incorporation of pharmacogenetic information into clinical practice must therefore be accurate, precise, and strictly regulated.

Pharmacogenomics will play a large role in the development of current and future compounds. Pharmacogenomic analysis is currently being applied to both the preclinical and clinical phases of drug development. The Food and Drug Administration has published guidance on its use in the drug development process.[7,8] There are many issues that healthcare professionals and regulatory authorities need to identify and develop before this technology is widely accepted.

Pharmacogenetic studies are geared toward the understanding of the genes that code for pharmacokinetic (absorption, distribution, and metabolism) and pharmacodynamic (therapeutic effect at the receptor level) processes. The pharmacokinetic phenotype is more easily measured and less complex than the pharmacodynamic one is. Pharmacokinetic measurements of bodily fluids are relatively easy, the number of genes involved is limited, and the amount of genetic variation and penetrance is usually high (analogous to single gene disorders).[2] Analysis of pharmacodynamic properties is far more complex and has only recently become available through emerging technologies. Another area in genomic studies is toxicology, where potentially a researcher could determine a compound's toxicity early in the discovery phase before being tested in humans.

Being able to understand the predictability of a drug's response in certain populations allows the pharmaceutical industry to make better preclinical selections of compounds that have a greater likelihood of being safe and efficacious. This will allow the pharmaceutical industry to reduce expenses. In addition companies can conduct smaller, more rapid, and population-focused clinical trials that may result in more effective tailor-made prescribing and therapeutics.[9,10]

A critical challenge for the pharmaceutical industry is to increase its productivity and focus on introducing novel strategies aimed at enhancing early stage discovery as well as the efficiency of decision making throughout the research process.[11] Novel approaches for high-throughput experiments to discern associations between disease and disease traits with large numbers of drug targets are now available.[12] In drug development, understanding of pharmacogenetic contribution to drug response may generate data that can be used to streamline phase 2 and phase 3 clinical trials; saving a company time, effort, and money.[3] This has been held out as a significant hope to help drive greater efficiency in the clinical trial process.[3]

Pharmacogenetics can be applied either retrospectively or prospectively.[2] Retrospectively, pharmacogenetics can look back over the results of clinical trials, using genotype data to generate insights into issues such as the kinetic and dynamic properties of drug efficacy and adverse events.[2] Prospectively, pharmacogenetics allows proactive identification of patient subgroups that would or would not produce the desired therapeutic response.[2] Pharmacogenetic analysis can also be incorporated into postmarketing surveillance programs to help identify subjects who may experience rare but serious adverse reactions that were not apparent during the clinical phase of testing.

Industry is a profit-driven entity; therefore, initially, the cost of such testing will be geared to developing drugs that are targeted toward large, genetically homogeneous populations and diseases.[13] The development of pharmacogenetics applicable to personalization of medicines is proceeding at such a pace that it is not a matter of *if* these technologies affect medicine prescription, but *when* and to what extent.[14] This is not to say the number of new drugs coming from industry will increase because of a better understanding of disease and what the opportunity will be for each class target.[3] Drugs will not be made for each individual, but rather the best drug from our current armamentarium will be chosen for each individual patient. Blockbuster drugs may eventually lessen in importance, but that will be caused by the lack of suitable therapeutic targets and differentiable drugs, not pharmacogenetics.[3]

■ Nanotechnology

Most of today's drugs are delivered by the various routes: orally, intramuscularly, intravenously, subcutaneously, ocularly, transdermally, buccally, rectally, vaginally, or by inhalation. These are not always the most efficient routes for a particular therapy. New biologic drugs such as proteins and nucleic acids require novel delivery technologies that will minimize side effects and lead to better compliance.[15,16] Similarly, the success of DNA and RNA therapies will depend on such innovative drug delivery techniques.[17] Market forces are also driving the need for new, effective drug delivery methods.[18] In many cases, the success of a drug is dependent on the delivery method and this is exemplified by the presence of more than 300 companies based in the United States involved with developing drug delivery systems.[19,20]

The delivery and targeting of pharmaceutical and therapeutic agents is the forefront of nanomedicine. Nanomedicine involves the identification of precise targets related to specific clinical conditions and choice of the appropriate nanocarriers to achieve the acquired responses while minimizing side effects.[21] Nanomedicine is a large area and includes nanoparticles, nanomachines, nanofibers, polymeric nanoconstructs, and nanoscale microfabrication-based devices.[21] What does this all mean? It means nanotechnology is quite complex, involving a host of disciplines including physics, physiology, chemistry, engineering, and a whole host of others. Its application in treating diseases is mindboggling and at the present seems limitless.

The delivery to various parts of the body is limited by the particle size. Most nanoparticles are very, very small, often less than 100 nanometers—smaller than the head of a pin. Nanoparticles can be used as a vehicle or carrier for drug delivery into the body. The majority if these particles can be delivered with one of the following drug delivery technologies: biologic, polymeric, silicon based, carbon based, or metallic. Therapeutic agents can be attached to nanoparticles by encapsulation, absorption, or chemically, allowing the therapeutic agent to be delivered to its target destination (ie, tumor). This in turn may improve therapeutic effectiveness of drugs and cause even fewer side effects. These particles can be injected into the body either by intravenous or subcutaneous routes. There is also the possibility of designing nanocarriers that are multifunctional, such as those that target specific cells, deliver a drug product, and act as a biological sensor.[22]

Anatomic features such as the blood–brain barrier, the branching pathways of the pulmonary system, and the tight epithelial junctions of the skin make it difficult for many drugs to reach desired physiologic targets. Nanostructured drug carriers, however, can penetrate or overcome these barriers to drug delivery.[19] When injected intravenously, nanoparticles are cleared rapidly from the circulation predominantly by the liver and spleen macrophages.[22]

As nanomedicine/nanotechnology progresses, a multidisciplinary approach involving expertise from many different fields will likely be of great benefit to the future of this growing field. Complex issues relating to future FDA approval of nanomedical materials, devices, and even the possibility of nano robots are already being addressed in mainstream legal journals.[23,24] The outlook for the applications of nanomedicine in patient care is very promising.

■ Discussion and Conclusions

In an effort to maintain full drug development pipelines, larger firms will attempt to "license in" future products being developed by other companies. These other companies are likely to be smaller, second- or third-tier companies or foreign firms doing business elsewhere, but not in the United States. When the small number of promising future products dries up, the next logical reaction step is for the larger firms to buy entire smaller firms to obtain the desired products that their developers were unwilling to sell.

Given the existing trend in consolidation, it would appear that the industry will be composed of 20 to 30 or so intermediate or larger companies that will merge into 6 to 8 groups, with European and Asian partners. Such consolidation creates some economies of scale and fills the development pipelines. Within the past decade, we have seen the beginning phase of this trend:

- Ciba, Geigy, and Sandoz became Novartis.
- Rhone-Poulenc, Rorer, and Marion became Aventis.
- Searle, Pharmacia, Upjohn, Warner-Lambert, and Parke-Davis became part of Pfizer.

- Syntex became part of Roche.
- Burroughs-Wellcome, Glaxo, and SmithKline became GSK.

In addition, there have been numerous smaller acquisitions and mergers. When that reaches a steady state, it is likely that we will see purchases of biotechnology firms by traditional synthetic chemistry (small molecule) firms. Most of the biotechnology firms remain small with the exception of Amgen and Genentech and a few others.

The pot of gold at the end of the R&D rainbow has been taking longer to materialize than the experts had originally imagined. Some of the biotech firms that are recent startups will have run out of working capital before the FDA approves any product and might be forced to sell their assets such as R&D work or even the entire company to a traditional pharma company.

The pharmaceutical industry has been known to take some inexplicable actions over the years. In the 1950s and 1960s, pharmaceutical manufacturers purchased fragrance and cosmetics concerns. What one did, the other emulated. Perhaps the original thinking was that cosmetics and pharmaceuticals are both sold through pharmacy outlets. Only later did they realize that although the distribution channels were partially similar, totally different pricing, promotion, and marketing paths were followed. It would be safe to say that just about all of the cosmetics companies once owned by big pharma have been sold. Then, in 1980s and 1990s, big pharma purchased Pharmacy Benefit Management (PBM) firms, all of which were sold within several years. To this day, it is difficult to find a rationale that makes sense as to why a drug manufacturer would want to own a PBM.

Diversification takes many routes. Johnson & Johnson operates nearly 200 separate companies making bandages, stents, prosthetic joints, sutures, diagnostics, and so forth. Others have gone into generic drugs, overseas expansion, OTCs, private label, and custom or private manufacturing.

If present trends continue, pharma manufacturers will continue to invest in new technologies. But in addition to that, we shouldn't be surprised if pharma companies buy liquor manufacturers or other highly regulated industry firms. Some have experimented with clinical labs and diagnostic products.

For the foreseeable future, we see a healthy and profitable pharmaceutical industry, as greater numbers of patients reach old age, and as the lesser developed countries become wealthier and are able to participate in the drug market. Society seems to be accepting $20,000 drugs that add only a few months to patients' life expectancy. And then there is the enormous market of lifestyle drugs. People appear willing to pay large sums of money to hide their facial wrinkles and other signs of aging. They are willing to pay dearly for "quick-fix" drugs that resolve problems effortlessly. Investors have high hopes for patients swallowing massive quantities of anti-obesity agents, hair restorers, libido stimulants, and drugs against sexual dysfunction, social phobias, cigarette addiction, and so forth.

Yes, biotech will make the drugs we know rather superfluous, but that change could be 20 or more years from now.

■ References

1. Mager J, Glaser G, Razin A, et al. Metabolic effects of pyrimidines derived from fava bean glycosides on human erythrocytes deficient in glucose-6-phosphate dehydrogenase. *Biochem Biophys Res Commun.* 1965;20:235–240.
2. McCarthy A, Kennedy J, Middleton L. Pharmacogenetics in drug development. *Phil Trans R Soc B.* 2005;360:1579–1588.
3. Johnson K, Thompson J, Power A. Pharmacogenomics: integration into drug discovery and development. *Curr Top Med Chem.* 2005;5:1039–1046.
4. Hakonarsson H, Stefansson K. Role of pharmacogenomics in drug development. *Drug Dev Res.* 2004;62:86–96.
5. Stoughton R, Friend S. How molecular profiling could revolutionize drug discovery. *Nat Rev Drug Disc.* 2005;4:345–350.
6. Weinshilboum R. Inheritance of drug response. *N Eng J Med.* 2003;348:529–537.
7. Food and Drug Administration. *Challenge and Opportunity on the Critical Path to New Medicinal Products.* March 2004. Available at: http://www.fda.gov/oc/initiatives/criticalpath/whitepaper.pdf. Accessed December 15, 2008.
8. US Department of Health and Human Services, Food and Drug Administration, Center for Drug Evaluation and Research (CDER), Center for Biologics Evaluation and Research (CBER), and Center for Devices and Radiologic Health (CDRH). *Guidance for Industry: Pharmacogenomic Data Submissions.* March 2005. Available at: http://www.fda.gov/Cber/gdlns/pharmdtasub.pdf. Accessed December 15, 2008.
9. Regalado A. Inventing the pharmacogenomics business. *Am J Health Syst Pharm.* 1999;56:40–50.
10. Rothstein MA, Epps PG. Ethical and legal implications of pharmacogenomics. *Nat Rev Genet.* 2001;2:228–231.
11. Roses AD. Genome-based pharmacogenetics and drug development: the path to safer and more effective drugs. *Nat Rev Drug Disc.* 2004;3:645–656.
12. Roses AD, Burns DK, Chissoe S, Middleton L. St Jean P. Disease specific target selection: a critical first step down the right road. *Drug Disc Today.* 2005;10:177–189.
13. Mahlknecht U, Voelter-Mahlknecht S. Pharmacogenomics: questions and concerns. *Curr Med Res Opin.* 2005;(21)7:1041–1047.
14. Lesko LJ, Woodcock J. Translation of pharmacogenomics and pharmacogenetics: a regulatory perspective. *Nat Rev Drug Disc.* 2004;3:763–769.
15. Kefalides PT. New methods for drug delivery. *Ann Intern Med.* 1998;128:1053–1055.
16. Bradbury J. Beyond pills and jabs. *Lancet.* 2003;362:1984–1985.
17. El-Aneed A. An overview of the current delivery systems in cancer gene therapy. *J Controlled Release.* 2004;94:1–14.
18. Henry CM. New wrinkles in drug delivery. *Chem Eng News.* 2004;82:37–42.
19. Hughes GA. Nanostructure-mediated drug delivery. *Nanomed: Nanotech, Bio, Med.* 2005;1:23–30.
20. D'Aquino R. Good drug therapy: it's not just the molecule—it's the delivery. *CEP Magazine.* 2004;100:15S–17S.

21. Moghimi S, Hunter A, Murray J. Nanomedicine: current status and future prospects. *FASEB J.* 2005;19:311–330.

22. Moghimi S, Hunter A, Murray J. Long-circulating and target-specific nanoparticles: theory to practice. *Pharmacol Rev.* 2001;53:283–318.

23. Fiedler FA, Reynolds GH. Legal problems of nanotechnology: an overview. *S Cal Interdisciplinary Law J.* 1994;3:593–629.

24. Miller J. Beyond biotechnology: FDA regulation on nanomedicine. *Columbia Sci Technol Law Rev.* 2002–2003:4.

Index

non-compendial non-novel excipients, 83–85
nonmanpower promotion elements, 223
not approvable letter, FDA, 147
novel excipients, 83–85
nucleotides, receptors for, 25
nucleotide sequences, 7
Nuremberg code, 102–104

O

ocular ointments, 96
Official Trademark Gazette, 212
off-label uses, 166–167, 169
Ogston three-point attachment, 15
ointments, 43–44, 96, 98
oligonucleotides, 18
oligosaccharides, 18
ophthalmic drug products, 95–96, 275
oral absorption, 14
oral bioavailability, 14
oral dosage forms, 37–41, 91–92
Orange Book, 144
organ-targeted therapy, 96–97
orphan receptors, 25–28
OTC. *See* over-the-counter medications
OTC Review, 285
outcomes research
    drug effectiveness and cost, 254–255
    overview, 247–251
    reasons for, 253–254
    study designs, 252–253
out-of-specifications (OOS), 77
outsourcing, 171–172, 295
overdose, 192
over-the-counter (OTC) medications
    advertising, 287–290
    public relations organizations, 259
    regulation of, 282–285
    retail environment, 290–293
    Rx-to-OTC switch, 285–290
oxidation, 68–69
oxidation process, 41
oxygen scavenger packets, 41

P

package insert, 140
packaging
    container closure systems, 70, 88–89, 274
    final print labeling (FPL), 140
    general controls, 77–78
    generic drug applications, 274
    Investigational New Drug (IND) application, 135
    ophthalmic drug products, 96
    over-the-counter medications, 282–284

overview, 88–89
oxidation and, 41
parenteral products, 94–95
patents, 206
stability testing, 68–69
paddle apparatus, 72
parallel studies, 124
parallel synthesis, 18–20
parenterals, 92–95
particle size, formulation and, 40
partition coefficient, 35
Partnership for Quality Medical Donations, 261
passive diffusion, 35
pastes, 98
patches, transdermal, 43–44, 97–98
patents, 143, 144, 203–208, 272
patients, drug effectiveness, 254–255
patient satisfaction, 250–251
PBM (pharmacy benefit managers), 242
PCAOB (Public Company Accounting Oversight Board), 244–245
PCR machines, 7
pediatric populations, 113, 143
peer-reviewed journals, 128
peptide chains, 16
peptide ligands, 25
performance qualification, 50, 53–54
permeability, formulation, 35
Perutz, Max, 3
pH, 36, 59–61, 96
Pharmaceutical Research and Manufacturers Accountability Act (2005), 199
Pharmaceutical Research and Manufacturers of America, 161, 259
pharmacists, role in industry, 155–160
pharmacodynamic processes, 298
pharmacoeconomics
    clinical trials and, 256
pharmacoeconomics (*cont.*)
    drug effectiveness and cost, 254–255
    evaluation types, 251–252
    outcomes research study designs, 252–253
    overview, 247–251
    reasons for, 253–254
pharmacogenetics/genomics, 296–299
pharmacokinetic processes, 298
pharmacology studies, 135
pharmacy benefit managers (PBMs), 242
photolysis, stability testing, 68–69
photostability, 68–69
Pichia pastoris, 9
pilot batches, 42–45
pivotal trials, 121
placebo controlled trials, 116, 126, 135

solubility, formulation, 35, 40
solutions, 43–44, 92–95, 95
specifications
    components, 52
    drug product, 86–88
    general controls, 77–78
    Investigational New Drug (IND) application, 135
    pilot batches, 43
    release, defined, 71
    shelf life, defined, 71
specificity, analytical testing, 86–88
SPL (Structured Product Labeling), 150
stability studies, defined, 70
stability testing
    degradation studies, 37
    excipients, 83
    formulation, 41–45
    general controls, 78
    generic drug applications, 274
    Investigational New Drug (IND) application, 135
    overview, 67–69, 90–91
    parenteral products, 93
stabilizing polymer, 40
standard written responses, 167–169
starch, 41
state discount pricing, 243–244
statistical genetics, 10
sterile products, 89, 92–96
steroid hormones, 2
stomach, 36, 37–41
storage, 68, 76, 90–91. *See also* stability testing
strategic planning, finance, 234–237
stressed conditions, process validation, 50
stress testing, defined, 71
structural genomics, 9–11
Structured Product Labeling (SPL), 150
subcutaneous (SC) products, 92–95
sublingual tablets, 37
sugar, stability testing, 41
support group, research, 127
suppositories, 44
surfactants, 40
surveys, 178
susceptibility genes, 10
suspensions, 38, 43–44, 92–96
SWOT analysis, 235
symposia, marketing at, 222
synthons, 14–15

T
tablets
    dosage form design, 37–41
    manufacturing, 91–92
    pilot batches, 42–45

process equipment, 44
    stability testing, 41–42
tackiness, tablets, 42
target receptors, 28–29
target selection, 21–22
tax accounting, 232
TEAS (Trademark Electronic Application System), 212
technical transfer issues, 49
telemarketing, 223
television advertising, 221, 290
temperature
    formulation and, 39–40
    stability testing, 41–45, 68–69, 90–91
testing. *See also* stability testing
    compatibility studies, 39–40
    degradation studies, 37
    general controls, 77–78
    in-process materials, 51
    Investigational New Drug (IND) application, 135
    preclinical, 35–37
    preformulation, 35–37
    process validation, 49–54
    validation, 78–80
thalidomide, 190
therapeutic failures, 192
therapeutic misconception, 113
think tanks, 265
three-dimensional molecule structure, 3–4
three-point attachment, 15
time, manufacturing, 43
tonicity, 93, 96
topical drug products, 97–98
toxicity studies, 36, 89, 135, 141
trade dress, 210
Trademark Electronic Application Systems (TEAS), 212
trademarks, 208–213
Trademark Trial and Appeal Board (TTAB), 212
training, clinical researchers, 129
training, sales representatives, 173, 175–176
transdermal patches, 43–44, 97–98
transfected cell array (TCA), 23, 24–25
transfection, 27–28
transmissible spongiform encephalopathy (TSE), 85
tray drying, 44, 46
trials, scale up, 47–49
TTAB (Trademark Trial and Appeal Board), 212

U
ultraviolet spectrophotometers, 20–21
unexpected adverse events, 137, 148–149
unfairness policy, advertising claims, 289–290
United States Adopted Names (USAN) Council, 209
United States Patent and Trademark Office (USPTO),
    204–205, 211